INTERPRETATION

A Handbook Synopsis of Laboratory Medicine

OF DIAGNOSTIC

Second Edition

TESTS

Bert Spilker

Anion Gap $Na - (Cl + CO_2) = 4-12$

Osmolality $2\{Na\} + \dfrac{glucose}{18} + \dfrac{BUN}{3} = 288-300$

INTERPR

A Handbook Synopsis

OF DIA

Second Edition

TESTS

Jacques Wallach, M.D.
Clinical Associate Professor of Pathology,
College of Medicine and Dentistry of New Jersey,
Rutgers Medical School, New Brunswick;
Visiting Assistant Professor of Pathology,
Albert Einstein College of Medicine, New York

Library of Congress catalog card No. 73-10612

ISBN-0-316-92043-6

Printed in the United States of America

INTERPRETATION OF DIAGNOSTIC TESTS: A HANDBOOK SYNOPSIS OF LABORATORY MEDICINE, First Edition, is published in the following translations:

INTERPRETACIÓN DE LOS DIAGNÓSTICOS DE LABORATORIO: MANUAL SINÓPTICO DE BIOLOGÍA MÉDICA

Ἑρμηνεία τῶν Διαγνωστικῶν Ἐξετάσεων καί Δοκιμασιῶν: Συνοπτικὸν Ἐγχειρίδιον Ἐργαστηριακῆς Ἰατρικῆς

INTERPRETAÇÃO DOS DIAGNÓSTICOS DE LABORATÓRIO

ETATION

of Laboratory Medicine

GNOSTIC

LITTLE, BROWN AND COMPANY   BOSTON

To Doris

and

To Kim, Lisa, and Tracy

Preface to the Second Edition

A new edition is indicated to keep the contents current with the medical literature as well as with daily clinical experience and needs. Much of the material has been amplified or altered to provide the latest information, and several new sections have been added to meet the clinical awareness of new problems (e.g., the Alteration of Laboratory Test Values by Drugs) and to better deal with older problems (e.g., Bacterial Cultures). In addition, the index has been improved and expanded to facilitate the use of the book.

The book's features of size, format, organization, style, and content have been deemed successful in meeting the needs of pathologists as well as of practicing clinicians, medical students, and occasional technologists. Its usefulness may be increased by such current trends as the frequent lack of easily available assistance in clinical pathology, greater demands for the physician's time, the development of many new tests, and the routine performance of more "routine" and "screening" tests.

The widespread acceptance of this book confirms the underlying premise of the first edition and has been most gratifying. As with the preparation of the previous edition, I have been rewarded by learning much more than I could compress into this small volume. Colleagues and patients have always stimulated my efforts.

My wife, Doris, has been the source of wisdom, good sense, and certain rare special qualities that have made possible so much that I could not otherwise have done.

J. W.

Cranford, New Jersey

Preface to the First Edition

Results of laboratory tests may aid in:
  discovery of occult disease
  prevention of irreparable damage (e.g., phenylketonuria)
  early diagnosis after onset of signs or symptoms
  differential diagnosis of various possible diseases
  determining the stage of the disease
  estimating the activity of the disease
  detecting the recurrence of disease
  measuring the effect of therapy
  genetic counseling in familial conditions
  medicolegal problems such as paternity suits
This book is written to help the physician achieve these purposes
with the least amount of:
  duplication of tests
  waste of patient's money
  overtaxing of laboratory facilities and personnel
  loss of physician's time
  confusion caused by the increasing number, variety, and com-
    plexity of tests currently available. Some of these tests may
    be unrequested but performed as part of routine surveys or
    hospital admission multitest screening.
In order to provide quick reference and maximum availability and
usefulness, this handy-sized book features:
  tabular and graphic style of concise presentation
  emphasis on serial time changes in laboratory findings in
    various stages of disease
  omission of rarely performed, irrelevant, esoteric, and out-
    moded laboratory tests
  exclusion of discussion of physiologic mechanisms, metabolic
    pathways, clinical features, and nonlaboratory aspects of
    disease
  discussion of only the more important diseases that the physi-
    cian encounters and should be able to diagnose
This book is not:
  an encyclopedic compendium of clinical pathology
  an all-inclusive textbook
  a technical manual
  a substitute for good clinical judgment and basic knowledge of
    medicine
Deliberately omitted are:
  technical procedures and directions
  photographs and illustrations of anatomic changes (e g., blood
    cells, karyotypes, isotope scans)

discussions of quality control
selection of a referral laboratory
performance of laboratory tests in the clinician's own office
bibliographic references except for the most general reference
    texts in medicine, hematology, and clinical pathology and for
    some very recent references to specific conditions

The contents of this book are oriented toward the questions posed by physicians and the assistance they sometimes request and often need from the pathologist. There is no other such single adequate source of information presented in this fashion.

A perusal of the table of contents and index will quickly show the reader the general organization of the material by type of laboratory test or organ system or certain special chapters. In order to maintain a concise format, separate chapters have not been organized for such categories as pediatric, newborn, and geriatric periods or for primary psychiatric or dermatologic diseases. A complete index provides maximum access to this information.

Obviously these data are not original but have been adapted from many sources referred to over the years. Only the selection, organization, manner of presentation, and emphasis are original. I have formulated this point of view during my 20 years as clinician and pathologist, viewing with pride the important and growing role of the laboratory but deeply regretting its inadequate utilization.

This book is written to improve laboratory utilization by making it simpler for the physician to select the most useful laboratory tests for his clinical problems.

J. W.

Cranford, New Jersey

Acknowledgments

I thank those colleagues whose trust and loyalty have made this book possible. They have stimulated me to find answers to their laboratory questions and clinical needs and to provide these in a format that will be most useful to them.

> Ah, if my brush could only catch the faint
> Scent of the white plum-blossoms that I paint!*
> —Shôha

In particular, I am grateful to patients who have always taught me so much when I have listened. Special thanks are due the staff of Little, Brown and Company, especially Phyllis Ehrlich and Lin Richter, for their unfailing encouragement and assistance.

J. W.

* Haiku poem reprinted from Harold Stewart, trans., *A Chime of Windbells*. Rutland, Vt.: Tuttle, 1969.

Contents

Tables

Normal Values

1
Blood

A review of the texts, reference books, and current literature in Clinical Pathology often reveals surprising and considerable discrepancy between well-known sources. The following pages of normal laboratory values were summarized from what seemed to be the best and most current sources of data available.

I have used my own experience and clinical judgment in selecting the most useful data to be included.

Table 1. Normal Leukocyte

Age	Segmented Neutrophils		Band* Neutrophils		Eosinophils	
	%	No. per cubic millimeter	%	No. per cubic millimeter	%	No. per cubic millimeter
At birth	47 ± 15	8,400	14.1 ± 4	2,540	2.2	400
12 hr.	53	12,100	15.2	3,460	2.0	450
24 hr.	47	8,870	14.2	2,680	2.4	450
1 wk.	34	4,100	11.8	1,420	4.1	500
2 wk.	29	3,320	10.5	1,200	3.1	350
4 wk.	25 ± 10	2,750	9.5 ± 3	1,150	2.8	300
2 mo.	25	2,750	8.4	1,100	2.7	300
4 mo.	24	2,730	8.9	1,000	2.6	300
6 mo.	23	2,710	8.8	1,000	2.5	300
8 mo.	22	2,680	8.3	1,000	2.5	300
10 mo.	22	2,600	8.3	1,000	2.5	300
12 mo.	23	2,680	8.1	990	2.6	300
2 yr.	25	2,660	8.0	850	2.6	280
4 yr.	34 ± 11	3,040	8.0 ± 3	710	2.8	250
6 yr.	43	3,600	8.0	670	2.7	230
8 yr.	45	3,700	8.0	660	2.4	200
10 yr.	46 ± 15	3,700	8.0 ± 3	645	2.4	200
12 yr.	47	3,700	8.0	640	2.5	200
14 yr.	48	3,700	8.0	640	2.5	200
16 yr.	49 ± 15	3,800	8.0 ± 3	620	2.6	200
18 yr.	49	3,800	8.0	620	2.6	200
20 yr.	51	3,800	8.0	620	2.7	200
21 yr.	51 ± 15	3,800	8.0 ± 3	620	2.7	200

*Note that these values are higher than those found in other references. They have been obtained by using strict criteria in differentiating segmented from band forms. We do not classify a neutrophil as a segmented form unless a typical threadlike filament is visible.

Differential Count in Peripheral Blood

Basophils		Lymphocytes		Monocytes		
%	No. per cubic milli-meter	%	No. per cubic milli-meter	%	No. per cubic milli-meter	Age
0.6	100	31 ± 5	5,500	5.8	1,050	At birth
0.4	100	24	5,500	5.3	1,200	12 hr.
0.5	100	31	5,800	5.8	1,100	24 hr.
0.4	50	41	5,000	9.1	1,100	1 wk.
0.4	50	48	5,500	8.8	1,000	2 wk.
0.5	50	56 ± 15	6,000	6.5	700	4 wk.
0.5	50	57	6,300	5.9	650	2 mo.
0.4	50	59	6,800	5.2	600	4 mo.
0.4	50	61	7,300	4.8	580	6 mo.
0.4	50	62	7,600	4.7	580	8 mo.
0.4	50	63	7,500	4.6	550	10 mo.
0.4	50	61	7,000	4.8	550	12 mo.
0.5	50	59	6,300	5.0	530	2 yr.
0.6	50	50 ± 15	4,500	5.0	450	4 yr.
0.6	50	42	3,500	4.7	400	6 yr.
0.6	50	39	3,300	4.2	350	8 yr.
0.5	40	38 ± 10	3,100	4.3	350	10 yr.
0.5	40	38	3,000	4.4	350	12 yr.
0.5	40	37	2,900	4.7	380	14 yr.
0.5	40	35 ± 10	2,800	5.1	400	16 yr.
0.5	40	35	2,700	5.2	400	18 yr.
0.5	40	33	2 500	5.0	380	20 yr.
0.5	40	34 ± 10	2,500	4.0	300	21 yr.

Source: J. B. Miale, *Laboratory Medicine – Hematology,* 4th ed.
St. Louis: Mosby, 1972.

Table 2. Normal Values for Red Corpuscles at Various Ages

Age	Red Cell Count (millions/cu mm)	Hemoglobin (gm/100 ml)	Vol. Packed RBC (ml/100 ml)	Corpuscular Values			
				MCV (cu μ)	MCH ($\gamma\gamma$)	MCHC (%)	MCD (μ)
First day	5.1 ± 1.0	19.5 ± 5.0	54.0 ± 10.0	106	38	36	8.6
2–3 days	5.1	19.0	53.5	105	37	35	
4–8 days	5.1	18.3 ± 4.0	52.5	103	36	35	
9–13 days	5.0	16.5	49.0	98	33	34	
14–60 days	4.7 ± 0.9	14.0 ± 3.3	42.0 ± 7.0	90	30	33	8.1
3–5 mo.	4.5 ± 0.7	12.2 ± 2.3	36.0	80	27	34	7.7
6–11 mo.	4.6	11.8	35.5 ± 5.0	77	26	33	7.4
1 yr.	4.5	11.2	35.0	78	25	32	7.3
2 yr.	4.6	11.5	35.5	77	25	32	
3 yr.	4.5	12.5	36.0	80	27	35	7.4
4 yr.	4.6 ± 0.6	12.6	37.0	80	27	34	
5 yr.	4.6	12.6	37.0	80	27	34	
6–10 yr.	4.7	12.9	37.5	80	27	34	7.4
11–15 yr.	4.8	13.4	39.0	82	28	34	
Adults							
Females	4.8 ± 0.6	14.0 ± 2.0	42.0 ± 5.0	87 ± 5	29 ± 2	34 ± 2	7.5 ± 0.3
Males	5.4 ± 0.8	16.0 ± 2.0	47.0 ± 5.0	87 ± 5	29 ± 2	34 ± 2	7.5 ± 0.3

MCV = mean corpuscular volume; MCH = mean corpuscular hemoglobin; MCHC = mean corpuscular hemoglobin concentration; MCD = mean corpuscular diameter.
Source: M.M. Wintrobe, *Clinical Hematology*, 6th. ed. Philadelphia: Lea & Febiger, 1967.

NORMAL HEMATOLOGIC VALUES

Fetal hemoglobin	Less than 2% of total
Methemoglobin	Less than 3% of total
Carboxyhemoglobin	Less than 5% of total
Haptoglobins	Adults: 40–180 mg/100 ml
	Age 1–6 months: gradual increase to 30 mg/100 ml
	Newborn: absent in 90%; 10 mg/100 ml in 10%
	Genetic absence in 1% of population
Osmotic fragility of RBC	Begins in 0.45–0.39% NaCl
	Complete in 0.33–0.30% NaCl
Erythrocyte sedimentation rate	
Wintrobe	Males: 0–10 mm in 1 hour
	Females: 0–15 mm in 1 hour
Westergren	Males: 0–15 mm in 1 hour
	Females: 0–20 mm in 1 hour
Blood volume	Males: 75 ml/kg of body weight
	Females: 67 ml/kg of body weight
Plasma volume	Males: 44 ml/kg of body weight
	Females: 43 ml/kg of body weight
Red blood cell volume	Males: 30 ml/kg of body weight
	Females: 24 ml/kg of body weight
RBC survival time (^{51}Cr)	Half-time: 25–35 days
Reticulocyte count	0.5–1.5% of erythrocytes
Plasma iron turnover rate	38 mg/24 hours (0.47 mg/kg)

BLOOD COAGULATION TESTS

Platelet count	140,000–340,000/cu mm (Rees-Ecker)
Bleeding time	
Ivy	Less than 4 minutes
Duke	1–4 minutes
Clot retraction qualitative	Begins in 30–60 minutes
	Complete within 24 hours; usually within 6 hours
Coagulation time (Lee-White)	6–17 minutes (glass tubes)
	19–60 minutes (siliconized tubes)
Fibrinolysins	0
Prothrombin time (one stage)	Same as control (control should be 11–16 seconds)
Prothrombin content	100% (calculated from prothrombin time)
Prothrombin consumption	Over 80% consumed in 1 hour
Thromboplastin generation test	Compared to normal control
Thrombin time	Within 5 seconds of control

The lists of normal blood chemistries are arranged both alphabetically and by type of chemical component (e.g., enzymes, electrolytes, blood gases, pH) for greatest convenience.

BLOOD CHEMISTRIES

The normal values will vary depending upon the individual laboratory as well as the methods used.

Acetone	0.3–2.0 mg/100 ml
Aldolase (ALD)	3–8 (Sibley-Lehninger) units/ml
Ammonia	30–70 μg/100 ml
Amylase	60–180 Somogyi units/100 ml
Barbiturates	0
	Coma level: phenobarbital approximately 11 mg/100 ml; most other barbiturates 2–4 mg/100 ml
Total base	145–160 mEq/L
Bilirubin	
Direct	0.1–0.4 mg/100 ml
Indirect (=total minus direct)	0.1–0.5 mg/100 ml
Total	0.2–0.9 mg/100 ml
Bromides	0
	Toxic levels above 17 mEq/L (150 mg/100 ml)
Calcium	8.5–10.5 mg/100 ml (higher in children)
Carbon dioxide	
Content	26–28 mEq/L (20–26 mEq/L in infants)
Tension pCO_2	35–45 mm Hg
Carbon monoxide	Symptoms with over 20% saturation
Ceruloplasmin	20–35 mg/100 ml
Chloride	98–106 mEq/L
Cholesterol	

Cholesterol Total:

Age (years)	Cholesterol (mg/100 ml)
1–19	120–230
20–29	120–240
30–39	140–270
40–49	150–310
50–59	160–330

Esters	60–75% of total
Cholinesterase (Michel method)	
Plasma	0.44–1.63 for men; 0.24–1.54 for women (Δ pH/hr)
RBC	0.39–1.02 for men; 0.34–1.10 for women (Δ pH/hr)
Copper	65–170 μg/100 ml
Creatine phosphokinase (CPK)	0–12 Sigma units/ml
Creatinine	0.7–1.5 mg/100 ml
Cryoglobulins	0

Dilantin	Therapeutic levels 1–11 μg/ml
	Toxic levels 20 μg/ml
Ethanol	
Marked intoxication	0.3–0.4%
Alcoholic stupor	0.4–0.5%
Coma	Above 0.5%
Fibrinogen	200–400 mg/100 ml
Gamma-glutamyl transpeptidase	Females: 4–18 mU/ml at 25°C
	5.3–24 mU/ml at 30°C
	Males: 6–28 mU/ml at 25°C
	8–37 mU/ml at 30°C
Glucose (fasting)	
O-toluidine	60–100 mg/100 ml
True	70–110 mg/100 ml
Folin	80–120 mg/100 ml
Icterus index	4–7 units
Iodine	
Butanol-extractable (BEI)	3.0–6.5 μg/100 ml
Protein-bound (PBI)	3.5–8.8 μg/100 ml
Iron	80–160 μg/100 ml in men; 60–135 μg/100 ml in women
Iron-binding capacity	250–350 μg/100 ml
% saturation	20–55%
Transferrin	300–359 mg/100 ml
Isocitric dehydrogenase (ICD)	50–180 Sigma units/ml
Lactic acid	6–16 mg/100 ml
Lactic dehydrogenase (LDH)	200–680 units/ml
Lead	0–50 μg/100 ml
Leucine aminopeptidase (LAP)	75–230 (Goldbarg-Rutenburg) units/ml
Lipase	Less than 1.5 units (ml of N/20 NaOH)
Lipids, total	450–850 mg/100 ml
Lipid fractionation	

Lipid fractionation — Cholesterol

Age (years)	Cholesterol (mg/100 ml)
1–19	120–230
20–29	120–240
30–39	140–270
40–49	150–310
50–59	160–330

    Phospholipids   60–350 mg/100 ml

Triglycerides

Age (years)	Triglyceride (mg/100 ml)
1–19	10–140
20–29	10–140
30–39	10–150
40–49	10–160
50–59	10–190

Magnesium	1.5–2.5 mEq/L
	(1.8–3.0 mg/100 ml)
Nonprotein nitrogen (NPN)	16–35 mg/100 ml
Osmolality	285–295 mOsm/L

Oxygen
    Capacity   16–24 vol% (varies with Hb)
    Content
        Arterial   15–23 vol%
        Venous   10–16 vol%
    Saturation
        Arterial   94–100% of capacity
        Venous   60–85% of capacity
    Tension, pO_2 Arterial   95–100 mm Hg
pH, arterial   7.35–7.45
Phenylalanine   0–2 mg/100 ml
Phosphatase
    Acid   1.0–5.0 King-Armstrong units
        0.5–2.0 Bodansky units
        0.5–2.0 Gutman units
        0–1.1 Shinowara units
        0.1–0.73 Bessey-Lowry units
    Alkaline   5.0–13.0 King-Armstrong units (10–20*)
        2.0–4.5 Bodansky units (3–13*)
        3.0–10.0 Gutman units
        2.2–8.6 Shinowara units
        0.8–2.3 Bessey-Lowry units (3.4–9.0*)
Phosphorus   2.0–4.5 mg/100 ml (4.0–7.0 mg/100 ml*)
Potassium   3.5–5.5 mEq/L
Proteins, serum
    Total   6.0–8.0 gm/100 ml
        Albumin   3.5–5.5 gm/100 ml
        Globulin   1.5–3.0 gm/100 ml
    Paper electrophoresis
        Albumin   45–55% of total
        Globulin
            Alpha$_1$ 5–8% of total
            Alpha$_2$ 8–13% of total
            Beta   11–17% of total
            Gamma   15–25% of total
Alpha$_1$ antitrypsin   47–153% normal
Haptoglobin   30–160 mg/100 ml
Transferrin   205–374 mg/100 ml
C3   100–200 mg/100 ml
Immunoglobulins

	IgG (mg/100 ml)	IgA (mg/100 ml)	IgM (ml/100 ml)
Newborn	900–1500	0–5	5–20
1–3 months	250–550	5–50	20–40
4–6 months	300–600	10–55	30–60
7–12 months	400–900	20–60	35–75
2 years	550–1000	35–75	40–80
3 years	550–1100	50–110	40–85
4–5 years	550–1100	60–150	40–95
6–8 years	550–1200	60–170	40–95
12 years	550–1400	60–200	40–110
Adult	550–1900	60–330	45–145

* = values in children.

	IgE (mean units/ml)	*IgE* (range units/ml)
Cord serum	1.6	0.7– 3.4
6 weeks–3 months	4.4	1.1– 17
3 months–9 months	16	4.2– 60
9 months–2 years	18	6.4– 53
2 years–5 years	65	21 –198
5 years–10 years	89	18 –451
10 years–20 years	86	12 –618
20 years–70 years	71	10 –506

The level of IgE in normal sera is extremely low. For the Phadebas IgE Test, the above normal values have been recorded.

Salicylate	0
Therapeutic range	20–25 mg/100 ml
Toxic range	Over 30 mg/100 ml
Sodium	136–145 mEq/L
Transaminase	
SGOT (glutamic-oxalacetic)	5–40 units/ml (Sigma-Frankel units)
SGPT (glutamic-pyruvic)	5–35 units/ml (Sigma-Frankel units)
Urea nitrogen (BUN)	10–20 mg/100 ml
Uric acid	3.0–7.5 mg/100 ml in females; up to 8.5 mg/100 ml in males

BLOOD CHEMISTRIES BY TYPE OF COMPONENT

The normal values will vary depending upon the individual laboratory as well as the methods used.

General

Glucose (fasting)	
O-toluidine	60–100 mg/100 ml
True	70–110 mg/100 ml
Folin	80–120 mg/100 ml
Uric acid	3.0–7.5 mg/100 ml; up to 8.5 mg/100 ml in males
Urea nitrogen (BUN)	10–20 mg/100 ml
Creatinine	0.7–1.5 mg/100 ml
Bilirubin	
Direct	0.1–0.4 mg/100 ml
Indirect	0.1–0.5 mg/100 ml
Total	0.2–0.9 mg/100 ml

Icterus index   4–7 units
Iodine
    Butanol-extractable (BEI)   3.0–6.5 µg/100 ml
    Protein-bound (PBI)   3.5–8.8 µg/100 ml
Ammonia   30–70 µg/100 ml
Cholesterol

Total	Age (years)	Cholesterol (mg/100 ml)
	1–19	120–230
	20–29	120–240
	30–39	140–270
	40–49	150–310
	50–59	160–330

    Esters   60–75% of total
Lipids, total   450–850 mg/100 ml
Lipid fractionation

Cholesterol	Age (years)	Cholesterol (mg/100 ml)
	1–19	120–230
	20–29	120–240
	30–39	140–270
	40–49	150–310
	50–59	160–330

    Phospholipids   60–350 mg/100 ml

Triglycerides	Age (years)	Triglyceride (mg/100 ml)
	1–19	10–140
	20–29	10–140
	30–39	10–150
	40–49	10–160
	50–59	10–190

Nonprotein nitrogen (NPN)   16–35 mg/100 ml

Enzymes
Amylase   60–180 Somogyi units/100 ml
Lipase   Less than 1.5 units (ml of N/20 NaOH)

Transaminase
    SGOT (glutamic-oxalacetic)   5–40 units/ml (Sigma-Frankel units)
    SGPT (glutamic-pyruvic)   5–35 units/ml (Sigma-Frankel units)

Phosphatase
    Acid   1.0–5.0 King-Armstrong units
                               0.5–2.0 Bodansky units
                               0.5–2.0 Gutman units
                               0–1.1 Shinowara units
                               0.1–0.73 Bessey-Lowry units
    Alkaline   5.0–13.0 King-Armstrong units (10–20*)
                               2.0–4.5 Bodansky units (3–13*)
                               3–10 Gutman units
                               2.2–8.6 Shinowara units
                               0.8–2.3 Bessey-Lowry units (3.4–9*)

---

* = values in children.

Gamma-glutamyl transpeptidase	Females: 4–18 mU/ml at 25°C 5.3–24 mU/ml at 30°C Males: 6–28 mU/ml at 25°C 8–37 mU/ml at 30°C
Leucine aminopeptidase (LAP)	75–230 (Goldbarg-Rutenburg) units/ml
Lactic dehydrogenase (LDH)	200–680 units/ml
Hydroxybutyric dehydrogenase (α-HBD)	120–260 Rosalki units/ml
Isocitric dehydrogenase (ICD)	50–180 Sigma units/ml
Creatine phosphokinase (CPK)	0–12 Sigma units/ml
Cholinesterase (Michel method)	
Plasma	0.44–1.63 for men; 0.24–1.54 for women (Δ pH/hr)
RBC	0.39–1.02 for men; 0.34–1.10 for women (Δ pH/hr)
Aldolase (ALD)	3–8 (Sibley-Lehninger) units/ml
Malic dehydrogenase (MDH)	25–100 units/ml
Ornithine carbamyl transferase (OCT)	0–500 Sigma units/ml
5'-Nucleotidase	0.3–2.6 Bodansky units

Erythrocyte Enzymes

Glucose-6-phosphate dehydrogenase	5–15 units
6-Phosphogluconate dehydrogenase	2–5 units
Glutathione reductase	9–13 units
Pyruvate kinase	2–3 units

Electrolytes

Sodium	136–145 mEq/L
Potassium	3.5–5.5 mEq/L
Chloride	100–106 mEq/L
Calcium	8.5–10.5 mg/100 ml (higher in children)
Phosphorus	2.0–4.5 mg/100 ml (4.0–7.0 mg/100 ml*)
Magnesium	1.5–2.5 mEq/L (1.8–3.0 mg/100 ml)

Blood Gases and pH

Total base	145–160 mEq/L
Carbon dioxide	
Content	26–28 mEq/L (20–26 mEq/L in infants)
Tension, pCO_2	35–45 mm Hg
Oxygen	
Capacity	16–24 vol% (varies with Hb)
Content	
Arterial	15–23 vol%
Venous	10–16 vol%
Saturation	
Arterial	94–100% of capacity
Venous	60–85% of capacity

---

* = values in children.

Tension, pO$_2$, arterial	95–100 mm Hg
Carbon monoxide	Symptoms with over 20% saturation
Osmolality	285–295 mOsm/L
Arterial pH	7.35–7.45
Lactic acid	6–16 mg/100 ml

Blood Proteins

Proteins, serum	
Total	6.0–8.0 gm/100 ml
Albumin	3.5–5.5 gm/100 ml
Globulin	1.5–3.0 gm/100 ml
Electrophoresis	
Albumin	45–55% of total
Globulin	
Alpha$_1$	5–8% of total
Alpha$_2$	8–13% of total
Beta	11–17% of total
Gamma	15–25% of total
Fibrinogen	200–400 mg/100 ml
Cryoglobulins	0
Alpha$_1$ antitrypsin	47–153% normal
Haptoglobin	30–160 mg/100 ml
Transferrin	205–374 mg/100 ml
C3	100–200 mg/100 ml
Immunoglobulins	

	IgG (mg/100 ml)	*IgA* (mg/100 ml)	*IgM* (mg/100 ml)
Newborn	900–1500	0–5	5–20
1–3 months	250–550	5–50	20–40
4–6 months	300–600	10–55	30–60
7–12 months	400–900	20–60	35–75
2 years	550–1000	35–75	40–80
3 years	550–1100	50–110	40–85
4–5 years	550–1100	60–150	40–95
6–8 years	550–1200	60–170	40–95
12 years	550–1400	60–200	40–110
Adult	550–1900	60–330	45–145

	IgE (mean units/ml)	*IgE* (range units/ml)
Cord serum	1.6	0.7– 3.4
6 weeks–3 months	4.4	1.1– 17
3 months–9 months	16	4.2– 60
9 months–2 years	18	6.4– 53
2 years–5 years	65	21 –198
5 years–10 years	89	18 –451
10 years–20 years	86	12 –618
20 years–70 years	71	10 –506

(The level of IgE in normal sera is extremely low. For the Phadebas IgE Test, the above normal values have been recorded.)

Hematology

Iron	80–160 μg/100 ml in men; 60–135 μg/100 ml in women

Iron-binding capacity	250–350 μg/100 ml
% saturation	20–55%
Transferrin	300–359 mg/100 ml
Ceruloplasmin	20–35 mg/100 ml
Copper	65–170 μg/100 ml

Toxicology

Salicylate	0
Therapeutic range	20–25 mg/100 ml
Toxic range	Over 30 mg/100 ml
Dilantin	Therapeutic levels 1–11 μg/ml
	Toxic levels 20 μg/ml

Ethanol
Marked intoxication	0.3–0.4%
Alcoholic stupor	0.4–0.5%
Coma	Above 0.5%
Lead	0–50 μg/100 ml
Barbiturates	0

Coma level: phenobarbital approximately 11 mg/100 ml; most other barbiturates 1.5 mg/100 ml

Bromides   0

Toxic levels above 17 mEq/L (150 mg/100 ml)

Lithium   Therapeutic levels, 8 hours after administration

Acute	0.5–1.5 mEq/L
Long-term control	0.5–1.0 mEq/L
Toxic	1.5–2.5 mEq/L

2
Urine

Specific gravity	1.003–1.030
pH	4.6–8.0 (average 6.0), depends on diet
Total solids	30–70 gm/L (average 50). To estimate: multiply last two figures of specific gravity by 2.66 (Long's coefficient)
Osmolality	50–1200 mOsm/kg urine water
Volume	600–2500 ml/24 hours (average 1200); night volume usually less than 700 ml with specific gravity more than 1.018; ratio of night to day volume 1:2 to 1:4
Protein	Qualitative = 0
	0–0.1 gm/24 hours
Glucose	Qualitative = 0
	Up to 0.3 gm/24 hours
Ketones	Qualitative = 0
Calcium	Less than 150 mg/24 hours on low-calcium (Bauer-Aub) diet
Phosphorus	1 gm/24 hours (average); depends on diet
Urobilinogen	0–4 mg/24 hours
Porphyrins	50–300 μg/24 hours; 0–75 μg/24 hours in children weighing less than 80 pounds
Amylase	260–950 Somogyi units/24 hours
Lead	Less than 0.08 μg/ml or 120 μg/24 hours
Delta-aminolevulinic acid	1.3–7.0 mg/24 hours
Homogentisic acid	0
Hemoglobin and myoglobin	0
Creatinine	1.0–1.6 gm/24 hours (15–25 mg/kg of body weight/24 hours)
Creatine	Less than 100 mg/24 hours (less than 6% of creatinine); higher during childhood and pregnancy

Cystine or cysteine	0
Phenylpyruvic acid	0
Microscopical examination	Up to 1–2 RBC, WBC, epithelial cells/hpf; occasional hyaline cast/lpf
Addis count	RBC up to 1,000,000/24 hours
	Casts up to 100,000/24 hours
	WBC + epithelial cells, up to 2,000,000/24 hours

3

Stool

Bulk	100–200 gm
Water	Up to 75%
Color	Brown
	Clay color (gray white) in biliary obstruction
	Tarry if more than 100 ml of blood in upper GI tract
	Red—blood in large intestine or undigested beets or tomatoes
	Black—blood or iron or bismuth medication
	Various colors depending on diet
pH	7.0–7.5 (may be acid with high lactose intake)
Microscopical examination	RBCs absent
	Epithelial cells present (increased with GI tract irritation)
	Few WBCs present (increased with GI tract inflammation)
	Crystals of calcium oxalate, fatty acid, and triple phosphate commonly present
	Hematoidin crystals sometimes found after GI tract hemorrhage
	Charcot-Leyden crystals sometimes found in parasitic infestation (especially amebiasis)
	Some undigested vegetable fibers and muscle fibers sometimes found normally
	Neutral fat globules (stained with Sudan) normal 0 to 2+
Nitrogen	Less than 2.5 gm/day
Urobilinogen	40–280 mg/24 hours (100–400 Ehrlich units/100 gm)

Coproporphyrin	400–1000 mg/24 hours
Fat	Less than 7 gm/24 hours during 3-day period
	Less than 30% of dry weight (on diet of more than 50 gm of fat/day)
Calcium	About 0.6 gm/24 hours

4

Cerebrospinal Fluid

Simultaneous measurement of blood level should always be performed.

Appearance	Clear, colorless; no clot
Total cell count	0–10/cu mm (all mononuclear cells) in adults
	0–20/cu mm in infants
Glucose	45–80 mg/100 ml (20 mg/100 ml less than blood level)
	Ventricular fluid 5–10 mg/100 ml higher than lumbar
Total protein	15–45 mg/100 ml (lumbar)
	15–25 mg/100 ml (cisternal)
	5–15 mg/100 ml (ventricular)
Gamma globulin	5–12% of total protein
Colloidal gold	Not more than 1 in any tube
Chloride	120–130 mEq/L (20 mEq/L higher than serum)
Sodium	142–150 mEq/L
Potassium	2.2–3.3 mEq/L
Carbon dioxide	25 mEq/L
pH	7.35–7.40
Transaminase (GOT)	7–49 units
Lactic dehydrogenase (LDH)	15–71 units
Creatine phosphokinase (CPK)	0–3 I.U.
Bilirubin	0
Urea nitrogen	5–25 mg/100 ml
Amino acids	30% of blood level

5

Serous Fluids
(*Pleural, Pericardial, and Ascitic*)

Specific gravity	1.010–1.026
Total protein	0.3–4.1 gm/100 ml
Albumin	50–70%
Globulin	30–45%
Fibrinogen	0.3–4.5%
pH	6.8–7.6

6

Synovial Fluid

Volume	1.0–3.5 ml
pH	Parallels serum
Appearance	Clear, pale yellow or straw-colored
	Viscous, does not clot
Fibrin clot	0
Mucin clot	Good
WBC (per cu mm)	Less than 200 (even in presence of leukocytosis in blood)
Neutrophils (%)	Less than 25
Crystals	
Free	0
Intracellular	0
Fasting glucose, uric acid, bilirubin	Approximately the same as serum
Total protein	Approximately 25–30% of serum protein
	Mean is 1.8 gm/100 ml
	Abnormal if more than 2.5 gm/100 ml; inflammation is moderately severe if more than 4.5 gm/100 ml
Culture	0

7

Semen

Volume	More than 3 ml
Liquefaction	Complete in 15 minutes
pH	7.2–8.0 (average 7.8)
Count	More than 50 million/ml; 250 million/ejaculation
Morphology	More than 60% of sperm motile and more than 50% of normal morphology
Smear	Usually no RBC or WBC present

8

Liver Function Tests

Bromsulphalein (BSP) test	Serum—less than 5% retained 45 minutes after IV injection of 5 mg/kg body weight
Cephalin-cholesterol floccula-tion test	0 to 2+ in 48 hours
Cholinesterase (pseudocholin-esterase)	0.5 pH units or more/hour
Galactose tolerance test (GTT)	Excretion of not more than 3 gm galactose in urine 5 hours after ingestion of 40 gm galactose
Prothrombin time	Same as control; if increased, IV administration of synthetic vi-tamin K returns prothrombin time to normal in obstructive liver disease (or other causes of malabsorption of vitamin K) but not in parenchymal liver disease
Thymol turbidity	0 to 5 units

Serum bilirubin, serum enzymes (e.g., SGOT, SGPT, LDH, alkaline phosphatase), urine bile and urobilinogen. See Differential Diag-nosis of Liver Disease (Tables 18, 19, and 20, pp. 181–183).

Serum proteins, protein electrophoresis, lipoprotein electrophoresis, fractionation of lipids, etc. See Chapter 27.

9

Renal Function Tests

Concentration and dilution	Specific gravity >1.025 Specific gravity <1.003
Phenolsulfonphthalein (PSP) excretion	$>25\%$ in urine in 15 minutes 55–75% in 2 hours

Clearances (corrected to 1.73 square meters body surface area)
To measure glomerular filtration rate (GFR)

Endogenous creatinine	90–130 ml/minute
Inulin	Males: 110–150 ml/minute Females: 105–132 ml/minute
Urea	Maximum: 60–100 ml/minute Standard: 40–65 ml/minute

To measure effective renal plasma flow (RPF) and tubular function

Para-aminohippurate (PAH) or Diodrast	Males: 560–800 ml/minute Females: 50–700 ml/minute
Filtration fraction (FF) = GFR/RPF	Males: 17–21% Females: 17–23%
Maximal PAH excretory capacity, Tm_{PAH}	80–90 mg/minute
Maximal Diodrast excretory capacity, Tm_D	Males: 43–59 mg/minute Females: 33–51 mg/minute
Maximal glucose reabsorptive capacity, Tm_G	Males: 300–450 mg/minute Females: 250–350 mg/minute
BUN, Creatinine, Addis Count. See pp. 38, 39, 17.	

10

Blood and Urine Hormone Levels

Measurement of Thyroid Function	Blood
Protein-bound iodine (PBI)	3.6–8.8 μg/100 ml
Butanol-extractable iodine (BEI)	3–6 μg/100 ml
T-3 (resin sponge uptake)	24–36%
T-4 (resin sponge)	4–11%
T-4 (thyroxine by column chromatography)	2.9–6.4 μg/100 ml
Free thyroxine index (T-3 × T-4)	96–396
"Free thyroxine"	1.0–2.1 mμg/100 ml
Thyroxine-binding globulin (TBG)	10–26 μg/100 ml thyroxine
Thyroid-stimulating hormone (TSH)	Up to 0.2 mU/ml
Long-acting thyroid stimulator (LATS)	None detectable
Radioactive iodine uptake (RAIU)	9–19% in 1 hour 7–25% in 6 hours 10–50% in 24 hours
Radioactive iodine excretion	40–70% of administered dose in 24 hours

Hormone	Blood	Urine
Pregnanediol		
Male		<1.5 mg/24 hours
Female		
Proliferative phase		0.5–1.5 mg/24 hours
Luteal phase		2–7 mg/24 hours
Postmenopausal		0.2–1.0 mg/24 hours
Pregnanetriol		<4 mg/24 hours

Hormone	*Blood*	*Urine*
Estrogens (total)		Male: 4–25 μg/24 hours Female: 4–60 μg/24 hours Marked increase during pregnancy
Testosterone		
Male (adult)	0.37–1.0 μg/100 ml (average = 0.7)	47–156 μg/24 hours (average = 70)
Male (adolescent)	>0.10 μg/100 ml	
Female	0–0.1 μg/100 ml (average = 0.04)	0–15 μg/24 hours (average = < 6)
Pituitary gonadotropins (FSH)		6–50 mouse uterine units/24 hours
Chorionic gonadotropin		0
Aldosterone	0.015 μg/100 ml	2–12 μg/24 hours
Catecholamines (adrenaline-noradrenaline)		Epinephrine—< 10 μg/24 hours Norepinephrine—< 100 μg/24 hours
Metanephrines, total		24–288 μg/24 hours
Metanephrine		24–96 μg/24 hours
Normetanephrine		72–288 μg/24 hours
Vanilmandelic acid (VMA)		Up to 9 mg/24 hours
Homovanillic acid		<15 mg/24 hours
Serotonin (as 5-hydroxyindoleacetic acid, 5-HIAA)	0.05–0.20 μg/ml	2–10 mg/24 hours (qualitative = 0)
17-Hydroxycorticoids	(cortisol) 5–25 μg/100 ml at 8 A.M. <10 μg/100 ml at 8 P.M. Falls to <10 μg/100 ml by 9 P.M.	
Glenn-Nelson		Males: 3–10 mg/24 hours Females: 2–6 mg/24 hours
17-Ketogenic steroids		Males: 5–23 mg/24 hours Females: 3–15 mg/24 hours

Hormone	*Blood*	*Urine*
17-Ketosteroids	25–125 units/100 ml	Under 8 years old: 0–2 mg/24 hours Adolescents: 2–18 mg/24 hours Male (adult): 8–18 mg/24 hours Female (adult): 5–15 mg/24 hours Beta:alpha ratio 0.2

11

Blood Vitamin Levels

Vitamin A	65–275 I.U./100 ml
	$> 20~\mu g/100$ ml
Carotene	100–300 I.U./100 ml
	40–300 $\mu g/100$ ml
Vitamin C	0.2–2.0 mg/100 ml
Ascorbic acid	> 0.20 mg/100 ml
Vitamin D	0.7–3.3 I.U./ml (procedure not generally available)
	Indirect estimate by measuring serum alkaline phosphatase, calcium, and phosphorus)
Vitamin E (tocopherol)	> 0.5 mg/100 ml
Vitamin B$_{12}$	300–1000 pg/ml
Folic acid	5–21 $\mu\mu g/100$ ml

12

Urine Vitamin Levels

Urinary Riboflavin Excretion

Age	Deficient	Low	Acceptable	High
(Unit of measurement: µg/6 hours)				
Adults	< 10	10–29	30–99	> 100
(Unit of measurement: µg/gm creatinine)				
Adults	< 27	27–79	80–269	> 270
1–3 yrs	< 150	150–499	500–900	> 900
4–6	< 100	100–299	300–600	> 600
7–9	< 85	85–269	270–500	> 500
10–15	< 70	70–199	200–400	> 400

Urinary Niacin Metabolite Excretion

	Deficient	Low	Acceptable	High
(Unit of measurement: mg N-methylnicotinamide/6 hours) *(affected by intake of tryptophan)*				
Adults	< 0.2	0.2–0.59	0.6–1.59	> 1.6
(Unit of measurement: mg N-methylnicotinamide/gm creatinine)				
Adults	< 0.5	0.5–1.59	1.6–4.29	> 4.3

Urinary Thiamine Excretion

	Deficient	Low	Acceptable	High
(Unit of measurement: µg/6 hours)				
Adults	< 10	10–24	25–49	> 50
(Unit of measurement: µg/gm creatinine)				
Adults	< 27	27–65	66–129	> 130
1–3 yrs	< 120	120–175	176–600	> 600
4–6	< 85	85–120	121–400	> 400
7–9	< 70	70–180	181–350	> 350
10–12	< 60	60–180	181–300	> 300
13–15	< 50	50–150	151–250	> 250

Urinary Pyridoxine and Pantothenic Acid

Microbiologic assay

13

Amniotic Fluid

COMPARISON OF VARIOUS CHEMICAL COMPONENTS IN AMNIOTIC FLUID, MATERNAL SERUM, AND FETAL SERUM DURING NORMAL PREGNANCY*

	Amniotic Fluid	Maternal Serum	Fetal Serum
Total protein (gm/100 ml)	0.28 (0.3)	6.5 (0.6)	5.8 (0.7)
Albumin (% by electrophoresis)	65.2 (4.8)	46.4 (3.1)	60.8 (4.8)
A/G ratio	1.9 (0.7)	0.8 (0.1)	1.5 (0.3)
Urea (mg/100 ml)	33.9 (11.7)	17.1 (8.7)	16.5 (8.14)
Uric acid (mg/100 ml)	7.5 (0.3)	3.1 (0.8)	2.6 (0.9)
Creatinine (mg/100 ml)	2.4 (0.3)	1.1 (0.2)	1.3 (0.3)
Glucose (mg/100 ml)	10.7 (5.2)	66.6 (8.7)	49.7 (10.4)
Lactic dehydrogenase (LDH) (units/ml)	112.3 (64.8)	199.5 (46.4)	328.2 (114.0)
Aldolase (units/ml)	10.1 (7.5)	9.5 (7.0)	23.3 (9.4)
Total cholesterol (mg/100 ml)	42.8 (3.2)	258.6 (47.2)	83.5 (39.7)
Triglycerides (mg/100 ml)	19.3 (9.4)	153.7 (51.4)	16.1 (10.7)

Values are mean values. Numbers in ( ) represent one standard deviation.

---

* L. Castelazo-Ayala, S. Karchmer, and V. Shor-Pinsker, "The Biochemistry of Amniotic Fluid During Normal Pregnancy Correlation with Maternal and Fetal Blood," in A. A. Hodari and F. Mariona (Eds.), *Physiological Biochemistry of the Fetus, Proceedings of the International Symposium.* Springfield, Ill.: Thomas, 1972, pp. 32-53.

COMPARISON OF VARIOUS CHEMICAL COMPONENTS IN AMNIOTIC FLUID DURING SECOND TRIMESTER OF NORMAL PREGNANCY AND AT TERM

	Second Trimester	At Term
Uric acid*	3.7 mg	9.9 mg (represents increased urinary output and increased muscle mass of fetus)
Creatinine*	0.9 mg	2.0 mg (represents increased muscle mass of fetus)
Total protein	0.6 gm	0.3 gm
Albumin	0.4 gm	0.05 gm
Transaminase (GOT)	17 I.U.	40 I.U.
Alkaline phosphatase	25 I.U.	80 I.U. (up to 350 I.U. in some cases)

Bilirubin†
Urea nitrogen
Calcium
Phosphorus   } Values do not change significantly during gestation
Glucose
Lactic dehydrogenase (LDH)
Cholesterol

---

* Could be useful in determining fetal age in utero.
† Useful in following course of hemolytic disease of newborn.

Values are mean values per 100 ml as determined by SMA-12 Autoanalyser (Technicon).

Source: T. Tsudaka, D. Bloch, and P. L. Wolf, An automated profile of amniotic fluid. *Lab. Med.* (1971), 32.

FETAL LUNG MATURITY

It has been reported that determination of lecithin and sphingomyelin in amniotic fluid (thin-layer chromatography) predicts fetal lung maturity.*

Immature lungs	Lecithin less than sphingomyelin
Lungs on threshold of maturity	Lecithin equal to sphingomyelin
Mature lungs	Lecithin greater than sphingomyelin
Postmature lungs	Large amounts of lecithin with only a trace or no sphingomyelin

---

* M. R. Knieser, R. Hurst, and C. R. Tuegel, *Amer. J. Clin. Path.* 58:579, 1972.

OTHER USES OF AMNIOTIC FLUID

Amniotic fluid can also be used for

Prenatal determination of sex of infant by detection of Barr bodies (see p. 137). May be useful when mother is heterozygous for X-linked recessive disorders (e.g., hemophilia A and B, muscular dystrophy). Fifty percent of male children will be affected but the fact that he is male does not establish the diagnosis in that infant.

Karyotyping (see p. 138) is useful principally in diagnosis of Down's syndrome. May be useful to screen when mother is over 40 or has previously had an affected child.

Diagnosis of some inborn errors of metabolism is made by detecting biochemical abnormality in fluid or in culture of cells, e.g., Tay-Sachs disease, Lesch-Nyham syndrome, mucopolysaccharidoses Types I and II, metachromatic leukodystrophy.

14

Other Functional Tests

Other tests to determine the functioning status of the various organ
systems appear under the appropriate specific diseases in each
chapter.

       Gastrointestinal Diseases
       Hepatobiliary Diseases and Disorders of the Pancreas
       Metabolic and Hereditary Diseases
       Endocrine Diseases

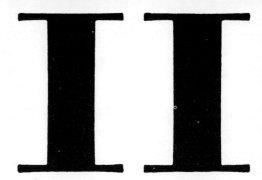

Specific Laboratory Examinations

15

Blood

CHEMISTRIES

SERUM GLUCOSE

May Be Increased In
Diabetes mellitus including
    Hemochromatosis
    Cushing's syndrome (with insulin-resistant diabetes)
    Acromegaly and gigantism (with insulin-resistant diabetes in
        early stages; hypopituitarism later)
Increased circulating adrenalin
    Adrenalin injection
    Pheochromocytoma
    Stress (emotion, burns, shock, anesthesia, etc.)
Acute pancreatitis
Chronic pancreatitis (some cases)
Wernicke's encephalopathy (vitamin B_1 deficiency)
Some CNS lesions (subarachnoid hemorrhage, convulsive states)
ACTH administration

May Be Decreased In
Pancreatic disorders
    Islet cell tumor, hyperplasia
    Pancreatitis
    Glucagon deficiency
Extrapancreatic tumors
    Carcinoma of adrenal
    Carcinoma of stomach
    Fibrosarcoma
    Others
Hepatic disease
    Diffuse severe disease (e.g., poisons, hepatitis, cirrhosis, primary
        or metastatic tumor)
Endocrine disorders
    Hypopituitarism and Addison's disease
    Hypothyroidism
    Adrenal medulla unresponsiveness
    Early diabetes mellitus

Functional disturbances
    Postgastrectomy, gastroenterostomy, autonomic nervous system disorders
Others
    Exogenous insulin
    Oral hypoglycemic medications
    Leucine sensitivity
    Malnutrition
    Hypothalamic lesions
Pediatric anomalies
    Prematurity
    Infant of diabetic mother
    Ketotic hypoglycemia
    Zetterstrom's syndrome
    Idiopathic leucine sensitivity
    Spontaneous hypoglycemia in infants
Enzyme diseases
    von Gierke's disease
    Galactosemia
    Maple syrup urine disease
    Fructose intolerance

SERUM UREA NITROGEN (BUN)

Increased In
Impaired kidney function. See Serum Creatinine, p. 39.
Prerenal azotemia. Any cause of reduced renal blood flow
    E.g., congestive heart failure
        salt and water depletion (vomiting, diarrhea, diuresis, sweating)
        shock
Postrenal azotemia. Any obstruction of urinary tract
    (Ratio of BUN : creatinine increases above normal 10 : 1.)
Increased protein catabolism (Serum creatinine remains normal.)
    Hemorrhage into gastrointestinal tract
    Acute myocardial infarction
    Stress

Decreased In
Severe liver damage (liver failure)
    Drugs, poisons, hepatitis, etc.
Increased utilization of protein for synthesis
    Late pregnancy
    Infancy
    Acromegaly
Diet
    Low protein and high carbohydrate
    IV feedings only
    Impaired absorption (celiac disease)
Nephrotic syndrome (some patients)

A low BUN of 6–8 mg/100 ml is frequently associated with states of overhydration.
A BUN of 10–15 mg/100 ml almost always indicates normal glomerular function.
A BUN of 50–150 mg/100 ml implies serious impairment of renal function.

Markedly increased BUN (150–250 mg/100 ml) is virtually conclusive of severely impaired glomerular function.

In chronic renal disease, BUN correlates better with symptoms of uremia than does the serum creatinine.

SERUM NONPROTEIN NITROGEN (NPN)

NPN is not as useful as BUN as an index of renal function because it represents a heterogeneous group of substances not all of which are excreted by the kidney. The increase parallels that of BUN.

SERUM CREATININE

Increased In
Diet
    Ingestion of creatinine (roast meat)
Muscle disease
    Gigantism
    Acromegaly
Prerenal azotemia. See Serum Urea Nitrogen, p. 38.
Postrenal azotemia. See Serum Urea Nitrogen, p. 38.
Impaired kidney function
A. Ratio of BUN : creatinine more than 10 : 1
    Excess intake of protein
    Blood in small bowel
    Excess tissue breakdown (cachexia, burns, high fever, corticosteroid therapy)
    Urinary tract obstruction (postrenal)
    Inadequate renal blood flow (prerenal congestive heart failure, dehydration, shock, etc.)
    Urinary reabsorption (e.g., ureterocolostomy)
B. Ratio of BUN : creatinine less than 10 : 1
    Low protein intake
    Repeated dialysis
    Severe diarrhea or vomiting
    Hepatic insufficiency

Serum creatinine is a more specific and sensitive indicator of renal disease than BUN. Use of simultaneous BUN and creatinine determinations provides more information.

Decreased In
Not clinically significant

SERUM CREATINE

Increased In
High dietary intake (meat)
Destruction of muscle
Hyperthyroidism (this diagnosis almost excluded by normal serum creatine)
Active rheumatoid arthritis
Testosterone therapy

Decreased In
Not clinically significant

SERUM URIC ACID

Levels are very labile and show day-to-day and seasonal variation in same individuals; also increased by emotional stress, total fasting.

Increased In
Gout
25% of relatives of patients with gout
Renal failure (does not correlate with severity of kidney damage; urea and creatinine should be used)
Increased destruction of nucleoproteins
  Leukemia, multiple myeloma
  Polycythemia
  Lymphoma, especially post–x-radiation
  Other disseminated neoplasms
  Hemolytic anemia
  Resolving pneumonia
  Toxemia of pregnancy (serial determinations to follow therapeutic response and estimate prognosis)
  Psoriasis (one-third of patients)
Diet
  High-protein weight reduction diet
  Excess nucleoprotein (sweetbreads, liver)
Asymptomatic hyperuricemia (incidental finding with no evidence of gout, etc.; clinical significance not known but these people should be rechecked periodically for gout) The higher the level of serum uric acid, the greater the likelihood of an attack of acute gouty arthritis.
Miscellaneous
  von Gierke's disease
  Lead poisoning
  Lesch-Nyham syndrome
  Calcinosis universalis and circumscripta
  Some drugs (e.g., thiazides, furosemide, ethacrynic acid)
  Hypoparathyroidism
  Primary hyperparathyroidism
  Sarcoidosis
  Chronic berylliosis
  Some patients with alcoholism
  Patients with arteriosclerosis and hypertension (*Serum uric acid is increased in more than 80% of patients with elevated serum triglycerides.*)
  Certain population groups (Blackfoot and Pima Indians, Filipinos, New Zealand Maoris, etc.)

Decreased In
Administration of ACTH
Administration of uricosuric drugs (high doses of salicylates, probenecid, cortisone, allopurinol, coumarins, etc.)
Wilson's disease
Fanconi's syndrome
Acromegaly (some patients)
Celiac disease (slight)
Pernicious anemia in relapse (some patients)
Xanthinuria

Administration of various other drugs (x-ray contrast agents, glyc-
eryl guaiacolate)
Neoplasms (occasional cases) such as carcinomas, Hodgkin's disease
Healthy adults with isolated defect in tubular transport of uric acid
(Dalmatian dog mutation)

Unchanged In
Colchicine administration

SERUM CHOLESTEROL

Increased In
Idiopathic hypercholesterolemia
Biliary obstruction
    Stone, carcinoma, etc., of duct
    Cholangiolitic cirrhosis
von Gierke's disease
Hypothyroidism
Nephrosis (due to chronic nephritis, renal vein thrombosis, amyloid-
osis, systemic lupus erythematosus, periarteritis, diabetic glomer-
ulosclerosis)
Pancreatic disease
    Diabetes mellitus
    Total pancreatectomy
    Chronic pancreatitis (some cases)
Pregnancy

Decreased In
Severe liver cell damage (due to chemicals, drugs, hepatitis)
Hyperthyroidism
Malnutrition (e.g., starvation, terminal neoplasm, uremia, malab-
sorption in steatorrhea)
Chronic anemia
    Pernicious anemia in relapse
    Hemolytic anemias
    Marked hypochromic anemia
Cortisone and ACTH therapy
A-beta-lipoproteinemia
Tangier disease

DECREASED ARTERIAL BLOOD OXYGEN (pO_2 TENSION) ASSOCIATED WITH NORMAL OR DECREASED ARTERIAL BLOOD CO_2 (pCO_2 TENSION)

Diffuse interstitial pulmonary infiltration
Pulmonary edema
Pulmonary embolism
Postoperative extracorporeal circulation

DECREASED ARTERIAL BLOOD OXYGEN ASSOCIATED WITH INCREASED ARTERIAL BLOOD CO_2

Chronic obstructive lung disease
Patients with respiratory complications postoperatively
Flail chest

Continued on page 44.

Table 3. Urine and Blood Changes in Electrolytes, pH, and Volume in Various Conditions

Measurement	Pulmonary Emphysema	Congestive Heart Failure	Excessive Sweating	Diarrhea	Pyloric Obstruction	Dehydration	Starvation	Malabsorption	Salicylate Intoxication	Primary Aldosteronism
Blood										
Sodium	N	N or D	D	D	D	I	N	D	N	I
Potassium	N	N	N	D	D	N	D	D	N or D	D
Bicarbonate	I	N	N	D	I	N or D	D	N or D	D	I
Chloride	D	D	D	D	D	I	N	N	I	D
Volume	N or I	I	N	D	D	D	N or D	D	N	N
Urine										
Sodium	D	D	D	D	D	I	N or I	D	I	D
Potassium	N	N	N	N or D	N	I	I or N	D	N or I	I
pH	D	N	N	D	I	D	D	N or D	I	N or D
Volume	N	D	N	D	D	D	I	N	N	I

Table 3. *(Continued)*

Measurement	Adrenal Cortical Insufficiency	Diabetes Insipidus	Diabetic Acidosis	Mercurial Diuretic Administration	Chlorothiazide Diuretic Administration	Ammonium Chloride Administration	Diamox Administration	Renal Tubular Acidosis	Chronic Renal Failure	Acute Renal Failure
Blood										
Sodium	D	N or I	D	D	D	D	D	D	D	D
Potassium	I	N	N or I	D	D	D	D	D	N or D	I
Bicarbonate	N or D	N	D	I	D	D	D	D	D	D
Chloride	D	I	D	D	D	I	I	I	D or N	I
Volume	D	D	D	D	D	D	D	D	V	I
Urine										
Sodium	I	N	I	I	I	I	I	I	I	D
Potassium	N or D	N	I	I	I	I	I	I	I	D
pH	N or I	N	D	D	N or I	I	I	I	I	N or I
Volume	N or D	I	I	I	I	I	I	I	V*	D

N = normal; D = decreased; I = increased; V = variable.
* = usually increased.

Decreased arterial blood oxygen   *(continued)*

Thoracic bellows defects (e.g., kyphoscoliosis, neuromuscular impairment)

Obesity hypoventilation

SERUM OSMOLALITY
(freezing point determination)

Hyperosmolality

(due to negative water balance [usually excessive water loss; may be exacerbated by decreased water intake, increased solute intake, and/or decreased solute excretion] or positive sodium balance)

Elderly patients who cannot take fluids ad lib.

Infants with mild diarrhea who may lose more fluid than solute

(Hyposmolality is more common when the diarrhea is more severe.)

Some cases of acute brain trauma and brain surgery (may be impaired secretion of antidiuretic hormone)

Chronic renal disease (due to increased BUN as well as increased sodium)

Diabetes mellitus (due to increased blood sugar; also, during recovery from acidosis, inadequate replacement with water rather than only saline therapy)

Diabetes insipidus (lack of antidiuretic hormone) (*Differentiate from psychogenic polydipsia and nephrogenic diabetes insipidus: simultaneous determination of serum and urine osmolality after 3 hours of water deprivation. Ratio of urine to serum osmolality is < 1 in diabetes insipidus and nephrogenic diabetes insipidus; > 1 in psychogenic polydipsia. After administration of antidiuretic hormone, ratio becomes > 1 in diabetes insipidus; ratio remains < 1 in nephrogenic diabetes insipidus.*)

Hyposmolality

(due to low serum sodium often combined with excess water)

Treatment with diuretic drugs and low-salt diet in patients with heart failure, cirrhosis, etc.

Adrenal disease (e.g., Addison's disease, adrenogenital syndrome)

"Inappropriate secretion of antidiuretic hormone" (e.g., in bronchogenic carcinoma; severe hypothyroidism; porphyria; cerebral disease such as tumor, trauma, infection, vascular; idiopathic cases)

Postoperative state—especially with excessive water replacement therapy

SERUM MAGNESIUM

Increased In

Renal failure

Diabetic coma before treatment

Hypothyroidism

Addison's disease and after adrenalectomy

Controlled diabetes mellitus in older age groups

Administration of antacids containing magnesium

Decreased In

GI disease showing malabsorption and abnormal loss of GI fluids (e.g., nontropical sprue, small bowel resection, biliary and intesti-

nal fistulas, abdominal irradiation, prolonged aspiration of intestinal contents, celiac disease and other causes of steatorrhea)
Acute alcoholism and alcoholic cirrhosis
Insulin treatment of diabetic coma
Hyperthyroidism
Aldosteronism
Hyperparathyroidism
Hypoparathyroidism
Lytic tumors of bone
Diuretic drug therapy
Some cases of renal disease (e.g., glomerulonephritis, pyelonephritis, renal tubular acidosis)
Excessive lactation
Idiopathic cases

Magnesium deficiency may cause apparently unexplained hypocalcemia and hypokalemia; the patients may have neurologic and GI symptoms.

SERUM CALCIUM
(also see Table 47, p. 321)

Increased In
Hyperparathyroidism due to hyperplasia or adenoma of parathyroids
Excess vitamin D intake
Bone tumor
    Metastatic carcinoma (some cases)
Acute osteoporosis
Milk-alkali (Burnett's) syndrome
Idiopathic hypercalcemia of infants
Infantile hypophosphatasia
Berylliosis
Hyperthyroidism (some cases)
Hyperproteinemia
    Sarcoidosis
    Multiple myeloma (some cases)

Decreased In
Hypoparathyroidism
    Surgical
    Idiopathic
    Pseudohypoparathyroidism
Malabsorption of calcium and vitamin D
    Obstructive jaundice
Hypoalbuminemia
    Cachexia
    Nephrotic syndrome
    Sprue
    Celiac disease
    Cystic fibrosis of pancreas
Chronic renal disease with uremia and phosphate retention
Acute pancreatitis with extensive fat necrosis
Insufficient calcium, phosphorus, and vitamin D ingestion
    Bone disease (osteomalacia, rickets)
    Starvation
    Late pregnancy

*Total serum protein should always be known for proper interpretation of
serum calcium levels.*

SERUM PHOSPHORUS
(also see Table 47, p. 321)

Increased In
Hypoparathyroidism
    Idiopathic
    Surgical
    Pseudohypoparathyroidism
Excess vitamin D intake
Secondary hyperparathyroidism (renal rickets)
Bone disease
    Healing fractures
    Multiple myeloma (some cases)
    Paget's (some cases)
    Osteolytic metastatic tumor in bone (some cases)
Addison's disease
Acromegaly
Childhood
Myelogenous leukemia
Acute yellow atrophy
High intestinal obstruction
Sarcoidosis (some cases)
Milk-alkali (Burnett's) syndrome (some cases)

Artifactual increase by hemolysis of blood

Decreased In
Hyperparathyroidism due to hyperplasia or adenoma of parathy-
    roids
Vitamin D deficiencies
    Rickets, osteomalacia, steatorrhea
Malabsorption
    Celiac disease
    Sprue
Hyperinsulinism
    Adenoma of islets of Langerhans
    Insulin administration
Diabetes mellitus
Administration of glucose
Loss of phosphate in urine
    Fanconi's syndrome
Primary hypophosphatemia

SERUM ALKALINE PHOSPHATASE
(also see Table 47, p. 321)

Increased In
Increased deposition of calcium in bone
    Osteitis fibrosa cystica (hyperparathyroidism)
    Paget's disease (osteitis deformans)
    Healing fractures (slightly)
    Osteoblastic bone tumors (osteogenic sarcoma, metastatic car-
        cinoma)

Osteogenesis imperfecta
Familial osteoectasia
Osteomalacia
Rickets
Polyostotic fibrous dysplasia (occasionally)
Pregnancy, late. Reverts to normal level by 20th day postpartum.
Childhood
Administration of ergosterol
Liver disease—any obstruction of biliary system (see pp. 188–190)
  Nodules in liver (metastatic tumor, abscess, cyst, parasite, amyloid, tuberculosis, sarcoid, or leukemia)
  Biliary duct obstruction (stone, carcinoma, etc.)
  Cholangiolar obstruction in hepatitis
  Progressive elevation may be first indication of adverse reaction to therapeutic drug (e.g., chlorpropamide) and indicates that drug administration should be halted.
Marked hyperthyroidism
Hyperphosphatasia
Primary hypophosphatemia (often increased)
Intravenous injection of albumin; sometimes marked increase (e.g., 10 times normal level) lasting for several days
Some patients with myocardial or pulmonary infarction, usually during phase of organization

Decreased In
Excess vitamin D ingestion
Milk-alkali syndrome
Scurvy
Hypophosphatasia
Hypothyroidism
Pernicious anemia in one-third of patients
Celiac disease
Malnutrition

Alkaline phosphatase isoenzyme determinations are not clinically useful.

SERUM LEUCINE AMINOPEPTIDASE (LAP)

Parallels serum alkaline phosphatase except that
  LAP is usually normal in the presence of bone disease or malabsorption syndrome.
  LAP is a more sensitive indicator of choledocholithiasis and of liver metastases in anicteric patients.
When serum LAP is increased, urine LAP is almost always increased; but when urine LAP is increased, serum LAP may have already returned to normal.

5'-NUCLEOTIDASE (5'-N)

Increased Only In
Obstructive type of hepatobiliary disease

May be an early indication of liver metastases in the cancer patient, especially if jaundice is absent.

Normal In
Pregnancy and postpartum period (in contrast to serum LAP and
  alkaline phosphatase); therefore may aid in differential diagnosis
  of hepatobiliary disease occurring during pregnancy.

*Whenever the alkaline phosphatase is elevated, a simultaneous elevation
of 5'-N establishes biliary disease as the cause of the elevated alkaline phosphatase. If the 5'-N is not increased, the cause of the elevated alkaline phosphatase must be found elsewhere, e.g., bone disease.*

SERUM GAMMA-GLUTAMYL TRANSPEPTIDASE

Increased In
Liver disease. Generally parallels changes in serum alkaline phos-
  phatase, LAP, and 5'-nucleotidase but is more sensitive.
  Acute hepatitis. Elevation is less marked than that of other liver
    enzymes, but it is the last to return to normal and therefore
    is useful to indicate recovery.
  Chronic hepatitis. Increased more than in acute hepatitis. More
    elevated than SGOT and SGPT. In dormant stage, may be
    the only enzyme elevated.
  Cirrhosis. In inactive cases, average values are lower than in
    chronic hepatitis. Increases greater than 10 to 20 times in
    cirrhotic patients suggest superimposed primary carcinoma
    of the liver.
  Primary biliary cirrhosis. Elevation is marked.
  Fatty liver. Elevation parallels that of SGOT and SGPT but is
    greater.
  Obstructive jaundice. Increase is faster and greater than that of
    serum alkaline phosphatase and LAP.
  Liver metastases. Parallels alkaline phosphatase; elevation pre-
    cedes positive liver scans.
Pancreatitis. Always elevated in acute pancreatitis. In chronic
  pancreatitis is increased when there is involvement of the biliary
  tract or active inflammation.
Renal disease. Increased in lipoid nephrosis and some cases of renal
  carcinoma.
Acute myocardial infarction. Increased in half the patients. Elevation begins on fourth to fifth day, reaches maximum at 8–12 days.
  With shock or acute right heart failure, may have early peak
  within 48 hours with rapid decline followed by later rise.

Normal In
Pregnancy (in contrast to serum alkaline phosphatase and LAP);
  therefore may aid in differential diagnosis of hepatobiliary disease
  occurring during pregnancy.
Bone disease or patients with increased bone growth (children and
  adolescents).
Renal failure.

SERUM ACID PHOSPHATASE

Increased In
Carcinoma of the prostate (see p. 371)
Infarction of the prostate (sometimes to high levels)

Operative trauma or instrumentation of the prostate (may cause transient increase)

Gaucher's disease (only when certain substrates are used in the laboratory determination)

Excessive destruction of platelets as in idiopathic thrombocytopenic purpura *with* megakaryocytes in bone marrow

Thromboembolism, hemolytic crises (e.g., sickle cell disease) due to hemolysis (only when certain substrates are used in the laboratory determination)

In the absence of prostatic disease, increased acid phosphatase is seen occasionally in

> Partial translocation trisomy 21
>
> Diseases of bone, e.g.,
>> Advanced Paget's disease
>> Metastatic carcinoma of bone
>> Multiple myeloma (some patients)
>> Hyperparathyroidism
>
> Various liver diseases (up to 9 King-Armstrong units), e.g.,
>> Hepatitis
>> Obstructive jaundice
>> Laennec's cirrhosis
>
> Acute renal impairment (not related to degree of azotemia)
>
> Other diseases of the reticuloendothelial system with liver or bone involvement, e.g.,
>> Niemann-Pick disease

Decreased In

Not clinically significant

SERUM AMYLASE

Increased In*

Acute pancreatitis. Increase begins in 3–6 hours; reaches maximum in 20–30 hours; may persist for 48–72 hours. May increase up to 40 times normal. Level should be at least 500 Somogyi units/100 ml to be significant of acute pancreatitis. Urine levels reflect serum changes by a time lag of 6–10 hours.

Acute exacerbation of chronic pancreatitis

Perforated or penetrating peptic ulcer especially with involvement of pancreas

Postoperative upper abdominal surgery, especially partial gastrectomy (up to twice normal in one-third of patients)

Obstruction of pancreatic duct by

> Stone or carcinoma
>
> Drug-induced spasm of sphincter (e.g., opiates, codeine, methyl choline, chlorothiazide)
>
> Partial obstruction + drug stimulation (see Pancreozymin-Secretin Test, p. 121)

Acute alcohol ingestion or poisoning

Salivary gland disease (mumps, suppurative inflammation, duct obstruction due to calculus)

---

* It has been suggested that more than 1000 Somogyi units is usually due to surgically correctable lesions (most frequently stones in biliary tree), and pancreas shows only edema or is negative; but 200–500 units is usually associated with pancreatic lesions that are not surgically correctable (e.g., hemorrhagic pancreatitis, necrosis of pancreas).

Advanced renal insufficiency. Often increased even without pancreatitis
Macroamylasemia

May also be increased in acute cholecystitis, intestinal obstruction with strangulation, mesenteric thrombosis, ruptured aortic aneurysm, ruptured tubal pregnancy.

Decreased In
Extensive marked destruction of pancreas (e.g., acute fulminant pancreatitis)
Severe liver damage (hepatitis, poisons, toxemia of pregnancy, severe thyrotoxicosis, severe burns, etc.)

Decreased levels are clinically significant only in occasional cases of fulminant pancreatitis.

SERUM LIPASE

Increased In
Acute pancreatitis. May remain elevated for as long as 14 days after amylase returns to normal
Perforated or penetrating peptic ulcer, especially with involvement of pancreas
Obstruction of pancreatic duct by
  Stone
  Drug-induced spasm of sphincter (e.g., by opiates, codeine, methyl choline)
  Partial obstruction + drug stimulation

Usually Normal In
Mumps

SERUM BILIRUBIN

Increased In (see Chapter 27, p. 177 and following)
Hepatic cellular damage
Biliary duct obstructions
Hemolytic diseases
Prolonged fasting

N.B. 48-hour fast produces a mean increase of 240% in normal patients and 194% in those with hepatic dysfunction.

SERUM TRANSAMINASE (SGOT)

Increased In
Acute myocardial infarction
Liver disease
Musculoskeletal diseases including trauma and intramuscular injections
Acute pancreatitis
Others
  Myoglobinuria
  Intestinal injury (e.g., surgery, infarction)
  Local irradiation injury
  Pulmonary infarction (relatively slight)
  Cerebral infarction (increased in following week in 50% of cases)

Cerebral neoplasms (in occasional cases)
Renal infarction (in occasional cases)
"Pseudo-myocardial infarction" pattern. Administration of opiates to patients with diseased biliary tract or previous cholecystectomy causes increase in LDH and especially SGOT. SGOT increases by 2–4 hours, peaks in 5–8 hours, and increase may persist for 24 hours; elevation may be 2½ to 65 times normal.

Falsely Increased In
(because of activating enzymes during test)
Therapy with Prostaphlin, Polycillin, opiates, erythromycin
Calcium dust in air (e.g., due to construction in laboratory)

Falsely Decreased In
(because of increased serum lactate consuming enzyme during test)
Diabetic ketoacidosis
Beriberi
Severe liver disease
Chronic hemodialysis (reason unknown)

Normal In
Angina pectoris
Coronary insufficiency
Pericarditis
Congestive heart failure without liver damage

Varies less than 10 units/day in the same individual.

SGPT generally parallels SGOT, but the increase is less marked in myocardial necrosis, chronic hepatitis, cirrhosis, hepatic metastases, and congestive changes in liver, and more marked in liver necrosis and acute hepatitis.

SERUM LACTIC DEHYDROGENASE (LDH)

Increased In
Acute myocardial infarction. May remain elevated up to 10–14 days after onset; therefore is particularly useful when patient is first seen after sufficient time has elapsed for CPK and SGOT to become normal. Increase is due to LDH_1 and LDH_2; with small infarcts LDH_1 may be increased when total LDH remains normal. LDH_1 may remain elevated after total LDH has returned to normal.
Acute myocardial infarction with congestive heart failure. May show increase of LDH_1 and LDH_5
Congestive heart failure alone. LDH isoenzymes are normal.
Insertion of intracardiac prosthetic valves consistently causes chronic hemolysis with increase of total LDH and of LDH_1 and LDH_2. This is also often present before surgery in patients with severe hemodynamic abnormalities of cardiac valves.
Cardiovascular surgery. LDH is increased up to twice normal without cardiopulmonary bypass and returns to normal in 3–4 days; with extracorporeal circulation, it may increase up to 4–6 times normal; increase is more marked when transfused blood is older.

Hepatitis. Most marked increase is of LDH_5, which occurs during prodromal stage and is greatest at time of onset of jaundice. Total LDH is also increased in half the cases. LDH_5 is also increased with other causes of liver damage (e.g., chlorpromazine hepatitis, carbon tetrachloride poisoning, exacerbation of cirrhosis, biliary obstruction) even when total LDH is normal.

Untreated pernicious anemia. Total LDH (chiefly LDH_1) is markedly increased, especially with hemoglobin less than 8 gm/100 ml. Only slightly increased in severe hemolytic anemia. Normal in iron-deficiency anemia even when very severe.

Malignant tumors. Increased in about 50% of patients with carcinoma, especially in advanced stages. Increased in about 60% of patients with lymphomas and lymphocytic leukemias. Increased in about 90% of patients with acute leukemia; degree of increase is not correlated with level of WBC; relatively low levels in lymphatic type of leukemia. Increased in 95% of patients with myelogenous leukemia. (See also Chapter 30, Hematologic Diseases.)

Diseases of muscle. See pp. 219–225.

Pulmonary embolus and infarction. See following section Serum Lactic Dehydrogenase (LDH) Isoenzymes.

Renal diseases. Occasional increase but to no clinically useful degree

Decreased In
X-ray irradiation

SERUM LACTIC DEHYDROGENASE (LDH) ISOENZYMES

This test must be correlated with clinical status of the patient. Do serial determinations to obtain maximum information.

Condition	LDH Isoenzyme Increased
Myocardial infarction	I and II
Pernicious anemia	I
Sickle cell crisis	I and II
Mother carrying erythro-blastotic child	IV and V
Acute myocardial infarction with acute congestion of liver	I and V
Early hepatitis	V (may become normal even when SGPT is still rising) and IV (may even increase II) (also useful for following effect of chemotherapy
Malignant lymphoma	III
Disseminated lupus erythematosus	III and IV
Dermatomyositis	V
Prostate carcinoma	V
Pulmonary embolus and infarction	
Without hemorrhage into lung	III
With hemorrhage into lung	I, II, III
Embolus with acute cor pulmonale causing acute congestion of liver	III and V

Increased total LDH with normal distribution of isoenzymes may be seen in myocardial infarction, arteriosclerotic heart disease with chronic heart failure, various combinations of acute and chronic diseases (this may represent a general stress reaction).

About 50% of patients with carcinoma have altered LDH patterns. This change often is nonspecific and of no diagnostic value.

SERUM ALPHA-HYDROXYBUTYRIC DEHYDROGENASE (alpha-HBD)

Increased In
Acute myocardial infarction. Is more specific than SGOT and LDH but less specific than CPK and LDH isoenzymes.
Other conditions that cause elevation of fast-moving LDH in serum (e.g., muscular dystrophy, megaloblastic anemia)

Increase is always accompanied by increased LDH activity.

May Be Slightly Increased In
Heart failure
Nephrosis

Normal In
Angina pectoris

SERUM CREATINE PHOSPHOKINASE (CPK)

Increased In
Necrosis or acute atrophy of striated muscle
    Acute myocardial infarction
    Severe myocarditis
    Progressive muscular dystrophy
    Polymyositis
    Myoglobinuria
    Traumatic injury of muscle. Increase may last for 2 weeks, especially if associated with arterial obstruction.
    Severe or prolonged exercise (transient increase, some cases)
    Status epilepticus
    Postoperative state. Increase may last up to 5 days. Greater increase with use of electrocautery in surgery.
Half of patients with extensive brain infarction. Maximum levels in 3 days; increase may not appear before 2 days; levels usually less than in acute myocardial infarction and remain increased for longer time; return to normal within 14 days; high mortality associated with levels more than 300 I.U. Elevated serum CPK in brain infarction may obscure diagnosis of concomitant acute myocardial infarction.
Parturition and frequently last few weeks of pregnancy

Slight Increase Occasionally In
Hypothyroidism
Frequent intramuscular injections. Variable increase after intramuscular injection to 2–6 times normal level. Returns to normal 48 hours after cessation of injections.
Muscle spasms or convulsions in childhood
Electrical cardiac defibrillation or countershock in 50% of patients; returns to normal in 48–72 hours.

Normal In
Angina pectoris
Pericarditis
Pulmonary infarction
Renal infarction
Liver disease
Biliary obstruction
Neurogenic muscle atrophy
Pernicious anemia
Malignancies
Following cardiac catheterization and coronary arteriography unless
   myocardium has been injured by catheter

SERUM ISOCITRATE DEHYDROGENASE (ICD)

Increased In
Liver disease
   Early viral hepatitis, hepatitis of infectious mononucleosis and
      of liver poisons—ICD more than 25 I.U., becomes normal in
      2–3 weeks
   Metastatic carcinoma—ICD less than 20 I.U.
   Cirrhosis—normal or slightly increased
   Extrahepatic biliary obstruction—normal
   Neonatal biliary atresia—may be increased
   With protein malnutrition—may be increased
Active placental degeneration
   Placental infarction
   Preeclampsia

Normal In
Acute myocardial infarction
Pregnancy

SERUM ALDOLASE (ALD)

Increased In
Cell destruction
   Acute myocardial infarction
   Burns
   Acute hepatitis
   Muscular dystrophy
   Carcinoma of prostate
   20% of cancer patients—more frequent with liver involvement

Normal In
Neurogenic muscle atrophy
Cirrhosis (or may be slightly increased)
Obstructive jaundice (or may be slightly increased)

SERUM ORNITHINE CARBAMYL TRANSFERASE (OCT)

Increased In
Liver cell damage (e.g., hepatitis, metastatic carcinoma, cirrhosis,
   acute cholecystitis)
Alcohol consumption
Prolonged exercise (some patients)

SERUM CHOLINESTERASE

Decreased In
Poisoning with organic phosphate insecticides
Liver diseases

> Especially hepatitis. Lowest level corresponds to peak of disease and becomes normal with recovery.
>
> Cirrhosis with ascites or jaundice. Persistent decrease may indicate a poor prognosis.
>
> Some patients with metastatic carcinoma, obstructive jaundice, congestive heart failure

Some conditions which may have decreased serum albumin (e.g., malnutrition, anemias, infections, dermatomyositis, acute myocardial infarction, liver diseases—see above)

SERUM FRUCTOSE 1-PHOSPHATE ALDOLASE

Decreased In
Heterozygous carrier state for Tay-Sachs disease

SERUM PROTEIN GAMMOPATHIES
(localized or general increase in immunoglobulins demonstrated by serum immunoelectrophoresis)

Monoclonal   (Hyperproteinemia is very frequent.)

60% are IgG with or without Bence Jones protein.
16% are IgA.
15% are IgM.
9% are Bence Jones protein only (light-chain disease).
Very rare are IgE (heavy-chain disease).
Very rare are IgD.
Only two-thirds of patients with monoclonal gammopathy are symptomatic (IgG, IgA, IgD, and Bence Jones gammopathies are associated with classic picture of multiple myeloma—see p. 274; IgM gammopathy is associated with classic picture of macroglobulinemia—see p. 275).
Classic (associated with increased serum M-protein > 3 gm/100 ml and increased number of plasma cells in marrow > 25%)

> Multiple myeloma
> Waldenström's macroglobulinemia
> Certain malignant lymphomas

Idiopathic (not associated with diseases in classical group) (serum M-protein usually < 2 gm/100 ml; plasma marrow cells usually 5–25% of total marrow white cells)

> In apparently healthy persons
> Associated with various diseases (e.g., diabetes mellitus, cirrhosis, abnormalities of lipid metabolism, chronic infections, collagen diseases, myeloproliferative diseases and neoplasms not of lymphocyte or plasma cell origin)

Either type may be familial.

Polyclonal Gammopathy with Hyperproteinemia
Collagen diseases (e.g., systemic lupus erythematosus, rheumatoid arthritis, scleroderma)
Liver disease (e.g., chronic hepatitis, cirrhosis)

Continued on page 58.

Table 4. Serum Protein Electrophoretic Patterns in Various Diseases

Condition	Total Protein	Albumin	Alpha$_1$ Globulin	Alpha$_2$ Globulin	Beta Globulin	Gamma Globulin	Comment
Multiple myeloma	I	D		Dyscrasia of Beta$_{2A}$ or gamma$_2$ Ig			Total globulin, marked I; Variable location of M globulin
Macroglobulinemia	I	D		Dyscrasia of beta$_{2M}$		Marked I	Electrophoresis same as multiple myeloma
Hodgkin's disease	D	D	I	I		V	
Lymphatic leukemia and lymphoma	D	D			D	D	
Myelogenous and monocytic leukemia	D	D			D	I	Gamma globulin to differentiate types of acute leukemias
Hypogammaglobulinemia	D	N	N	N	N	D	
Analbuminemia	Marked D	Marked D	N	I	I	I	
Gastrointestinal diseases							
Peptic ulcer	D	D	May be I	May be I			
Ulcerative colitis	D	D	May be I	May be I	D		
Protein-losing enteropathy		Marked D	I	I	D	D	
Acute cholecystitis	D	D					
Nephrosis	D	D		I	D	D	Typical pattern
Chronic glomerulonephritis	D	D	N	I	N	N	
Laennec's cirrhosis	D	D	N	N	N	I	Characteristic pattern of beta-gamma "bridging"
Acute viral hepatitis		D	D (means acute hepatocellular damage)	D	N	V	

	Albumin	α₂-globulin	β-globulin	γ-globulin	Comments
Stress	D			I	"Three-fingered" pattern
Hypersensitivity				I	
Sarcoidosis	D	→ Stepwise increase of alpha₂, beta, and gamma			"Sarcoid steps" help differentiate from other lung disease
Collagen diseases					Gamma globulin levels of prognostic value
Lupus erythematosus (SLE)	D	I	I	I	
Polyarteritis nodosa	D	I	I	N	
Rheumatoid arthritis	D	I	I	I	
Scleroderma	D			V	No significant changes
Acute rheumatic fever	D	I			Albumin D due to hemodilution
Essential hypertension ⎱	D	No significant changes			(Hemodilution, diminished hepatic synthesis, and possible excessive enteric loss)
Congestive heart failure ⎰	D				
Metastatic carcinomatosis	D	I	D		Nonspecific pattern
Certain infections (meningitis, pneumonia, osteomyelitis)	D	I			
Myxedema	D				Changes due to hemodilution
Hyperthyroidism	D	N	N	N	
Diabetes mellitus	D	I	I	N	

I = increased or elevated; D = decreased or diminished; V = variable; N = normal; blank = no significant change.

Nonspecific changes of decreased albumin and increased globulin occur in many conditions (e.g., infections, neoplasms, metabolic diseases).

Source: Adapted from F. W. Sunderman, Jr., "Recent Advances in Clinical Interpretation of Electrophoretic Fractionations of the Serum Proteins," in *Serum Proteins and the Dysproteinemias*, eds. Sunderman and Sunderman. Philadelphia: Lippincott, 1964.

[57]

Serum protein gammopathies, polyclonal
(continued)

Chronic infection (e.g., chronic bronchitis and bronchiectasis, lung abscess, tuberculosis, osteomyelitis, subacute bacterial endocarditis, infectious mononucleosis, malaria)
Miscellaneous (e.g., sarcoidosis, malignant lymphoma, acute myeloid and monocytic leukemia, diabetes mellitus)
Idiopathic (family of patients with lupus erythematosus)

SERUM BETA$_{2M}$ GLOBULIN
(also called gamma$_{1M}$ globulin, 19S gamma globulin, gamma$_1$ globulin, beta$_2$ macroglobulin)

Increased In
Waldenström's macroglobulinemia (marked increase)
Symptomatic macroglobulinemia
      Cirrhosis
      Nephrosis
      Rheumatoid arthritis
      Eosinophilic granulomatosis
      Hyperglobulinemic purpura
      Etc.

SERUM BETA$_{2A}$ GLOBULIN
(also called gamma$_{1A}$ globulin)

Increased In
Multiple myeloma (occasionally)

Decreased In
Multiple myeloma
Lipoid nephrosis
Macroglobulinemia

IMMUNODIFFUSION OF SERUM PROTEIN

Diagnosis of Specific Diseases
Multiple myeloma
Waldenström's macroglobulinemia
Hypogammaglobulinemia
      Agammaglobulinemia
      Agamma-A-globulinemia
Analbuminemia
Bisalbuminemia
Afibrinogenemia
Atransferrinemia
Wilson's disease

Other Changes
Nonspecific changes in serum proteins
Protein pattern changes in urine, cerebrospinal fluid, peritoneal fluid, etc.

IMMUNOGLOBULIN A (IgA)

Increased In
      (in relation to other immunoglobulins)
γA myeloma (M component)
Cirrhosis of liver
Rheumatoid arthritis with high titers of rheumatoid factor

Systemic lupus erythematosus (some cases)
Sarcoidosis (some cases)
Wiskott-Aldrich syndrome
Others

Decreased In
(alone)
Normal persons (1:700)
Hereditary telangiectasia (4 out of 5)
Type III dysgammaglobulinemia
Malabsorption (some cases)
Systemic lupus erythematosus (occasional cases)
Cirrhosis of liver (occasional cases)
Still's disease (occasional cases)
Recurrent otitis media (occasional cases)

Decreased In
(combined with other immunoglobulin decreases)
Agammaglobulinemia
    Acquired
        Primary
        Secondary (multiple myeloma, leukemia, nephrotic syndrome, protein-losing enteropathy, etc.)
    Congenital
Hereditary thymic aplasia
Type I dysgammaglobulinemia (decreased IgG and IgA and increased IgM)
Type II dysgammaglobulinemia (absent IgA and IgM and normal levels of IgG)

IMMUNOGLOBULIN E (IgE)

Increased In
Atopic diseases
    Exogenous asthma in about 60% of patients
    Hay fever in about 30% of patients
    Atopic eczema
    Influenced by type of allergen, duration of stimulation, presence of symptoms, hyposensitization treatment
Parasitic diseases (e.g., ascariasis, visceral larva migrans, hookworm disease, schistosomiasis, *Echinococcus* infestation)
E-myeloma

IMMUNOGLOBULIN D (IgD)

Increased In
Chronic infection (moderately increased)
IgD myelomas (greatly increased)

SERUM LIPOPROTEINS

A-beta-lipoproteinemia. Low-density beta lipoproteins are absent; high-density lipoproteins are normal. Patients also have acanthotic RBCs and low serum carotene levels.

Continued on page 62.

Table 5. Serum Immunoglobulin Changes in Various Diseases

Disease	IgG	IgA	IgM
Immunoglobulin disorders (see Table 38, pp. 276–277)			
Lymphoid aplasia	D	D	D
Agammaglobulinemia	D	D	D
Type I dysgammaglobulinemia (selective IgG and IgA deficiency)	D	D	N or I
Type II dysgammaglobulinemia (absent IgA and IgM)	N	D	D
IgA globulinemia	N	D	N
Ataxia-telangiectasia	N	D	N
Multiple myeloma, macroglobulinemia, lymphomas (see pp. 273–275)			
Heavy-chain disease	D	D	D
IgG myeloma	I	D	D
IgA myeloma	D	I	D
Macroglobulinemia	D	D	I
Acute lymphocytic leukemia	N	D	N
Chronic lymphocytic leukemia	D	D	D
Acute myelogenous leukemia	N	N	N
Chronic myelogenous leukemia	N	D	N
Hodgkin's disease	N	N	N
Liver diseases			
Hepatitis	I	I	I
Laennec's cirrhosis	I	I	N
Biliary cirrhosis	N	N	I
Hepatoma	N	N	D
Miscellaneous			
Rheumatoid arthritis	I	I	I
Systemic lupus erythematosus (SLE)	I	I	I
Nephrotic syndrome	D	D	N
Trypanosomiasis	N	N	I
Pulmonary tuberculosis	I	N	N

N = normal; I = increased; D = decreased.

Table 6. Changes in Serum Immunoproteins in Various Conditions

Condition	Albumin	Alpha₁ Antitrypsin	Haptoglobin	Transferrin	C3
Acute inflammation	D	I	I	D	Slight I
Chronic inflammation	D	V I	V I	D	Slight I
Chronic liver disease	D	V I	V	D	V D
Obstructive jaundice	N	N	V I	N	I
Hemolytic anemia	N	N	D	N	N
Iron deficiency	N	N	N	I	N
Acute glomerulonephritis	N	N	N	N	D
Systemic lupus erythematosus (SLE)	D	I	D*	D	V D†
Alpha₁ antitrypsin deficiency	N	D	N	N	N
Analbuminemia	D	N	N	N	N
Agammaglobulinemia	N	N	N	N	N
IgG myeloma	D	N	N	N	N
IgA myeloma	D	N	N	N	N
Waldenström's macroglobulinemia	D	N	N	N	N

*D if associated hemolytic anemia.
†N if immunosuppressive treatment is effective.
N = normal; D = decreased; I = increased; V= variable.

Serum lipoproteins   *(continued)*

Tangier disease. There is marked decrease (heterozygous) or absence (homozygous) of high-density lipoprotein. Pre-beta is absent.
Familial lipoprotein abnormalities. See Table 42.

TRIGLYCERIDES

Increased In (see section on lipoprotein electrophoresis, pp. 295-296)
Familial hyperlipidemia
Liver diseases
Nephrotic syndrome
Hypothyroidism
Diabetes mellitus (higher values correlate with hyperglycemia and poorer control of diabetes; reduced by insulin therapy)
Pancreatitis
von Gierke's disease
Acute myocardial infarction (rise to peak in 3 weeks; increase may persist for 1 year)

Decreased In
Congenital a-beta-lipoproteinemia (rare disease characterized by acanthocytes, absence of serum low-density lipoproteins, very low serum triglyceride values—e.g., less than 6 mg/100 ml—excess fat in villous absorptive cells in biopsy of small intestine)
Malnutrition

THYMOL TURBIDITY

Increased In
Active liver disease (e.g., in acute hepatitis thymol turbidity becomes positive later than transaminase elevation; may remain positive after cephalin flocculation has become negative. In cirrhosis may be normal.)
Altered serum proteins (e.g., multiple myeloma, sarcoidosis, lupus erythematosus)
Lipemic serum (e.g., postprandial lipemia)

CEPHALIN FLOCCULATION TEST

Parallels thymol turbidity test. See preceding section.

SERUM TRIIODOTHYRONINE (T-3) UPTAKE (see Table 45, pp. 316-317)

Increased In
Hyperthyroidism
Certain drugs (e.g., testosterone, androgens, anabolic steroids, prednisone; heparin, Dicumarol; salicylates, Butazolidin, penicillin, Dilantin)
Threatened abortion

Infancy (up to about 2 months of age)
Severe nephrosis
Metastatic neoplasms

Decreased In
Hypothyroidism
Pregnancy (from about tenth week of pregnancy until up to twelfth week postpartum)
Certain drugs (e.g., estrogens alone or in birth control pills; large amounts of iodine; propylthiouracil in hyperthyroidism)

Normal In
Pregnancy with hyperthyroidism
Nontoxic goiter
Carcinoma of thyroid
Diabetes mellitus
Addison's disease
Anxiety
Certain drugs (mercurials, iodine)

Variable In
Liver disease

SERUM PROTEIN-BOUND IODINE (PBI)
(see Table 45, pp. 316-317)

Usually Increased In
Hyperthyroidism
Hereditary increase in thyroxine-binding protein and other causes of increased TBG
Pregnancy (from about fourth week of pregnancy until up to sixth week postpartum)
Infancy
Certain drugs (especially iodine-containing, e.g., radiopaque substances for x-ray studies, expectorants, estrogens, levothyroxine, birth control pills; also iodine-containing products, e.g., toothpaste, suntan lotion, antidandruff preparation, food coloring)
About half of very ill euthyroid patients

Occasionally Increased In
Certain tumors (dermoid cyst of ovary, hydatidiform mole, metastatic choriocarcinoma, breast carcinoma, embryonal carcinoma of testicle)
Hashimoto's thyroiditis
Acute intermittent porphyria
Certain drugs (e.g., Bromsulphalein in BSP test, barium sulfate as in x-ray studies of GI tract)

Usually Decreased In
Hypothyroidism
Hereditary decrease in thyroxine-binding protein and other causes of decreased TBG
Nephrosis
Dietary iodine deficiency
Certain drugs (e.g., Dilantin, salicylates, thiouracil, thiocyanates, therapeutic ^{131}I)

Occasionally Decreased In
Starvation
Hypothermia
Certain drugs (e.g., ACTH, corticosteroids, androgens, PAS)

Normal In
Leukemia; polycythemia
Diabetes mellitus; acromegaly, Addison's disease
Certain drugs (diuretics, digitalis, antibiotics, gonadotropins, desiccated thyroid, etc.)

In hypothyroidism, PBI level attained with sufficient therapy to make patient euthyroid depends upon the particular thyroid hormone product:

Levothyroxine (Synthroid)	PBI higher than normal
Liothyronine (Cytomel)	Low PBI
U.S.P. thyroid	PBI normal to low normal
Thyroglobulin (Proloid)	PBI may be low

SERUM BUTANOL-EXTRACTABLE IODINE (BEI)

Altered in same conditions as listed for PBI, above, except that
    BEI is not affected by the presence of excess *inorganic* iodine.
    BEI measures thyroxine-like compounds.
BEI may be as falsely increased as PBI by organic iodine compounds.
BEI is lower than simultaneous PBI in thyroiditis.

SERUM TOTAL THYROXINE ASSAY (T-4)
(see Table 45, pp. 316-317)

Increased In
Hyperthyroidism
Pregnancy
Certain drugs (estrogens, birth control pills)

Decreased In
Hypothyroidism
Hypoproteinemia
Certain drugs (Dilantin, triiodothyronine, testosterone)

Not Affected By
Radiopaque substances for x-ray studies
Mercurial diuretics
Nonthyroidal iodine

FREE THYROXINE FACTOR (T-7)

This is the product of T-3 and T-4 (or T-3 and PBI).
It permits correction of misleading results of T-3 and T-4 (or PBI) determinations caused by pregnancy, estrogens (including especially contraceptive pills), and other conditions that alter the thyroxine-binding protein concentration.

Condition	T-3	T-4	Free Thyroxine Factor (T-7) (T-3 × T-4)
Normal			
Range	24–36	4–11	96–396
Mean	31	7	217
Hypothyroid	22	3	66
Hyperthyroid	38	12	456
Pregnancy, estrogens (especially contraceptive pills)	20	12	240*

FREE THYROXINE ASSAY
(see Table 45, pp. 316-317)

This is a useful determination because it gives normal values in about 5% of the cases in which the T-3 or PBI is altered on account of changes in serum proteins or in binding sites.
    Pregnancy
    Drugs (e.g., androgens, estrogens, birth control pills, Dilantin)
    Altered levels of serum proteins (e.g., nephrosis)

It is paralleled by the free thyroxine factor.

Increased In
Hyperthyroidism
Hypothyroidism treated with thyroxine
Very ill euthyroid patients (many cases)

Decreased In
Hypothyroidism
Hypothyroidism treated with triiodothyronine

SERUM THYROXINE-BINDING GLOBULIN (TBG)
(see Table 45, pp. 316-317)

Increased In
Pregnancy
Excess TBG, genetic or idiopathic
Hypothyroidism (some cases)
Certain drugs (estrogens, birth control pills)
Gross iodine contamination
Acute intermittent porphyria

Decreased In
Nephrosis and other causes of marked hypoproteinemia
Deficiency of TBG, genetic or idiopathic
Certain drugs (androgenic and anabolic steroids)

---

* Normal even though T-3 and T-4 alone are abnormal.

An increase of TBG is associated with an increase in PBI, BEI, and T-4 by column and a decrease in T-3; converse association for decrease of TBG.

SERUM THYROTROPIN
(hormone secreted by anterior pituitary; measured by radioimmunoassay)

Primary usefulness is in diagnosis of hypothyroidism and in differentiation of primary and secondary hypothyroidism.

Increased In
Primary untreated hypothyroidism. Decreases when therapy is initiated; if still elevated in 3–4 weeks, treatment is inadequate.
Hashimoto's thyroiditis including those with clinical hypothyroidism and about one-third of those patients who are clinically euthyroid
Other conditions (test is not clinically useful)
    Iodide deficiency goiter
    Iodide-induced goiter
    External neck irradiation
    Post–subtotal thyroidectomy

Decreased In
Secondary (pituitary) hypothyroidism
Hyperthyroidism (not useful for diagnosis because there is no lower limit of normal)

Normal In
Cushing's syndrome
Acromegaly
Pregnancy at term

SERUM LONG-ACTING THYROID STIMULATOR (LATS)

Normal Condition
None detectable

Increased In
    (frequently but not invariably)
Graves' disease
Exophthalmos (some euthyroid patients)
Pretibial myxedema

THYROID ANTIBODIES TEST

Precipitin test
    High titers in Hashimoto's disease
    May be positive but with lower titers in other thyroid diseases
        (e.g., primary myxedema)
Tanned red cell titers
    1:250,000 or more—Hashimoto's disease
    May be this high in primary myxedema
    Up to 1:250 in hyperthyroidism, carcinoma of thyroid, and
        simple goiter
Fluorescent antibody studies

BLOOD AMMONIA

Increased In
Liver failure (e.g., acute hepatic necrosis, terminal cirrhosis, hepa-
tectomy)

*In cirrhosis, blood ammonia may be increased after portacaval anasto-
mosis.*
Not all cases of hepatic coma show increased blood ammonia.

Some aminoacidurias (see Table 43, pp. 298-300)

BLOOD LACTIC ACID

Increased Because of
Alkalosis
Hypoxia due to respiratory or circulatory problems of oxygen
transport

May be of some prognostic value in shock.
Patient management is not determined by the degree of hyperlact-
acidemia.

SERUM CAROTENOIDS

Increased In
Excessive intake (especially carrots)
Postprandial hyperlipemia
Hyperlipemia (e.g., essential hyperlipemia)
Diabetes mellitus
Hypothyroidism

Decreased In
Carotenoid-poor diet—blood level falls within 1 week (*vitamin A
level unaffected by dietary change for 6 months because of much
larger body stores*)
Malabsorption syndromes (*a very useful screening test for malabsorp-
tion*)
Liver disease
High fever

PLASMA RENIN ACTIVITY (PRA)

*Blood should be drawn only after overnight recumbency and after 10
days of normal-sodium diet with no diuretic drugs.*

PRA is particularly useful to distinguish between primary and
secondary aldosteronism and to diagnose unilateral renal artery
stenosis.

Increased In
Reduced plasma volume due to low-sodium diet, diuretics, hemor-
rhage, Addison's disease
Secondary aldosteronism (usually very high levels)
Normal pregnancy

Last half of menstrual cycle (twofold increase)
Erect posture for 4 hours (twofold increase)
Ambulatory patients compared to bed patients

Decreased In
Increased plasma volume due to high-sodium diet, administration of
salt-retaining steroids
20% of patients diagnosed at the present time as having "essential
hypertension"
Primary aldosteronism. Usually absent or low and can be increased
less or not at all by sodium depletion and ambulation in contrast
to secondary aldosteronism. *PRA may not always be suppressed in
primary aldosteronism; repeated testing may be necessary to establish
the diagnosis.*

In diagnosis of renal hypertension, renin is assayed in blood from
each renal vein, inferior vena cava, and aorta. The test is
considered diagnostic when the level from the ischemic kidney is
at least 1½ times greater than the level from the normal kidney
(which is equal to or less than the level in the aorta that serves as
the standard). Maximum renin stimulation accentuates the difference between the two kidneys and should *always* be obtained by
pretest conditions (avoid antihypertensive and oral contraceptive
drugs for at least 1 month if possible; low-salt diet for 7 days;
administer thiazide diuretic for 1–3 days; upright posture for at
least 2 hours). This is the most useful diagnostic test in renovascular hypertension as judged by surgical results but is not a
sufficiently reliable guide to nephrectomy in patients with hypertension due to parenchymal renal disease. *In renovascular hypertension, if renal plasma flow is impaired in the "normal" kidney,
surgery often fails to cure the hypertension.**

PLASMA INSULIN

Not clinically useful for diagnosis of diabetes mellitus because of the
very wide range in both normal and diabetic patients and the fact
that results may be influenced by many other factors.

Increased In
Insulinoma. Fasting blood insulin level over 50 microunits/ml in
presence of low or normal blood glucose level. Intravenous
tolbutamide or administration of leucine causes rapid rise of
blood insulin to very high levels within a few minutes with rapid
return to normal.
Untreated obese diabetics (mild cases); fasting level often increased
Acromegaly (especially with active disease) after ingestion of glucose
Reactive hypoglycemia after glucose ingestion, particularly when
diabetic type of glucose tolerance curve is present

Absent In
Severe diabetes mellitus with ketosis and weight loss. In less severe
cases, insulin is frequently present but only at lower glucose
concentrations.

---

* E. F. Fraley and B. H. Feldman, Current concepts: Renal hypertension.
New Eng. J. Med. 287:550, 1972.

Normal In
Hypoglycemia associated with nonpancreatic tumors
Idiopathic hypoglycemia of childhood except after administration of leucine

PLASMA TESTOSTERONE

Male hypogonadism—levels lower than in normal male
Klinefelter's syndrome—levels lower than in normal male but higher than in normal female and orchiectomized male
Stein-Leventhal syndrome—variable; increased when virilization is present
Adrenogenital syndrome—with virilization (due to tumor or hyperplasia), level much higher than in normal female; falls following adrenal suppression
Idiopathic hirsutism—inconclusive
Ovarian stromal hyperthecosis

BLOOD CORTICOSTEROIDS

See Urinary Corticosteroids, p. 115.

SERUM ALPHA-FETOPROTEIN (AFP)

Normal
Absent after first several weeks of life

Present In
Primary cancer of liver (hepatoma) in 50% of whites and 75–90% of nonwhites
Embryonal carcinoma (in 27% of cases) or malignant teratoma (in 60% of cases) of ovary and testis
Some patients with liver metastases from carcinoma of stomach or pancreas
Pregnancy
Ataxia-telangiectasia

Actual serum concentration is not clinically useful.

Absent In
Various types of cirrhosis and hepatitis
Seminoma of testis
Choriocarcinoma, adenocarcinoma, and dermoid cyst of ovary

This is a rather recently developed test which may not be available locally. The disease states in which this test is clinically useful are subject to continuing redefinition.

SERUM CARCINOEMBRYONIC ANTIGEN (CEA)
(radioimmune assay detection in serum or plasma)

Usually Increased In
Carcinoma of colon (more than 80% of patients) or pancreas (virtually 100% of patients)
Adenocarcinoma of stomach
Carcinoma of lung (70% of patients), prostate (30% of patients), disseminated carcinoma of breast (70% of patients)

Neuroblastoma in children
Severe active alcoholic cirrhosis (50% of patients)
Advanced renal insufficiency (50% of patients)
A few patients with active ulcerative colitis
Few false positives

Increased serum levels correlate with amount of tumor and disappear after successful resection of tumor.

Negative assay does not exclude diagnosis of early cancer, but widespread metastatic cancer is considered highly unlikely. Negative assay in a patient with known colon cancer suggests a relatively favorable prognosis; i.e., cancer has not widely metastasized.

This is a recently developed test which may not be available locally. The disease states in which this test is clinically useful are subject to continuing redefinition.

SERUM GASTRIN
(determined by radioimmunoassay of serum)

Normal: from absent up to 300 pg gastrin/ml serum
Elevated level: over 500 pg/ml

	Serum Gastrin	Serum Gastrin After Intragastric Administration of 0.1N HCl
Peptic ulcer without Zollinger-Ellison syndrome	Normal range	—
Zollinger-Ellison syndrome	Very high	No change
Pernicious anemia	High level may approach that in Z-E syndrome	Marked decrease

This is a recently developed test which may not be available locally. The disease states in which this test is clinically useful are subject to continuing redefinition.

FUNCTIONAL TESTS

BROMSULPHALEIN (BSP) RETENTION IN SERUM

This test measures the rate of removal of dye from blood by the liver. It is a very sensitive and specific test of hepatic function. *It must be performed while the patient is fasting because postprandial increased hepatic blood flow produces increased excretion and falsely normal result.*

Increased In
Fever (without liver disease)
Liver disease of any type (e.g., chronic hepatitis, cirrhosis, chronic congestion)
Acute cholecystitis
Ingestion (without liver damage) of certain drugs and dyes (e.g., morphine, methadone, monoamine oxidase inhibitors, barbiturates, probenecid, Telepaque, phenolphthalein, phenolsulfonphthalein (PSP), Pyridium)

Upper GI tract hemorrhage. *BSP retention of more than 20% suggests presumptive diagnosis of cirrhosis. BSP retention up to 20% suggests absence of cirrhosis.*

False Values In
Albuminuria. *BSP dye may be lost in urine.* Results may falsely appear normal.
Ascites. *BSP dye may be lost into abdomen.* Results may falsely appear normal.
Any appreciable jaundice

ORAL GLUCOSE TOLERANCE TEST (GTT)

An appropriate prior diet of at least 250 gm of carbohydrate daily for 3 days before the test should be prescribed.
For older persons without elevated fasting levels, without glycosuria (alone or during oral GTT), without positive family history of diabetes, limits of normal at 1 and 2 hours should be increased 10 mg/100 ml at age 50 and an additional 10 mg for each subsequent decade (e.g., 30 mg/100 ml at age 70).
To detect early diabetes in pregnancy, upper limits of normal are 165 at 1 hour, 145 at 2 hours, 125 at 3 hours. If results are indecisive, confirm with IV GTT. If suggestive diagnosis of diabetes is not definite during pregnancy, do additional workup after delivery.

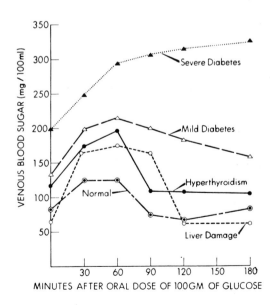

Fig. 1. Sample Oral Glucose Tolerance Curves in Various Conditions

Decreased Tolerance In

Excessive peak
 Increased absorption (normal IV GTT curve) with normal
  return to fasting level
   Mechanical (gastrectomy, gastroenterostomy, etc.)
   Hyperthyroidism
   Excess intake of glucose
 Decreased utilization with slow fall to fasting level
   Diabetes mellitus
   Hemochromatosis
   Steroid effect (Cushing's disease, administration of ACTH
    or steroids)
   CNS lesions
 Decreased formation of glycogen with low fasting levels and
  subsequent hypoglycemia
   von Gierke's disease
   Severe liver damage
   Hyperthyroidism (normal return to fasting level)
   Increased adrenalin (stress, pheochromocytoma) (normal
    return to fasting level)
   Pregnancy (normal return to fasting level)

Increased Tolerance In

Flat peak
 Pancreatic islet cell hyperplasia or tumor
 Poor absorption from GI tract (normal IV GTT curve)
   Intestinal diseases (steatorrhea, sprue, celiac disease, Whip-
    ple's disease, etc.)
   Hypothyroidism
   Addison's disease
   Hypoparathyroidism
Late hypoglycemia
 Pancreatic islet cell hyperplasia or tumor
 Hypopituitarism
 Liver disease

INTRAVENOUS GLUCOSE TOLERANCE TEST

Administer 20% glucose (0.5 gm/kg body weight) intravenously over
 30 minutes.
Normal
 Peak 200–250 mg/100 ml immediately
 Return to fasting level by 90 minutes
 Below fasting level by 2 hours
 Return to fasting level by 3 hours
Intestinal disease and hypothyroidism—normal (in contrast to oral
 GTT)
Liver disease—delayed fall after peak; return to fasting level in 3–5
 hours (variable in oral GTT)
Addison's disease and hypopituitarism—normal peak (flat peak in
 oral GTT); severe hypoglycemia later
Acromegaly—IV GTT abnormal more frequently than oral GTT

Oral GTT is more useful for diagnosis of diabetes mellitus and
 pancreatic cell hyperactivity. IV GTT is useful to clarify or rule
 out the influence of absorption factors in the curve.

SOSKIN'S INTRAVENOUS GLUCOSE TOLERANCE TEST

Administer 50% glucose (0.3 gm/kg body weight) intravenously within 3–5 minutes.

Normal. Blood sugar returns to fasting level in less than 60 minutes.

Diabetes. Blood sugar returns to fasting level in more than 120 minutes.

Liver disease. Blood sugar returns to fasting level in less than 120 minutes. In 25% of patients with liver disease blood sugar returns to fasting level in less than 60 minutes.

TOLBUTAMIDE TOLERANCE TEST

Administer 1 gm sodium tolbutamide intravenously within 2 minutes. *Always keep IV glucose available to prevent severe reaction.*

Table 7. Serum Glucose Change Induced by Tolbutamide in Various Conditions

Disease	% of Fasting Serum Glucose At	
	20 Minutes	30 Minutes
Islet cell tumor	17–50	40–60
Normal functional hyperinsulinism	50–80	60–76
Borderline diabetes	80–84	77–81
Probable diabetes	85–89	82–86
Diabetes	90 or more	87 or more

Adrenal insufficiency—normal or low curve
Severe liver disease—low curve

Test is most useful for diagnosis of secreting islet cell tumor and to rule out functional hyperinsulinism.

In islet cell tumor the fall in blood sugar is usually more marked than in functional hypoglycemia; more important, the blood sugar fails to recover even after 2–3 hours.

In functional hypoglycemia, return of blood sugar to normal is usually complete by 90 minutes.

INSULIN TOLERANCE TEST

Administer 0.1 unit insulin/kg body weight intravenously. *Use smaller dose if hypopituitarism is suspected. Always keep IV glucose available to prevent severe reaction.*

Normal
Blood glucose falls to 50% of fasting level within 20–30 minutes; returns to fasting level within 90–120 minutes.

Increased Tolerance
Blood glucose falls < 25% and returns rapidly to fasting level.

Hypothyroidism
Acromegaly
Cushing's syndrome
Diabetes mellitus (some cases; especially older, obese patients)

Decreased Tolerance
Increased sensitivity to insulin (excessive fall of blood glucose)
Hypoglycemic irresponsiveness (lack of response by glycogenolysis)
    Pancreatic islet cell tumor
    Adrenal cortical insufficiency
    Adrenal cortical insufficiency secondary to hypopituitarism
    Hypothyroidism
    von Gierke's disease (some cases)
    Starvation (depletion of liver glycogen)

INSULIN GLUCOSE TOLERANCE TEST

Administer simultaneously 0.1 unit insulin/kg body weight intravenously and 0.8 gm glucose/kg body weight orally.

Insulin-sensitive diabetics show little change in blood sugar.
Insulin-resistant diabetics show a diabetic glucose tolerance curve.
Other changes parallel those in the insulin tolerance test.

INTRAVENOUS GLUCOSE PHOSPHORUS TOLERANCE TEST

This test is indicated in diabetic suspects who also show evidence of liver disease. Liver disease and diabetes have a more prolonged decline than normal.

Normal. Serum phosphorus falls *to* 60–90% (average 75%) of fasting level by 1 hour after IV glucose administration
Liver disease. Serum phosphorus falls to average 63% of fasting level. Minimum level occurs in 90 minutes.
Diabetes mellitus. Serum phosphorus falls to average 88% of fasting level. Minimum level occurs in 120 minutes.

CORTISONE GLUCOSE TOLERANCE TEST

Cortisone increases the sensitivity of the oral GTT, but its clinical status is still uncertain.
Administer 50 mg cortisone acetate orally (62.5 mg if body weight is over 160 lb) at 8½ and 2 hours before test. Oral glucose of 1.75 gm/kg ideal weight is given as a 25% solution.

Upper limit of normal at 2 hours = 140 mg/100 ml.
Correct for age of patient: Add 18 mg at age 40 (158 mg/100 ml); add an additional 18 mg/100 ml for each decade over 40.

ORAL DISACCHARIDE TOLERANCE TEST

Administer 1 gm/kg body weight of the test carbohydrate (disaccharide). Determine blood glucose at fasting, ½-, 1-, 2-, and 3-hour intervals.

Normal. Blood glucose rises more than 24 mg/100 ml above fasting level.
Abnormal in disaccharide malabsorption. Blood glucose rises 0–21 mg/100 ml above fasting level. False abnormal test may be due to delayed gastric emptying or delayed blood collection.

Confirm disaccharide malabsorption by
> Repeating tolerance test using constituent monosaccharides
> Testing stool for
>> pH: 5 or less is abnormal.
>> Sugar: more than 0.5% is abnormal; 0.25–0.5% is suspicious; less than 0.25% is normal.
>
> Taking intestinal biopsy for histologic study and disaccharidase activity assay

D-XYLOSE TOLERANCE TEST

Give 25 gm D-xylose in water orally. Collect a total 5-hour urine specimen (normal is more, and abnormal is less, than 5 gm in 5 hours). Blood may also be taken at fasting, ½-, 1-, and 2-hour intervals (normal is more than 25 mg/100 ml). The test reflects intestinal malabsorption.

Decreased In
Malabsorption in jejunum (e.g., celiac disease, sprue)—less than 2–3 gm in 5-hour urine
Elderly persons
Renal disease and myxedema—normal absorption but decreased urinary excretion
Patients with ascites (urine values are low)

Normal In
Regional ileitis
Enterocolitis
Steatorrhea due to pancreatic disease
Cirrhosis of liver
Postgastrectomy state
Malnutrition

GALACTOSE TOLERANCE TEST

Use an oral dose of 35 gm of galactose/square meter of body area.

Normal. Serum galactose rises to 30–50 mg/100 ml, returns to normal within 3 hours.
Galactosemia. Serum increase is greater, and return to baseline level is delayed.
Heterozygous carrier. Response is intermediate.

The test is not specific or sensitive enough for genetic studies.

Beware of hypoglycemia in von Gierke's disease.

CAROTENE TOLERANCE TEST

Low values for serum carotene levels are usually associated with steatorrhea.
Measure serum carotene following daily oral loading of carotene for 3–7 days.

Normal
Increase of serum carotene by more than 35 μg/100 ml indicates previously low dietary intake of carotene and/or fat.

Decreased In
Steatorrhea. Serum carotene rises less than 30 μg/100 ml. Patients with sprue in remission with normal fecal fat excretion may still show low carotene absorption.

Mineral oil interferes with carotene absorption; on a fat-free diet only 10% is absorbed.

IODINE TOLERANCE TEST

A fasting patient who has received no iodine for 1 week is given 0.3–0.5 ml of strong iodine solution in milk. Blood iodine determinations are made every half-hour for 2½ hours.

Normal. Blood iodine rises from 10 up to 160 or 170 μg/100 ml in half an hour; by 2½ hours it falls to only 150 μg.
Hyperthyroidism. Blood iodine rises from 15 μg to only 40 μg after 1 hour.

CREATINE TOLERANCE TEST
(ingestion of 1–3 gm creatine)

Normal. Creatine is not increased in blood or urine.
Decreased muscle mass. Blood and urine creatine increases in
    Neurogenic atrophy
    Polymyositis
    Addison's disease
    Hyperthyroidism
    Male eunuchoidism
    Etc.

TRYPTOPHAN TOLERANCE TEST

The test demonstrates pyridoxine deficiency. It may be positive in pyridoxine-responsive anemia or it may be normal.
A positive test produces abnormally large urinary excretion of xanthurenic acid.

ELLSWORTH-HOWARD TEST

Determine urinary phosphorus before and after injection of *potent* parathyroid extract.
Hypoparathyroidism. Urinary phosphorus is increased more than 10 times.
Pseudohypoparathyroidism. Urinary phosphorus is increased less than 2 times (i.e., poor or no response to parathormone injection).
Pseudopseudohypoparathyroidism. Response to parathormone injection is normal. Urinary phosphorus is increased 5–6 times.
Basal cell nevus syndrome. Decreased response to parathormone injection is often shown.

RESPONSE OF ELEVATED SERUM CALCIUM TO CORTICOIDS

Corticoids do not suppress elevated serum calcium in hyperparathyroidism.

Corticoid administration does suppress the elevated serum calcium level in
  Sarcoidosis
  Metastatic neoplasm
  Vitamin D excess
  Multiple myeloma
  Hyperthyroidism

CALCIUM TOLERANCE

Constant diet. Measure phosphorus in three 24-hour urines. On second day, administer calcium intravenously (15 mg/kg body weight).

Normal. Calcium infusion causes marked decrease in urine phosphorus on second day followed by rebound increase on third day.
Hyperparathyroidism. Only slight changes appear in urine phosphorus.

PHOSPHATE DEPRIVATION

Low-phosphate diet (430 mg phosphate and 700 mg calcium/day) for 3–6 days causes low serum phosphate and increased serum calcium in persons with hyperparathyroidism but not in normal individuals.

The test is clinically useful when blood chemistries are at borderline levels.

PHOSPHATE CLEARANCE

After a diet of 800 mg phosphate/day, determine serum phosphorus and BUN and 12-hour urine phosphorus.

Normal: 6–17 ml/minute
Hyperparathyroidism: higher (even with renal dysfunction)
Hypoparathyroidism; lower (e.g., < 6 ml/minute) even when hypocalcemia has been corrected

TUBULAR REABSORPTION OF PHOSPHATE (TRP)

After a constant dietary intake of moderate calcium and phosphorus for 3 days, phosphorus and creatinine are determined in fasting blood and 4-hour urine specimens to calculate TRP.

$$TRP = 100\left(1 - \frac{\text{urine phosphorus} \times \text{serum calcium}}{\text{urine calcium} \times \text{serum phosphorus}}\right)$$

Normal: TRP = $> 78\%$ on normal diet; higher on low-phosphate diet (430mg/day)
Hyperparathyroidism: TRP = $< 74\%$ on normal diet; $< 85\%$ on low-phosphate diet
False positive result may occur in uremia, renal tubular disease (some patients), osteomalacia, sarcoidosis.

URINE CONCENTRATION TEST

Restrict water intake for 14–16 hours; then collect three urines at 1-, 2-, and 4-hour intervals and measure specific gravity.

Normal. Urine specific gravity is 1.025 or more.

With decreased renal function, specific gravity is < 1.020. As renal impairment is more severe, specific gravity approaches 1.010.

The test is sensitive for early loss of renal function, but a normal finding does not necessarily rule out active kidney disease.

The test is unreliable in the presence of any severe water and electrolyte imbalance (e.g., adrenal cortical insufficiency, edema formation), low-protein or low-salt diet, chronic liver disease, pregnancy, lack of patient cooperation.

Fluid deprivation may be contraindicated in heart disease or early renal failure.

VASOPRESSIN (PITRESSIN) CONCENTRATION TEST

The bladder is emptied and urine is collected 1 and 2 hours after subcutaneous injection of 10 units of vasopressin. Water intake is not restricted but no diuretics should be administered.

Normal. The specific gravity should reach 1.020 or more.

Interpretation is the same as in the urine concentration test.

In diabetes insipidus, urine specific gravity becomes normal after vasopressin administration but not after fluid restriction.

The test may be used in the presence of edema or ascites. It is contraindicated in coronary artery disease and pregnancy.

See Diabetes Insipidus, p. 349.

URINE OSMOLALITY

Measurement of urine osmolality during water restriction is an accurate, sensitive test of decreased renal function.

The patient is on a high-protein diet for 3 days; takes a dry supper and no fluids on the evening before the test; empties the bladder at 6 A.M., discards urine, and returns to bed. Test urine specimen is collected at 8 A.M.

Normal: concentration of more than 800 mOsm/kg

Minimal impairment of renal concentrating ability: 600–800 mOsm/kg

Moderate impairment: 400–600 mOsm/kg

Severe impairment: less than 400 mOsm/kg

Urine osmolality may be impaired when other tests are normal (Fishberg concentration test, BUN, PSP excretion, creatinine clearance, IV pyelogram); may be especially useful in diabetes mellitus, essential hypertension, silent pyelonephritis.

It may be well also to measure serum osmolality and calculate urine: serum ratio (normal is > 3).

See Diabetes Insipidus, p. 349.

URINE DILUTION TEST

No breakfast is allowed; 1500 ml of water is taken within 30–45 minutes, and urine is collected every hour for 4 hours.

Normal. Urine volume is over 80% of ingested amount (1200 ml). Specific gravity is 1.003 in at least one specimen.

With decreased renal function there is a smaller volume of urine. Specific gravity may not fall below 1.010.

Loss of dilution ability occurs later than loss of concentrating ability.

Water loading may be contraindicated in kidney and heart disease.

PHENOLSULFONPHTHALEIN (PSP) EXCRETION TEST

Administer an IV injection of 1 mg/kg body weight or usually 6 mg in 1 ml volume. Collect urine and sometimes blood samples at 15-, 30-, and 60-minute intervals.

The test is useful to detect slight to moderate decrease in renal function. It is not useful in chronic azotemia with fixed specific gravity (serum creatinine and creatinine clearance are more useful then).

It is hazardous in severe renal insufficiency or heart failure because adequate prior hydration is required to obtain sufficient urine volume. Using small urine volumes magnifies errors.

The test is distorted by residual bladder urine, abnormal drainage sites (e.g., fistulas), and interfering substances (e.g., hematuria).

Hepatic disease may give falsely elevated values (because 20% of the dye is normally removed by the liver). False results may also occur in multiple myeloma (because of excessive protein binding) and in hypoalbuminemia. Certain drugs may interfere with PSP excretion (e.g., salicylates, penicillin, some diuretic and uricosuric drugs, and some x-ray contrast media).

The 15-minute PSP excretion correlates with the glomerular filtration rate (GFR); a normal 15-minute value indicates normal GFR. Progressive decrease of 15-minute value is proportional to decreased GFR (e.g., 15% PSP excretion in 15 minutes approximates a 45% GFR). If the GFR is normal, the PSP test indicates renal blood flow or tubular function; there are better tests available for measuring these two functions.

Increased dye excretion in later time periods compared to the initial 15-minute period suggests increased residual urine due to obstructive uropathy or incomplete bladder emptying; the latter can be ruled out by indwelling catheterization during the test.

PSP that is normal with increased BUN and serum creatinine and decreased GFR suggests acute glomerulonephritis. PSP parallels these parameters in most chronic renal diseases.

OTHER RENAL FUNCTION TESTS*

Glomerular filtration rate (GFR) is measured with urea clearance or creatinine clearance or inulin clearance.

Renal plasma flow (RPF) is measured with para-aminohippurate (PAH) clearance or Diodrast clearance.

$$\text{Filtration fraction (FF)} = \frac{\text{GFR}}{\text{RPF}} \qquad (\text{normal} = 0.2)$$

---

* See standard laboratory texts for technical performance of clearance tests.

Urea clearance is normal until more than 50% of renal parenchyma is inactivated. With renal insufficiency, the clearance test parallels the parenchymal destruction.

Urinary acidification is impaired in chronic renal disease with azotemia. It is decreased without parallel impairment of GFR in renal tubular acidosis, some cases of Fanconi syndrome, and some cases of acquired nephrocalcinosis.

Proximal tubular malfunction is indicated by urinary excretion of substances normally reabsorbed by tubules: renal glycosuria (blood glucose < 180 mg/100 as in Fanconi syndrome, heavy-metal poisoning), aminoaciduria, phosphaturia.

See also Serum BUN (p. 38), Serum Creatinine (p. 39), PSP Excretion Test (preceding section), Urine Concentration Test (p. 77) and Urine Dilution Test (p. 78).

Table 8. Laboratory Guide to Evaluation of Renal Impairment

Condition	Renal Clearance of Endogenous Creatinine (glomerular filtration rate)	Urinary Excretion of IV PSP in 15 Minutes (renal tubular transport mechanisms)
Normal	Men: 130–200 L/24 hours (90–139 ml/min) Women: 115–180 L/24 hours (80–125 ml/min)	25% or more
Slight impairment	75–90 L/24 hours (52.0–62.5 ml/min)	15–25%
Mild impairment	60–75 L/24 hours (42–52 ml/min)	10–15%
Moderate impairment	40–60 L/24 hours (28–42 ml/min)	5–10%
Marked impairment	Less than 40 L/24 hours (less than 28 ml/min)	Less than 5%

If there is a discrepancy between these two tests, additional studies may be performed (e.g., concentration and dilution tests, urinalyses, biochemical studies of serum and urine, urine cultures, renograms and scans, biopsy).

Impairment may be more severe than indicated by laboratory studies if signs and symptoms are more disabling.

SPLIT RENAL FUNCTION TESTS
(for aid in diagnosis of renal artery stenosis)

Affected kidney shows decreased urine volume and sodium excretion, and decreased urine concentration of creatinine, inulin, or PAH.

The tests are not useful in presence of urinary tract obstruction (e.g., in men over age 50).

RENAL BIOPSY

May Be Indicated In
Acute renal failure to differentiate
   Acute glomerulonephritis—to be treated with immunosuppressive agents and dialysis

Drug-induced (e.g., methicillin) acute interstitial nephritis with eosinophilia—to be treated with prednisone

Interstitial nephritis and papillary necrosis due to analgesic drug abuse—to be treated with dialysis and cessation of analgesics (see p. 440)

Systemic lupus erythematosus (SLE), necrotizing angiitis, and Goodpasture's syndrome (to be treated with prednisone or hydrocortisone) are to be distinguished from ischemic or nephrotoxic renal failure (to be treated with dialysis and does not need drug therapy).

Lipoid nephrosis to differentiate
  SLE—to be treated with prednisone
  Amyloid nephropathy—to be treated by therapy of underlying infection
  Occult bacterial endocarditis—to be treated with antibiotics
  Renal vein thrombosis—to be treated with anticoagulants

  Characteristic lipoid nephrosis of children and young adults is prednisone-responsive.
  Diffuse generalized membranous glomerulonephritis is steroid-resistant.
  Proliferative glomerulonephritis (e.g., poststreptococcal, anaphylactoid purpura) is to be treated with immunosuppressive agents.

Fixed and persistent proteinuria that does not respond to trial of prednisone therapy; routine biopsy not indicated in childhood or adolescence
Diagnosis of unsuspected disease (e.g., nephrocalcinosis of hyperparathyroidism)
Diagnosis of renal disease of unknown etiology
Evaluation of therapeutic effect (e.g., SLE, polyarteritis nodosa)
Complete diagnosis prior to renal transplantation or chronic dialysis
Culture of organism in some cases of pyelonephritis
Others

Contraindicated In
Patient with bleeding tendencies
Patient with unilateral kidney
Uncooperative patient

CYTOLOGIC EXAMINATION OF VAGINAL SMEAR (PAPANICOLAOU SMEAR) FOR EVALUATION OF OVARIAN FUNCTION

Maturation index (MI) is the proportion of parabasal, intermediate, and superficial cells in each 100 cells counted.
  Lack of estrogen effect shows predominance of parabasal cells (e.g., MI = 100/0/0).
  Low estrogen effect shows predominance of intermediate cells (e.g., MI = 10/90/0).
  Increased estrogen effect shows predominance of superficial cells (e.g., MI = 0/0/100), as in hormone-producing tumors of ovary, persistent follicular cysts.

Karyopyknotic index (KI) is the percent of cells with pyknotic nuclei.

Increased estrogen effect (e.g., KI=85% or more) is seen, as in cystic glandular hyperplasia of the endometrium.

Eosinophilic index is the percent of cells showing eosinophilic cytoplasm; it may also be used as a measure of estrogen effect.

Combined progesterone-estrogen effect. No quantitative cytologic criteria are available. Endometrial biopsy should be used for this purpose.

The pattern may be obscured by cytolysis (e.g., infections, excess bacilli), increased red or white blood cells, excessively thin or thick smears, or drying of smears before fixation (artificial eosinophilic staining).

HEMATOLOGY

CAUSES OF LEUKOPENIA

Infections, especially
> Bacterial (e.g., overwhelming bacterial infection, septicemia, miliary tuberculosis, typhoid, paratyphoid, brucellosis, tularemia)
> Viral (e.g., infectious mononucleosis, hepatitis, influenza, measles, rubella, psittacosis)
> Rickettsial (e.g., scrub typhus, sandfly fever)
> Others (e.g., malaria, kala-azar)

Drugs and chemicals, especially
> Sulfonamides
> Antibiotics
> Analgesics
> Marrow depressants
> Arsenicals
> Antithyroid drugs
> Many others

Ionizing radiation

Hematopoietic diseases
> Pernicious anemia
> Aleukemic leukemia
> Aplastic anemia and related conditions
> Hypersplenism
> Gaucher's disease
> Felty's syndrome

Anaphylactic shock

Cachexia

Miscellaneous
> Disseminated lupus erythematosus
> Severe renal injury
> Various neutropenias

CAUSES OF LEUKOCYTOSIS

Acute infections
> Localized (e.g., pneumonia, meningitis, tonsillitis, abscess)
> Generalized (e.g., acute rheumatic fever, septicemia, cholera)

Intoxications
> Metabolic (uremia, acidosis, eclampsia, acute gout)

Poisoning by chemicals, drugs, venoms, etc. (e.g., mercury, epinephrine, black widow spider)
Parenteral foreign protein and vaccines
Acute hemorrhage
Acute hemolysis of red blood cells
Myeloproliferative diseases
Tissue necrosis
 Acute myocardial infarction
 Necrosis of tumors
 Burns
 Gangrene
 Bacterial necrosis, etc.
Physiologic conditions (e.g., exercise, emotional stress, menstruation, obstetrical labor)

CAUSES OF LYMPHOCYTOSIS — *mostly viral, some bacterial*

Infections
 Pertussis
 Infectious lymphocytosis
 Infectious mononucleosis
 Infectious hepatitis
 Mumps
 German measles
 Chronic tuberculosis
 Undulant fever
 Convalescence from acute infection
 Thyrotoxicosis (relative)
 Neutropenia with relative lymphocytosis
 Lymphatic leukemia

CAUSES OF ATYPICAL LYMPHOCYTES

Lymphatic leukemia
Viral infections
 Infectious lymphocytosis
 Infectious mononucleosis
 Infectious hepatitis
 Mumps
 Chickenpox
 German measles
Pertussis
Brucellosis
Syphilis (in some phases)

CLUES TO DIAGNOSIS OF ATYPICAL OR LEUKOPENIC LEUKEMIA

Peripheral monocytosis
Peripheral cytopenia with normoblasts
Hypercellular marrow with hyperplasia of myeloid and/or erythroid elements
Acquired Pelger-Huët anomaly (see pp. 271-272)

BASOPHILIC LEUKOCYTES

Increased In
Chronic myelogenous leukemia
Polycythemia
Myeloid metaplasia

Hodgkin's disease
Postsplenectomy
Chronic hemolytic anemia (some cases)
Chronic sinusitis
Chickenpox
Smallpox
Myxedema
Nephrosis (some cases)
Foreign protein injection

Decreased In
Hyperthyroidism
Pregnancy
Period following radiation, chemotherapy, and glucocorticoids
Acute phase of infection

CAUSES OF MONOCYTOSIS
**(more than 10% of differential count; absolute count more than 500/
cu mm)**

Monocytic leukemia, other leukemias
Myeloproliferative disorders (myeloid metaplasia, polycythemia
   vera)
Hodgkin's disease and other malignant lymphomas
Lipid storage diseases (e.g., Gaucher's disease)
Tetrachlorethane poisoning
Recovery from agranulocytosis and subsidence of acute infection
Many protozoan infections (e.g., malaria, kala-azar, trypanosomia-
   sis)
Some rickettsial infections (e.g., Rocky Mountain spotted fever,
   typhus)
Certain bacterial infections (e.g., subacute bacterial endocarditis,
   tuberculosis, brucellosis)
Chronic ulcerative colitis and regional enteritis
Sarcoidosis
Collagen diseases (e.g., rheumatoid arthritis, SLE)

PLASMA CELLS

Increased In
Plasma cell leukemia
Multiple myeloma
Serum reaction
Infectious mononucleosis
Rubella
Measles
Chickenpox
Benign lymphocytic meningitis

Decreased In
Not clinically significant

CAUSES OF EOSINOPHILIA
Allergic diseases (e.g., bronchial asthma, hay fever, urticaria, drug
   therapy)
Parasitic infestation, especially with tissue invasion (e.g., trichinosis,
   echinococcus disease) (see Pulmonary Infiltrations Associated
   with Eosinophilia, p. 160).
Some infectious diseases (e.g., scarlet fever, erythema multiforme)

Some skin diseases (e.g., pemphigus, dermatitis herpetiformis)
Some hematopoietic diseases (e.g., pernicious anemia, chronic mye-
  logenous leukemia, polycythemia, Hodgkin's disease); postsple-
  nectomy
Postirradiation
Miscellaneous conditions
  Polyarteritis nodosa
  Certain tumors (ovary; involvement of bone or serosal surfaces)
  Sarcoidosis
  Familial condition
  Poisoning (e.g., phosphorus, black widow spider bite)

Table 9. Some Common Causes of Leukemoid Reaction

Cause	Myelocytic	Lymphocytic	Monocytic
Infections	Endocarditis Pneumonia Septicemia Leptospirosis etc.	Infectious mono- nucleosis Infectious lympho- cytosis Pertussis Chickenpox Tuberculosis	Tuberculosis
Toxic conditions	Burns Eclampsia Poisons (e.g., mercury)		
Neoplasms	Carcinoma of colon Embryonal car- cinoma of kidney	Carcinoma of stomach Carcinoma of breast	
Miscellaneous	**Treatment of mega- loblastic anemia (of pregnancy, pernicious anemia)** Acute hemorrhage Acute hemolysis Recovery from agranulocytosis	Dermatitis herpetiformis	
Myeloprolifera- tive diseases			

LEUKOCYTE ALKALINE PHOSPHATASE STAINING REACTION
(in untreated diseases)

Usually Increased In
Leukemoid reaction
Polycythemia vera
Lymphoma (including Hodgkin's, reticulum cell sarcoma)
Acute and chronic lymphatic leukemia
Multiple myeloma
Myelosclerosis
Aplastic anemia
Agranulocytosis
Bacterial infections
Cirrhosis
Obstructive jaundice
Pregnancy and immediate postpartum period

Administration of Enovid
Mongolism (trisomy 21)
Klinefelter's syndrome (XXY)

Usually Decreased In
Chronic myelogenous leukemia
Paroxysmal nocturnal hemoglobinuria
Hereditary hypophosphatasia
Nephrotic syndrome
Progressive muscular dystrophy
Refractory anemia (siderotic)

Usually Normal In
Secondary polycythemia
Hemolytic anemia
Infectious mononucleosis
Viral hepatitis
Lymphosarcoma

Usually Variable In
Pernicious anemia
Idiopathic thrombocytopenic purpura
Iron-deficiency anemia
Acute myelogenous leukemia
Acute undifferentiated leukemia

*This test is clinically most useful to differentiate chronic myelogenous
    leukemia from leukemoid reaction.*

PLATELET COUNT

May Be Increased In (more than 500,000/cu mm)
Malignancy, especially disseminated, advanced, or inoperable
Myeloproliferative disease, e.g., polycythemia vera, chronic myelog-
    enous leukemia
Patients recently having surgery, especially splenectomy
Collagen disorders, usually rheumatoid arthritis
Iron-deficiency anemia
Miscellaneous disease states, e.g., acute infection, cardiac disease,
    cirrhosis of the liver, chronic pancreatitis

*Approximately 50% of patients with "unexpected" increase of platelet
    count are found to have a malignancy.*

Decreased In
See Thrombocytopenic Purpura (p. 282).

ERYTHROCYTE SEDIMENTATION RATE (ESR)

ESR is useful to
>   Detect occult disease (e.g., screening program)
>   Follow course of a certain disease (e.g., tuberculosis, rheumatic
>   fever, myocardial infarction)
>   Confirm a diagnosis or a differential diagnosis (e.g., acute
>   myocardial infarction versus angina pectoris; early acute
>   appendicitis versus ruptured tubal pregnancy or acute pelvic
>   inflammatory disease; rheumatoid arthritis versus osteoar-
>   thritis)

Table 10. Changes in ESR

Disease	Increased In	Not Increased In
Infectious	Tuberculosis (especially) Acute hepatitis	Typhoid fever Undulant fever Malarial paroxysm Infectious mononucleosis Uncomplicated viral diseases
Cardiac	Acute myocardial infarction Active rheumatic fever Postcommissurotomy syndrome	Angina pectoris Active renal failure with heart failure
Abdominal	Acute pelvic inflammatory disease Ruptured ectopic pregnancy **Pregnancy—third month to about 3 weeks postpartum** Menstruation	Acute appendicitis (first 24 hours) Unruptured ectopic pregnancy Early pregnancy
Joint	Rheumatoid arthritis Pyogenic arthritis	Degenerative arthritis
Miscellaneous	**Significant tissue necrosis especially neoplasms—** most frequently malignant lymphoma, cancer of colon and breast) Increased serum globulins (e.g., myeloma, cryoglobulinemia, macroglobulinuria) **Decreased serum albumin** **Hypothyroidism** **Hyperthyroidism** **Acute hemorrhage** Nephrosis, renal disease with azotemia Arsenic and lead intoxication Dextran and polyvinyl compounds in blood	Peptic ulcer Acute allergy Polycythemia vera Secondary polycythemia **Sickle cell anemia, spherocytosis, anisocytosis**

Extreme elevation of ESR is found particularly in association with malignancy (most frequently malignant lymphoma, carcinomas of colon and breast), hematologic diseases (most frequently myeloma), collagen diseases (rheumatoid arthritis, SLE, etc.), renal diseases (especially with azotemia), infections, and others (e.g., cirrhosis).

Low ESR: Sickle Cell, Hypofibrinogenemia, Trichinosis, CHF!

SERUM C-REACTIVE PROTEIN (CRP)

Normally CRP is not detected in serum.

Increased In
Any acute inflammatory change or necrosis. CRP precedes the rise in ESR; with recovery, disappearance of CRP precedes the return to normal of the ESR. CRP disappears when inflammatory process is suppressed by steroids or salicylates.
Acute myocardial infarction. CRP appears within 24–48 hours, begins to fall by third day and becomes negative after 1–2 weeks.

Acute rheumatic fever. CRP reflects rheumatic activity more promptly than ESR.
Bacterial infections
Neoplasm with widespread metastases

Increased Inconsistently In
Active tuberculosis
Viral infections
Rheumatoid arthritis

PERIPHERAL BLOOD SMEAR IN DIFFERENTIAL DIAGNOSIS OF ANEMIAS

Basophilic or polychromatophilic macrocytes—shows increased erythropoiesis in hemorrhage or hemolysis
Oval macrocytes with increased number of lobules of polynuclear leukocytes—in megaloblastic anemia
Target cells—in hemoglobinopathies (especially Hgb C); also thalassemia, iron-deficiency anemia, liver disease
Abnormally shaped RBC—ovalocytes, sickle cells, spherocytes, poikilocytes, schistocytes
Microcytes with stippling—in thalassemia, lead poisoning

The smear may also indicate leukemia, etc.
Confirm the RBC indices.

CONDITIONS ASSOCIATED WITH RBC INCLUSIONS

Reticulocytes*	Any condition with increased reticulocyte count
Basophilic stippling (multiple dark dots)	Lead poisoning; heavy metal poisoning and severe anemia
Cabot's rings	Occasionally seen in severe hemolytic anemias and pernicious anemia
Howell-Jolly bodies (dark purple spherical bodies)	Occasionally seen in severe hemolytic anemias and pernicious anemia
	Occasionally seen in leukemia, thalassemia, postsplenectomy
Pappenheimer bodies (siderotic granules) (purple coccoid granules at periphery)	Anemias with defect of incorporating iron into hemoglobin; show hypochromic microcytic anemia with increased serum iron and total iron-binding capacity (e.g., thalassemia, lead poisoning, di Guglielmo's disease, pyridoxine-responsive anemia, pyridoxine-unresponsive anemia)
Heinz-Ehrlich bodies*	Congenital G-6-PD deficiencies; other drug-induced hemolytic anemias
Plasmodium trophozoites	Malaria

---

* Not seen with Wright's stain; requires supravital cresyl violet stain.

RETICULOCYTES

Increased In
Blood loss or increased RBC destruction—normal response is 3–6 times increase
After iron therapy in iron-deficiency anemia
After specific therapy in megaloblastic anemias

Increase indicates effective RBC production mechanisms. It is a useful index of therapeutic response in these diseases.

Possibly other conditions, e.g., hematologic (polycythemia, metastatic carcinoma in bone marrow, di Guglielmo's disease, etc.)

Decreased In
(ineffective erythropoiesis or decreased RBC formation)
Severe autoimmune type of hemolytic disease
Aregenerative crises

SICKLING OF RBCs

Occurs In
Sickle cell disease
Sickle cell trait

False Positive In
Transfusion within 4 months with RBCs having sickle cell trait
Mixture on slide with fibrinogen, thrombin, gelatin (glue)
Excessive concentration of sodium metabisulfite (e.g., 4% or more instead of 2%)
Drying of wet coverslip preparation
Poikilocytosis

False Negative In
Transfusion within 4 months with normal RBCs
Heating, bacterial contamination, or prolonged washing with saline of RBCs
Newborn

Confirm sickling with hemoglobin electrophoresis and genetic studies.

SEVERELY DISTORTED RBCs (BURR, HELMET, TRIANGLE, ACANTHOID FORMS) IN PERIPHERAL BLOOD SMEARS
These may be found in some acquired hemolytic disorders (some cases with mechanical factors causing RBC damage and distortion with secondary hemolysis; some cases with consumption coagulopathy [defibrination syndrome]):
    Prosthetic heart valves
    Severe rheumatic valvular disease
    Hemolytic anemia in uremia
    Thrombotic thrombocytopenic purpura
    Gastric carcinoma and peptic ulcer with bleeding
    Microangiopathic hemolytic anemia

Cirrhosis with hemolytic anemia (associated with thrombocytopenia, reticulocytosis, increased serum indirect bilirubin)
Hereditary acanthocytosis, pyruvate kinase deficiency, hexo-
kinase deficiency
Snakebite (see p. 445)

OSMOTIC FRAGILITY

Increased In
Hereditary spherocytic anemia (*This disease can be ruled out if there
is normal fragility after 24-hour sterile incubation.*)
Hereditary nonspherocytic hemolytic anemia
Acquired hemolytic anemia (*usually normal in paroxysmal nocturnal
hemoglobinuria*)
Hemolytic disease of newborn due to ABO incompatibility
Some cases of secondary hemolytic anemia (usually normal)
After thermal injury
Symptomatic hemolytic anemia in some cases of
    Malignant lymphoma
    Leukemia
    Carcinoma
    Pregnancy
    Cirrhosis
    Infection (e.g., tuberculosis, malaria, syphilis)

Decreased In
Early infancy
Iron-deficiency anemia
Thalassemia
Sickle cell anemia
Homozygous hemoglobin C disease
Nutritional megaloblastic anemia
Postsplenectomy
Liver disease
Jaundice

SERUM IRON

Increased In
Idiopathic hemochromatosis
Hemosiderosis of excessive iron intake (e.g., repeated blood transfu-
sions, parenteral iron therapy)
Decreased formation of RBCs (e.g., thalassemia, pyridoxine-defi-
ciency anemia, pernicious anemia in relapse)
Increased destruction of RBCs (e.g., hemolytic anemias)
Acute liver damage (degree of increase parallels the amount of
hepatic necrosis)

Decreased In
Iron-deficiency anemia
Normochromic (normocytic or microcytic) anemias of infection and
chronic diseases
Nephrosis (due to loss of iron-binding protein in urine)
Pernicious anemia in remission

SERUM TOTAL IRON-BINDING CAPACITY (TIBC)

Increased In
Iron-deficiency anemia
Acute and chronic blood loss
Hepatitis
Late pregnancy

Decreased In
Hemochromatosis
Cirrhosis of the liver
Thalassemia
Anemias of infection and chronic diseases (e.g., uremia, rheumatoid arthritis, some neoplasms)
Nephrosis

SERUM TRANSFERRIN SATURATION

Increased In
Hemochromatosis
Hemosiderosis
Thalassemia

Decreased In
Iron-deficiency anemia
Anemias of infection and chronic diseases (e.g., uremia, rheumatoid arthritis, some neoplasms)

STAINABLE IRON (HEMOSIDERIN) IN BONE MARROW

Increased In
Hemolytic anemias
Pernicious anemia
Hemochromatosis and hemosiderosis
Uremia (some cases)
Chronic infection (some cases)
Chronic pancreatic insufficiency

Decreased In
Iron-deficiency anemia (e.g., inadequate dietary intake, chronic bleeding, malignancy)
Polycythemia vera (usually absent in polycythemia vera but usually normal or increased in secondary polycythemia)
Collagen diseases (especially rheumatoid arthritis, systemic lupus erythematosus)
Infiltration of marrow (e.g., malignant lymphomas, metastatic carcinoma, myelofibrosis, miliary granulomas)
Uremia
Chronic infection (e.g., pulmonary tuberculosis, bronchiectasis, chronic pyelonephritis)
Miscellaneous (e.g., old age, diabetes mellitus)

The presence of iron in marrow is the most reliable index of iron deficiency; it almost invariably rules out iron-deficiency anemia. Only individuals with decreased marrow iron are likely to benefit from iron therapy.

Marrow iron disappears before the peripheral blood changes. It rapidly disappears after hemorrhage.

One may have a normal serum iron and TIBC in iron-deficiency anemia, especially if Hb is less than 9 gm/100 ml.

EXCESSIVE IRON DEPOSITION IN DISEASES ASSOCIATED WITH IRON OVERLOAD

Idiopathic hemochromatosis

Hemochromatosis secondary to

Increased intake (e.g., Bantu siderosis, excessive medicinal ingestion)

Anemias with increased erythropoiesis (especially thalassemia major; also thalassemia minor, some other hemoglobinopathies, paroxysmal nocturnal hemoglobinuria, "sideroachrestic" anemias, refractory anemias with hypercellular bone marrow, etc.)

Liver injury (e.g., following portal shunt surgery)

Atransferrinemia

SERUM CERULOPLASMIN

Decreased In

Wilson's disease (deficient or absent in early stages)

Moderate transient deficiencies in some patients with

Nephrosis

Sprue

Kwashiorkor

Normal infants

Increased In

Pregnancy

Cases of patients taking estrogen

Rheumatoid arthritis (may cause green color of plasma)

SERUM COPPER

Increased In

Anemia

Pernicious anemia

Megaloblastic anemia of pregnancy

Iron-deficiency anemia

Aplastic anemia

Leukemia, acute and chronic

Infection, acute and chronic

Malignant lymphoma

Hemochromatosis

Collagen diseases (including systemic lupus erythematosus, rheumatoid arthritis, acute rheumatic fever, glomerulonephritis)

Hypothyroidism

Hyperthyroidism

Frequently associated with increased CRP

Decreased In
Nephrosis (ceruloplasmin lost in urine)
Wilson's disease
Acute leukemia in remission
Some iron-deficiency anemias of childhood (that require copper as
  well as iron therapy)
Kwashiorkor

SERUM VITAMIN B_{12}

Increased In
Leukemia—acute and chronic myelogenous (about one-third of the
  cases of chronic lymphatic; some cases of monocytic) (normal in
  stem cell leukemia, multiple myeloma, Hodgkin's disease)
Leukocytosis
Polycythemia vera
Some cases of carcinoma (especially with liver metastases)
Liver disease (acute hepatitis, chronic hepatitis, cirrhosis, hepatic
  coma)

Decreased In
Inadequate absorption
    Lack of intrinsic factor
        Pernicious anemia
        Loss of gastric mucosa (e.g., gastrectomy, cancer of stom-
          ach)
        Primary hypothyroidism (Almost half of patients have
          serum achlorhydria with intrinsic factor failure and low
          vitamin B_{12}; rarely megaloblastic anemia develops.)
    Malabsorption (e.g., sprue, celiac disease, idiopathic steator-
      rhea, regional ileitis, fistulas, resection of bowel)
    Loss of ingested vitamin B_{12}; fish tapeworm (*Diphyllobothrium
      latum*) infestation
    Inadequate intake due to severe dietary restrictions
Pregnancy—progressive decrease during pregnancy (*normal serum
B_{12} level in megaloblastic anemia of pregnancy*)

SERUM FOLIC ACID

Decreased In
Inadequate intake (e.g., megaloblastic anemia of pregnancy, megaloblastic anemia of infancy, nutritional megaloblastic anemia,
  some cases of liver disease)
Malabsorption (e.g., sprue, celiac disease, idiopathic steatorrhea)
Folic acid antagonist drugs (e.g., Aminopterin for treatment of
  leukemia, anticonvulsant drugs)
Excessive utilization due to marked cellular proliferation (e.g.,
  hemolytic anemias; myeloproliferative diseases, carcinomas)

Serum folic acid activity less than 3 mμg/ml is associated with a
  positive formiminoglutamic acid (FIGLU) test and positive hematologic findings.
Serum folic acid activity 3–6 mμg/ml is associated with a variable
  FIGLU test and variable hematologic findings.
Serum folic acid activity more than 6 mμg/ml is associated with a
  normal FIGLU test and normal hematologic findings.

FETAL HEMOGLOBIN
(alkali denaturation method; confirmed by examination of hemoglobin bands on starch-gel electrophoresis)

Normal
Less than 2% over age of 2 years
More than 50% at birth; gradual decrease to about 5% by age of 5 months

Increased In
Various hemoglobinopathies (see Table 36, p. 255). About 50% of patients with thalassemia minor have high levels of HbF; even higher levels are found in virtually all patients with thalassemia major. In sickle cell disease, HbF over 30% protects the cell from sickling; therefore, infants even with homozygous S have few problems before the age of 3 months.
Hereditary persistence of fetal hemoglobin
Nonhereditary refractory normoblastic anemia (one-third of patients)
Pernicious anemia (50% of untreated patients); increases after treatment and then gradually decreases during next 6 months; some patients still have slight elevation thereafter. Minimal elevation occurs in about 15% of patients with other types of megaloblastic anemia.
Some patients with leukemia, especially juvenile myeloid leukemia with HbF of 30–60%, absence of Philadelphia chromosome, rapid fatal course, more pronounced thrombocytopenia, and lower total WBC count
Multiple myeloma
Molar pregnancy
Patients with an extra D chromosome (13–15 trisomy, D_1 trisomy) or an extra G chromosome (21 trisomy, Down's syndrome, mongolism)
Acquired aplastic anemia (due to drugs, toxic chemicals, or infections, or idiopathic); returns to normal only after complete remission and therefore is reliable indicator of complete recovery. Better prognosis in patients with higher initial level—more than 400 mg/100 ml.

Decreased In
A rare case of multiple chromosome abnormalities (probably C/D translocation)

SERUM HEMOGLOBIN

Slight Increase In
Sickle cell thalassemia
Hemoglobin C disease

Moderate Increase In
Sickle cell–hemoglobin C disease
Sickle cell anemia
Thalassemia major
Acquired (autoimmune) hemolytic anemia

Marked Increase In
Any rapid intravascular hemolysis

SERUM HAPTOGLOBINS

Increased In
One-third of patients with obstructive biliary disease
Conditions associated with increased ESR and alpha$_2$ globulin (infection; inflammation; trauma; necrosis of tissue; collagen diseases such as rheumatic fever, rheumatoid arthritis, and dermatomyositis, scurvy; amyloidosis; nephrotic syndrome; disseminated neoplasms such as Hodgkin's disease, lymphosarcoma)
Therapy with steroids or androgens

Decreased In
Parenchymatous liver disease (especially cirrhosis)
Hemoglobinemia (related to the duration and severity of hemolysis) due to
>   Intravascular hemolysis
>   Extravascular hemolysis (e.g., large retroperitoneal hemorrhage, hereditary spherocytosis with marked hemolysis, pyruvate-kinase deficiency, autoimmune hemolytic anemia, some transfusion reactions)
>   Intramedullary hemolysis (e.g., thalassemia, megaloblastic anemias, sideroblastic anemias)
Genetically absent in 1% of general population

Haptoglobin determinations are useful
1. When splenectomy is being considered. Patients with chronic hemolysis (e.g., hereditary spherocytosis, pyruvate-kinase deficiency) should not have splenectomy when serum haptoglobin is more than 40 mg/deciliter if infection and inflammation have been ruled out. Increasing haptoglobin levels following splenectomy for these conditions indicate success of surgery; haptoglobin reappears at 24 hours and becomes normal in 4–6 days in hereditary spherocytosis treated with splenectomy.
2. In diagnosis of transfusion reaction by comparison of pretransfusion and posttransfusion levels: posttransfusion reaction serum haptoglobin level decreases in 6–8 hours; at 24 hours it is less than 40 mg/deciliter or less than 40% of pretransfusion level.
3. In paternity studies. May aid by determination of haptoglobin phenotypes.

BONE MARROW ASPIRATION

May Be Useful In
Nonhematologic diseases
>   Metastatic tumor
>   Parasitic infestations (e.g., malaria, kala-azar, histoplasmosis)
>   Infections (e.g., tuberculosis, brucellosis)
>   Granulomas (e.g., sarcoidosis, Hodgkin's disease)
>   Histiocytoses (Gaucher's disease, Niemann-Pick disease)
Hemosiderin staining of bone marrow
Hematologic diseases
>   With normal myeloid:erythroid ratio (in normal adult it is 3:1–4:1)
>>   Aplastic anemia
>>   Myelosclerosis

Multiple myeloma
Diseases of megakaryocytes
With increased myeloid:erythroid ratio
Most infections
Leukemoid reaction
Myeloid leukemias
Decreased number of nucleated red cells
With decreased myeloid:erythroid ratio
Decreased number of myeloid cells (agranulocytosis)
Hyperplasia of erythroid cells
Megaloblastic anemias (see, e.g., pernicious anemia, sprue, steatorrhea)
Normoblastic anemias (see, e.g., iron deficiency, hemorrhage, hemolysis, thalassemia)
Normoblastic hyperplasia (e.g., polycythemia vera)

NEEDLE ASPIRATION OF SPLEEN

May Be Useful In
Differential diagnosis of
Lymphocytic leukemia (> 90% lymphocytes, many of which are abnormal and have increased number of mitoses)
Myelocytic leukemia (20–60% of cells are myelocytes)
Myeloid metaplasia of spleen with myelofibrosis (50–60% of cells are lymphocytes that still persist)
Chronic inflammatory splenomegaly (myelocytes < 5% of cells)
Leukemoid reaction and leukemia
Parasitic infestations (e.g., malaria, leishmaniasis)
Infections (e.g., tuberculosis, brucellosis)
Histiocytoses
Hodgkin's disease
See Some Causes of Splenomegaly, p. 272.

SMEARS OF LYMPH NODE PUNCTURE

May Be Useful In Diagnosis Of
Metastatic carcinoma
Acute and chronic lymphatic leukemia
Lymphosarcoma
Hodgkin's disease
Lymphadenitis

COAGULATION

DUKE BLEEDING TIME

Usually Prolonged In
Thrombocytopenia
Defective platelet function (thrombocytopathies)
Minot–von Willebrand syndrome (2 hours after dose of 10 grains of aspirin; bleeding time is variable without this aspirin tolerance test)
Other coagulation defects—variable results

Usually Normal In
Hemophilia
Severe hereditary hypoprothrombinemia
Severe hereditary hypofibrinogenemia
Scurvy
Etc.

Normal = 1–4 minutes; up to 5.5 minutes is not necessarily pathologic.

The test is useful as part of a coagulation work-up.

COAGULATION (CLOTTING) TIME (CT) ("LEE-WHITE CLOTTING TIME")

Prolonged In
Severe deficiency of any known plasma clotting factors except XⁱII (fibrin-stabilizing factor) and VII
Afibrinogenemia
Marked hyperheparinemia

Normal In
Thrombocytopenia
Deficiency of Factor VII
Minot–von Willebrand syndrome
Mild coagulation defects due to any cause

This is the routine method for control of heparin therapy. It is not a reliable screening test for bleeding conditions because it is not sensitive enough to detect mild conditions but will only detect severe ones. Normal CT does not rule out a coagulation defect. There are many variables in the technique of performing the test.

TOURNIQUET TEST

Positive In
Thrombocytopenic purpuras
Nonthrombocytopenic purpuras
Thrombocytopathies
Scurvy

PROTHROMBIN TIME (PT)

Prolonged by Defect In
Factor I (fibrinogen)
Factor II (prothrombin)
Factor V (labile factor)
Factor VII (stable factor)
Factor X (Stuart-Prower factor)

Prolonged In
Inadequate vitamin K in diet
    Premature infants
    Newborn infants of vitamin K–deficient mother (hemorrhagic disease of the newborn)

Poor fat absorption (e.g., obstructive jaundice, fistulas, sprue, stea-
  torrhea, celiac disease, colitis, chronic diarrhea)
Severe liver damage (e.g., poisons, hepatitis, cirrhosis)
Drugs (e.g., coumarin-type drugs for anticoagulant therapy; salicy-
  lates)
Idiopathic familial hypoprothrombinemia
Circulating anticoagulants
Hypofibrinogenemia (acquired or inherited)

The test is very useful for control of long-term oral anticoagulant
  therapy.

PARTIAL THROMBOPLASTIN TIME (PTT)

Prolonged by Defect In
Factor I (fibrinogen)
Factor II (prothrombin)
Factor V (labile factor)
Factor VIII
Factor IX
Factor X (Stuart-Prower)
Factor XI
Factor XII (Hageman)

Normal In
Thrombocytopenia
Platelet dysfunction
von Willebrand's disease (may be prolonged in some cases)
Isolated defects of Factor VII

PTT is the best *single screening* test for disorders of coagulation; it
  is abnormal in 90% of patients with coagulation disorders when
  properly performed.
The test may not detect mild clotting defects (25–40% of normal
  levels), which seldom cause significant bleeding.

PROTHROMBIN CONSUMPTION

Impaired by any defect in phase I or phase II of blood coagulation
  Thrombocytopathies
  Thrombocytopenia
  Hypoprothrombinemia
  Hemophilias
  Circulating anticoagulants
  Etc.

THROMBOPLASTIN GENERATION TEST (TGT)

This test uses 3 components (BaSO$_4$-adsorbed plasma, serum,
  washed platelets) that are individually substituted in turn to
  mixtures of patient's blood to localize the defect in thromboplastin generation. It can be used to localize coagulation defects due
  to
  Factor VIII
  Factor IX (may not detect mild deficiencies)
  Factor X

Factor V
Factor VII
Thrombasthenia
Circulating anticoagulant

It may not detect disease after recent blood or plasma transfusion.

Table 11. Thromboplastin Generation Test

Components	Mixtures			
BaSO$_4$-adsorbed plasma (Factors V, VIII present; VII, IX, X absent) from	P	P	N	N
Serum (VII, IX, X present; V, VII absent) from	P	N	P	N
Washed platelets from	N	N	N	P
Abnormality				
Normal	+	+	+	+
Thrombocytopenia, thrombocytasthenia	+	+	+	0
von Willebrand's disease	0	0	+	+
Factor V deficiency (severe)	0	0	+	+
Factor VII deficiency	+	+	+	+
Factor VIII deficiency (hemophilia)	0	0	+	+
Factor IX deficiency (Christmas disease)	0	+	0	+
Factor X deficiency	0	+	0	+
Factor XI (PTA) deficiency	0	+	+	+
Factor XII deficiency	0	+	+	+
Circulating anticoagulant	0	0	0	+

P = patient; N = normal control; + = thromboplastin is generated (i.e., fibrin clot forms); O = thromboplastin is not generated (i.e., fibrin clot does not form).

POOR CLOT RETRACTION

Various thrombocytopenias
Thrombasthenia

COAGULATION TESTS

See Hematologic Diseases, Table 40, pp. 280–281, for specific diseases and altered test results.

SEROLOGY

"PREGNANCY" TEST
(immunoassay detection of human chorionic gonadotropin [HCG] in urine, serum, plasma)
(see also Urinary Chorionic Gonadotropins, p. 116)

Positive In
Pregnancy. Test becomes positive as early as 4 days after expected date of menstruation; it is more than 95% reliable by 10th–14th

day. HCG increases to peak at 60th–70th day, then drops progressively.

Hydatidiform mole, choriocarcinoma. Quantitative titers should be performed for diagnosis and for following the clinical course of patients with these conditions.

False negative results may occur in cases of missed abortion, dead fetus syndrome, ectopic pregnancy. False positive results may occur with protein or blood in urine or in patients on methadone therapy.

With the latex agglutination type of test, only urine should be used if patient has rheumatoid arthritis.

Older techniques used animals (e.g., mouse, rat, frog, toad, rabbit) for injection of specimen (usually concentrated urine) followed by examination of their ovaries after specific periods of time. These are more cumbersome and more subject to false positive reactions (e.g., due to high titers of pituitary gonadotropin or high titers of follicle-stimulating hormone in menopause or primary ovarian failure; aspirin, chlorpromazine, phenothiazines within 48 hours) and false negative reactions due to toxic substances in urine (e.g., drugs such as barbiturates and salicylates, excess electrolytes such as potassium, bacterial contamination).

Leukocyte alkaline phosphatase scoring may also be used as a test for pregnancy (see p. 85).

HETEROPHIL AGGLUTINATION
(agglutination of sheep RBCs by serum of patients with infectious mononucleosis)

Titers up to 1:56 may occur in normal individuals and patients with other illnesses.

A titer of 1:224 or higher is presumptive evidence of infectious mononucleosis but may also be caused by recent injection of horse serum or horse immune serum. Therefore, a differential absorption test should be performed using guinea pig kidney and beef cell antigens.

Guinea pig absorption will not reduce the titer in infectious mononucleosis to less than one-quarter of the original value; most commonly the titer is not reduced by more than 1 or 2 tube

Table 12. Sample Titers in Heterophil Agglutination

Presumptive Test	After Guinea Pig Kidney Absorption	After Beef RBC Absorption	Interpretation of Diagnosis of Infectious Mononucleosis
1:224	1:112	0	+
1:224	1:56	0	+
1:224	1:28	0	+
1:224	1:14 or less	0	−
1:224	1:56	1:56	−
1:224	0	1:112	−
1:56	1:56 to 1:7	0	+
1:56	1:56	1:28	−
1:28	1:28 to 1:7	0	+

dilutions. If more than 90% of the agglutination is removed by guinea pig absorption, the test is considered negative.

Beef red cell absorption takes most (90%) or all of the sheep agglutinations and does reduce the titer in infectious mononucleosis; failure to reduce the titer is against a diagnosis of infectious mononucleosis.

Heterophil agglutination may be negative when positive hematologic and clinical findings are present; a second heterophil agglutination in 1–2 weeks may become positive later in the course of the disease. The heterophil agglutination may have become negative even though some residual hematologic findings are still present.

False positives are very rare and occur in relatively low titers.

SEROLOGIC TESTS FOR SYPHILIS

| | % Reactive Patients with Syphilis in Different Stages | | | | |
	Primary	Secondary	Late	Latent	Presumably Normal
Fluorescent treponemal antibody absorbed (FTA-ABS)—most sensitive and specific tests. Reserve for problem cases. Test of choice for confirmation of diagnosis	85	99	95	95	1
Treponema pallidum immobilization (TPI)—specific but somewhat less sensitive than FTA-ABS. Antibodies appear later so test is less sensitive in early syphilis.	56	94	92	94	0
Venereal Disease Research Laboratory (VDRL)—simple test for routine screening at local level; frequent local requirement for premarital and prenatal serology. Does not become positive until 7–10 days after appearance of chancre. Reactive and weakly reactive tests should be confirmed with FTA-ABS.	78	97	77	74	0

Results of these tests are positive in presence of antibodies of related treponematoses, e.g., yaws, pinta, bejel. Once antibodies develop, the tests may thereafter remain positive despite therapy. (This is the mechanism for one type of BFP.) If therapy is given before antibodies develop, these tests may never be positive.

Biologic false positive (BFP) tests should be confirmed with FTA-ABS.

Up to 20% of reactive screening tests may be BFP. Two-thirds of these revert to normal within 6 months; patients have usually had recent infections or immunizations. The remaining third that do not become nonreactive in 6 months have serious underlying disease (e.g., SLE) in 25% or are shown to have syphilis in 50%. BFP occurs in 20–25% of narcotics addicts. Up to 10% of patients over age 70 may show BFP. More than 20% of patients with BFP also show positive tests for RA, antinuclear antibodies, antithyroid antibodies, cryoglobulins, elevated serum gamma globulins.

See Syphilis, pp. 389–390.

ANTISTREPTOCOCCAL ANTIBODY TITERS (ASOT)

A high or rising titer is indicative only of current or recent streptococcal infection.
>   Direct diagnostic value in
>   Scarlet fever
>   Erysipelas
>   Streptococcal pharyngitis and tonsillitis
>   Indirect diagnostic value in
>   Rheumatic fever
>   Glomerulonephritis

Serial determinations are most desirable since individual determinations depend upon various factors (e.g., duration and severity of infection, antigenicity). Even in severe streptococcal infection, there will be an elevated ASO titer in only 70–80% of patients.

Conditions	Usual ASO Titer (Todd Unit)
"Normal" individuals	12–166
Active rheumatic fever	500–5000
Inactive rheumatic fever	12–250
Rheumatoid arthritis	12–250
Acute glomerulonephritis	500–5000
Streptococcal upper respiratory tract infections	100–333
Collagen diseases	12–250

Other streptococcal antigens may be tested
>   Antistreptococcal hyaluronidase (ASH) (significant titer > 128)
>   Antideoxyribonuclease (ADNase) (significant titer > 10)

Useful In
Detecting subclinical streptococcal infection
Differential diagnosis of joint pains of rheumatic fever and rheumatoid arthritis

LUPUS ERYTHEMATOSUS (LE) CELL TEST

LE cells occur in
>   75% of patients with systemic lupus erythematosus (SLE)
>   10% of patients with rheumatoid arthritis (only half of these have multisystem disease)
>   10% of patients with scleroderma
>   100% of patients with lupoid hepatitis
>   Patients with drug-induced lupus-like syndrome (e.g., due to procainamide, hydralazine, isoniazid, various anticonvulsants)
>   Some infections

The test becomes negative in 4–6 weeks or more in 60% of patients treated successfully. It is not useful as a guide to therapy; it is not correlated with the clinical picture.
The test is positive when 2 typical LE cells are found; it may be repeated for verification. Because of gradual changes in LE cell factor, repetition in less than 3 weeks is not useful; instead a more

sensitive technique or a serologic test for antinuclear or anti-DNA antibodies should be used.

Rosettes (clusters of polynuclear leukocytes surrounding an extra-cellular hematoxylin body) are usually found in association with LE cells.

Hematoxylin bodies (homogeneous round extracellular material) may be found in SLE, rheumatoid arthritis, multiple myeloma, cirrhosis. In SLE, they may be found without LE cells in the same sample.

SEROLOGIC TESTS FOR SYSTEMIC LUPUS ERYTHEMATOSUS (SLE)

The Hyland "LE test" using latex nucleoprotein is quite specific but positive in only 30% of patients with LE.

Anti-DNA antibody is usually present only during the active stage of SLE; it is absent during sustained remission. It may be absent in SLE, in which case doubts should be raised about the diagnosis. It may be found in about 50% of patients with systemic sclerosis, dermatomyositis, and polyarteritis nodosa; 10% of patients with rheumatoid arthritis; variable number of patients with discoid lupus; 4–17% of patients with liver disease, thyroiditis, ulcerative colitis, myasthenia gravis.

Antinucleoprotein antibody is present in almost all patients in the active stage of SLE and sometimes during remission. Therefore a negative test is useful to rule out SLE. But the SLE test is positive in other diseases more frequently than the LE cell test (e.g., rheumatoid arthritis, drug reactions) or when the LE cell test is usually negative (e.g., infections, lymphoma).

Only the latex test is commercially available; other serologic tests are now available at certain laboratories.

TEST FOR RHEUMATOID FACTOR (RA TEST)

The test is negative in a third of patients with definite rheumatoid arthritis. It gives useful objective evidence of rheumatoid arthritis, but a negative RA test does not rule out rheumatoid arthritis.

It is positive in 5% of rheumatoid variants (arthritis associated with psoriasis, ulcerative colitis, regional enteritis, Reiter's syndrome, juvenile rheumatoid arthritis, rheumatoid spondylitis).

It is positive in up to 3% of normal persons.

It may be positive in up to one-third of patients with SLE.

It may be positive in syphilis.

COOMBS' (ANTIGLOBULIN) TEST

Positive Direct Coombs' Test
(using patient's RBCs coated with antibody)

1. Erythroblastosis fetalis
2. Most cases of autoimmune hemolytic anemia, including up to 15% of certain systemic diseases, especially acute and chronic leuke-mias, malignant lymphomas, collagen diseases
3. Three-quarters of patients receiving cephalothin therapy (blood level of 333–666 μg/ml) especially if azotemia is present

The test is negative in hemolytic anemias due to intrinsic defect in RBCs (e.g., G-6-PD deficiency, hemoglobinopathies).

Positive Indirect Coombs' Test
    (using patient's serum which contains antibody)
Specific antibody—usually isoimmunization from previous transfusion
"Nonspecific" autoantibody in acquired hemolytic anemia
Incompatible crossmatched blood prior to transfusion

Beware of false positive and false negative results due to poor quality test serum, not using fresh blood (must have complement), etc.

COLD AUTOHEMAGGLUTINATION

Increased In
Primary atypical (virus) pneumonia (30–90% of patients). Titer begins to rise during second week of illness and persists for 2 months or more (1:14 to 1:224 or more). Negative titer does not rule out primary atypical pneumonia.
Atypical hemolytic anemia
Paroxysmal hemoglobinuria
Raynaud's disease
Cirrhosis of the liver
Trypanosomiasis
Malaria
Mumps
Measles
Scarlet fever
Rheumatic fever

AUSTRALIA ANTIGEN (HEPATITIS-ASSOCIATED ANTIGEN) (Au, HAA, SH)

Occurs In
0.1% of normal Americans
3–20% of the population in many tropical parts of the world and Southeast Asia
63% of patients with acute viral hepatitis with a history of parenteral exposure
30% of patients with acute viral hepatitis without a history of parenteral exposure
2% of habitual drug users
Patients with chronic active hepatitis (10–30% in Americans) and persistent viral hepatitis
Patients with certain chronic diseases with impaired immune mechanisms; 30% of patients with Down's syndrome kept in large institutions (who also show mild abnormalities of SGPT, BSP retention, thymol turbidity, cephalin flocculation, liver biopsy evidence of hepatitis); patients with lymphocytic leukemia, Hodgkin's disease, lepromatous leprosy; patients undergoing hemodialysis therapy for chronic renal disease

Appears in blood a variable time after apparent infection (usually 2 weeks to 4 months) but precedes elevation of SGOT. Disappears within days or weeks of first detection.

Transfusion of blood containing Au caused hepatitis or appearance of Au in blood in more than 50% of recipients. Transfusion of blood not containing Au caused anicteric hepatitis in 16% and icteric hepatitis in 2% of recipients.

Au is probably responsible for about 25% of cases of posttransfusion hepatitis.

Hepatitis following transfusion of Au-negative blood tends to be clinically mild, and tests for Au are negative. Hepatitis following transfusion of Au-positive blood tends to be clinically severe, and tests for Au are positive in acute phase. Twenty percent of patients who develop Au antigen after transfusion become carriers; carriers tend to have mild or anicteric hepatitis. Patients with severe, icteric hepatitis tend to revert to Au-negative state.

OTHER PROCEDURES

See Chapter 34, Infectious Diseases, for specific serologic tests (e.g., complement fixation, hemagglutination, neutralizing antibody, precipitin antibody, latex particle agglutination, flocculation) that are applicable in the diagnosis of diseases due to various organisms (e.g., bacteria, viruses, *Rickettsia*, protozoa, etc.).

16

Urine

DETECTION OF BACTERIURIA

A colony count is significant if there are more than 100,000 bacteria/
cu mm under the following conditions: Periurethral area has first
been thoroughly cleaned with soap, a midstream, clean-catch first
morning specimen is submitted in a sterilized container, and the
specimen is refrigerated until the colony count is performed. A
positive result in a single specimen containing gram-negative rods
has an 85% chance of being the same in the next specimen (i.e.,
15% error in a single specimen determination). Colony counts less
than 10,000/cu mm in the absence of therapy largely rule out
bacteriuria. False low colony counts may occur with a high rate
of urinary flow, low urine specific gravity, low urine pH, presence
of antibacterial drugs, or inappropriate cultural techniques (e.g.,
tubercle bacilli, Mycoplasma, L-forms, anaerobes).
Direct microscopical examination of uncentrifuged urine unstained
or gram-stained has 80–95% of the reliability of a colony count. It
may show more than 10% false positive results. Microscopical
detection of pus cells is less sensitive and produces more false
positive results than detection of bacteria. Up to 50% of patients
with bacteriuria may not show significant numbers of WBC on
urine microscopical examination; however, 10 or more WBC/field
is associated with bacteriuria in about 90% of cases. Maximum
sensitivity is obtained with microscopical detection of both bacteria and pus cells. "Sterile" pyuria (i.e., pyogenic infection is
absent) may occur in renal tuberculosis, chemical inflammation,
mechanical inflammation (e.g., calculi, instrumentation), early
acute glomerulonephritis prior to appearance of hematuria or
proteinuria, extreme dehydration, hyperchloremic renal acidosis,
nonbacterial gastroenteritis and respiratory tract infections, and
after administration of oral polio vaccine.
Dye tests (bacterial reduction of nitrate to nitrite; tetrazolium
reduction) do not detect 10–50% of infections. Bacteria show great
variability in rate of dye reduction; some important bacteria do
not reduce dye at all. Dye tests are not to be recommended.

Decreased glucose in urine (less than 2 mg/100 ml) in properly collected first morning urine (no food or fluid intake after 10 P.M., no urination during night) correlates well with colony count.

A culture should be performed for identification of the organism and determination of sensitivity when these screening tests are positive. If culture shows a common gram-positive saprophyte, it should be repeated, as the second culture is often negative. *If* Pseudomonas *or* Proteus *is found, the patient may have an anatomic abnormality. If organism other than* E. coli *is found, patient probably has chronic pyelonephritis even if this is the first clinical episode of infection.*

Bacteriuria may be found in
    10% of patients who are pregnant
    15% of patients with diabetes mellitus
    20% of patients with cystocele
    70% of patients with prostatic obstruction
    95% of patients (untreated) with an indwelling catheter for more than 4 days

URINE SPECIFIC GRAVITY

Moderate increase of urine specific gravity results from
    Refrigeration of the urine
    Excretion of protein in urine
Marked increase of specific gravity results from
    Excretion of radiographic contrast medium (frequently up to 1.040–1.050)
None of these affect urinary osmolality.

See also urine concentration and dilution tests, pp. 77, 78.

DIFFERENTIATION OF URINARY PROTEINS

Precipitated by 5% Sulfosalicylic Acid

On boiling, precipitate remains	Albumin
	Globulin
	Pseudo–Bence Jones protein
On boiling, precipitate disappears	Bence Jones protein
	A "proteose"

Precipitated at 40–60°C
Resuspend precipitate in normal urine
and an equal volume of 5%
sulfosalicylic acid and boil:

Precipitate dissolves	Bence Jones protein
Precipitate does not dissolve	Pseudo–Bence Jones protein

POSITIVE BENEDICT REACTIONS IN URINE

Glycosuria
    Hyperglycemia
        Endocrine (e.g., diabetes mellitus, pituitary, adrenal, thyroid disease)
        Nonendocrine (e.g., liver, CNS diseases)
        Due to administration of hormones (e.g., ACTH, corticosteroids, thyroid, adrenalin) or drugs (e.g., morphine, anesthetic drugs, tranquilizers)

Renal tubular origin (low Tm_G)
  Renal diabetes
  Toxic renal tubular disease (e.g., due to lead, mercury, degraded tetracycline)
  Associated with defective amino acid transport
  Inflammatory renal disease (e.g., acute glomerulonephritis, nephrosis)
  Idiopathic
Melituria*
  Hereditary (e.g., galactose, fructose, pentose, lactose)
  Neonatal (e.g., physiologic lactosuria, sepsis, gastroenteritis, hepatitis)
  Lactosuria during lactation
Non-sugar-reducing substances (e.g., ascorbic acid, glucuronic acid, homogentisic acid, salicylates)

Galactosuria (in galactosemia) shows a positive urine reaction with Clinitest but negative with Clinistix and Tes-Tape.

False *negative* tests for glucose may occur in presence of ascorbic acid using glucose oxidase paper test (Labstix); found in more than 1% of routine urine analyses in hospital.

KETONURIA
(ketone bodies—acetone, beta-hydroxybutyric acid, acetoacetic acid—appear in urine)

Occurs In
Metabolic conditions
  Diabetes mellitus
  Renal glycosuria
  Glycogen storage disease
Dietary conditions
  Starvation
  High-fat diets
Increased metabolic requirements
  Hyperthyroidism
  Fever
  Pregnancy and lactation
  Etc.

False positive may occur after injection of Bromsulphalein (BSP test).

SUBSTANCES AND CONDITIONS THAT MAY CAUSE ABNORMAL COLOR OF URINE

Porphyrins. See p. 109.
Sickle cell crises produce a characteristic dark-brown color independent of volume or specific gravity that becomes darker on standing or on exposure to sunlight. Increase in total porphyrins, coproporphyrins, and uroporphyrins is routinely shown; increase

---

* 5% of cases of melituria in the general population are due to renal glycosuria (incidence is 1 in 100,000), pentosuria (incidence is 1 in 50,000), essential fructosuria (incidence is 1 in 120,000).

in the porphyrin precursors (delta-aminolevulinic acid and porphobilinogen) is occasionally shown.

Hemoglobin. See below.

Myoglobin. See p. 110.

Melanin. See p. 110.

Red urine may be caused by ingestion of beets, blackberries, certain cold-drink and food dyes, certain drugs (e.g., phenolphthalein in laxatives); presence of urates and bile may also cause red urine.

Darkening of urine on standing, alkalinization, or oxygenation is nonspecific and may be due to melanogen, hemoglobin, indican, urobilinogen, porphyrins, phenols, salicylate metabolites (e.g., gentisic acid), homogentisic acid (due to alkaptonuria; *if acid pH, may not darken for hours*), and may appear in tyrosinosis. Darkened urine may follow administration of metronidazole (Flagyl).

Biliverdin. Blue or green color is due to oxidation of bilirubin in poorly preserved specimens. *Gives negative diazo tests for bilirubin (Ictotest), but oxidative tests (Harrison spot test) may still be positive.*

Methylene blue ingestion may cause a similar urine color. Blue urine occurs very rarely in *Pseudomonas* infection.

Blue diaper syndrome results from indigo blue in urine due to familial metabolic defect in tryptophan absorption associated with idiopathic hypercalcemia and nephrocalcinosis.

Red diaper syndrome is due to a nonpathogenic chromobacterium (*Serratia marcescens*) that produces a red pigment when grown aerobically at 25–30°C.

White cloud is due to excessive oxalic acid and glycolic acid in urine; occurs in oxalosis (primary hyperoxaluria).

Chyluria. See p. 111.

Lipuria. See p. 111.

URINE UROBILINOGEN

Increased In

Increased hemolysis (e.g., hemolytic anemias)

Hemorrhage into tissues (e.g., pulmonary infarction, severe bruises)

Hepatic parenchymal cell damage (e.g., cirrhosis, acute hepatitis in early and recovery stages)

Cholangitis

Decreased In

Complete biliary obstruction

PORPHYRINURIA
(due mainly to coproporphyrin)

Lead poisoning

Cirrhosis

Infectious hepatitis

Passive in newborn of mother with porphyria; lasts for several days

Porphyria

HEMOGLOBINURIA

Renal threshold is 100–140 mg/100 ml plasma.

Infarction of kidney

Hematuria with hemolysis in urine

Intravascular hemolysis due to
  Parasites (e.g., malaria, Oroya fever due to *Bartonella bacilliformis*)
  Fava bean sensitivity
  Antibodies (e.g., transfusion reactions, acquired hemolytic anemia, paroxysmal cold hemoglobinuria, paroxysmal nocturnal hemoglobinuria)
  Hypotonicity (e.g., transurethral prostatectomy with irrigation of bladder with water)
  Chemicals (e.g., napthalene, sulfonamides)
  Thermal burns injuring RBCs
  Strenuous exercise and march hemoglobinuria

False positive (Occultest) results may occur in the presence of pus, iodides, bromides.

MYOGLOBINURIA

Renal threshold is 20 mg/100 ml plasma.

Hereditary
  Phosphorylase deficiency (McArdle syndrome)
  Metabolic defects (e.g., associated with muscular dystrophy)
Sporadic
  Ischemic (e.g., arterial occlusion, myocardial infarction)
  Crush syndrome
  Exertional (e.g., exercise, some cases of march hemoglobinuria, electric shock, convulsions, and seizures)
  Metabolic myoglobinuria (e.g., Haff disease, alcoholism, seasnake bite, carbon monoxide poisoning, diabetic acidosis, hypokalemia, fever and systemic infection, barbiturate poisoning)
  With progressive muscle disease

MELANOGENURIA

In some patients with malignant melanoma, when the urine is exposed to air for several hours, colorless melanogens are oxidized to melanin and urine becomes deep brown and later black.

Confirmatory tests
  Ferric chloride test
  Thormählen's test
  Ehrlich test
None of these is consistently more reliable or sensitive than observation of urine for darkening.

Melanogenuria occurs in 25% of patients with malignant melanoma; it is said to be more frequent with extensive liver metastasis. It is not useful for judging completeness of removal or early recurrence.

Beware of false positive red-brown or purple suspension due to salicylates.

CHYLURIA

Milky urine is due to chylomicrons recognized as fat globules by microscopy (this is almost entirely neutral fat). Protein is normal or low. Hematuria is common. Specific gravity is low and reaction is acid.

A test meal of milk and cream may cause chyluria in 1–4 hours.

Chyluria is due to obstruction of the lymphochylous system, usually filariasis.

Microfilariae appear in the urine for 6 weeks after acute infection, then disappear unless endemic.

Laboratory findings are due to the pyelonephritis that is usually present.

LIPURIA

Lipids in the urine include all fractions. Double refractile (cholesterol) bodies can be seen. There is a high protein content.

May Occur In
Nephrotic syndrome
Severe diabetes mellitus
Severe eclampsia
Phosphorus poisoning
Carbon monoxide poisoning

URINE CALCIUM

Increased In
Hyperparathyroidism
Idiopathic hypercalciuria
High-calcium diet
    Excess milk intake
Immobilization (especially in children)
Lytic bone lesions
    Metastatic tumor
    Multiple myeloma
    Osteoporosis (primary or secondary to hyperthyroidism, Cushing's syndrome, acromegaly)
Excess vitamin D ingestion
Drug therapy
    Mercurial diuretics
    Ammonium chloride
Fanconi's syndrome
Renal tubular acidosis

Decreased In
Hypoparathyroidism
Rickets, osteomalacia
Steatorrhea
Renal failure
Metastatic carcinoma of prostate

URINE CREATINE

Increased In
Physiologic states
    Growing children
    Pregnancy

Puerperium (2 weeks)
Starvation
Raw meat diet
Increased formation
Myopathy
Amyotonia congenita
Muscular dystrophy
Poliomyelitis
Myasthenia gravis
Crush injury
Acute paroxysmal myoglobinuria
Endocrine diseases
Hyperthyroidism
Addison's disease
Cushing's syndrome
Acromegaly
Diabetes mellitus
Eunuchoidism
Therapy with ACTH, cortisone, or DOCA
Increased breakdown
Infections
Burns
Fractures
Leukemia
Disseminated lupus erythematosus

Decreased In
Hypothyroidism

FERRIC CHLORIDE TEST OF URINE
(to be used as screening test)

Positive In
Phenylketonuria (unreliable for diagnosis)
Tyrosinuria—transient elevation in newborn infants
Maple syrup disease
Alkaptonuria
Histidinemia
Tyrosinosis
Oasthouse urine disease

A positive test should always be followed by chromatography of
blood and urine.

TYROSINE CRYSTALS IN URINE

Massive hepatic necrosis (acute yellow atrophy)

URINARY LACTIC DEHYDROGENASE (LDH) ACTIVITY

Increased In
Carcinoma of kidney, bladder, and prostate (high proportion of
cases—useful for detection of asymptomatic lesions or screening
of susceptible population groups, and differential diagnosis of
renal cysts)

Other renal diseases
> Active glomerulonephritis, SLE with nephritis, nephrotic syndrome, acute tubular necrosis, diabetic nephrosclerosis, malignant nephrosclerosis, renal infarction
>
> Active pyelonephritis (one-quarter of patients), cystitis, and other inflammations

Instrumentation of the GU tract (especially cystoscopy with retrograde pyelography) (transient increase—less than 1 week)

Myocardial infarction and other conditions with considerably increased serum levels.

Etc.

Normal In
Benign nephrosclerosis
Pyelonephritis (most cases)
Obstructive uropathy
Renal calculi
Polycystic kidneys
Renal cysts

The test is chiefly useful in screening for malignancy of kidney, renal pelvis, and bladder; increased values usually precede clinical symptoms. Increased levels suggest GU tract disease but do not indicate its nature.

Precautions: 8-hour overnight urine collection, clean voided to prevent bacterial and menstrual contamination. Refrigerate until analysis is begun. Specimen must be dialyzed to remove inhibitors in urine. Microscopical examination of urine should be performed first since false positive LDH may occur if there are more than 10 bacteria/hpf or RBCs are present. Results are false positive if hemolyzed blood is present.

URINARY EXCRETION OF FIGLU (FORMIMINOGLUTAMIC ACID)

Histidine loading is followed after 3 hours by a 5-hour urine collection.

Increased In
Folic acid deficiency occurring in
> Idiopathic steatorrhea (up to 80 mg/hour)
> Pregnancy, especially with toxemia and increased age, parity, and multiple pregnancy
> Administration of folic acid antagonists
> Malnutrition (some patients), chronic liver disease, use of anticonvulsant drugs, congenital hemolytic anemia

Normal = less than 2 mg/hour or 3 mg/100 ml

URINARY 5-HYDROXYINDOLEACETIC ACID (5-HIAA)

Increased In
Carcinoid syndrome
Ingestion of bananas, phenothiazine derivatives, Lugol's solution, etc.

Normal = 2-9 mg/day; carcinoid syndrome = > 40 mg/day; often 300-1000 mg/day.

URINARY ALDOSTERONE

Increased In
Primary and secondary aldosteronism (see pp. 335-336)

Decreased In
Hypoadrenalism
Panhypopituitarism

URINARY CATECHOLAMINES (NOREPINEPHRINE, NORMETANEPHRINE)*

Increased In
Pheochromocytoma
Neural crest tumors (neuroblastoma, ganglioneuroma, ganglioblastoma)
Progressive muscular dystrophy and myasthenia gravis (some cases)
May also be increased by vigorous exercise prior to urine collection (up to 7-fold)
False increase may be due to drugs that produce fluorescent urinary products (e.g., tetracyclines, Aldomet, epinephrine and epinephrine-like drugs, large doses of vitamin B complex. See p. 455).
Avoid such medications for 1 week before urine collection.

URINE VANILMANDELIC ACID (VMA)

VMA is the urinary metabolite of both epinephrine and norepinephrine.

Increased In
Pheochromocytoma
Neuroblastoma, ganglioneuroma, ganglioblastoma

Beware of false positive results due to certain foods, e.g., coffee, tea, chocolate, vanilla, some fruits and vegetables (especially bananas); certain drugs, e.g., vasopressor drugs, some antihypertensive drugs (methyldopa, etc.). Monamine oxidase inhibitors may increase metanephrine and decrease VMA. See pp. 455-456.

URINARY 17-KETOSTEROIDS (17-KS)

Increased In
Adrenal cortical hyperplasia (causing Cushing's syndrome, adrenogenital syndrome)
Adrenal cortical adenoma or carcinoma
Arrhenoblastoma and lutein cell tumor of ovary (if androgenic)
Interstitial cell tumor of testicle
Pituitary tumor or hyperplasia
ACTH administration
Severe stress
Third trimester of pregnancy
Testosterone administration
Nonspecific chromagens in urine

---

* Not all methods include dopamine in determination of total catecholamines.

Decreased In
Addison's disease
Panhypopituitarism
Hypothyroidism (myxedema)
Generalized wasting diseases
Nephrosis
Hypogonadism in men (castration)
Primary ovarian agenesis

*Urinary 17-ketosteroids may have a daily variation of 100% in the same
  individual.*

URINARY 17-KETOSTEROIDS BETA FRACTION

Increased In
Adrenal carcinoma

URINARY 17-KS BETA:ALPHA RATIO

(Beta fraction is largely dehydroepiandrosterone; alpha fraction is
  mostly androsterone and etiocholanolone.)
Normal. Beta:alpha ratio is usually less than 0.2.
Adrenal cortical hyperplasia. Ratio is usually normal; even when it
  is increased it is rarely more than 0.3.
Adrenal carcinoma. Ratio is usually 0.28 to 0.4. In adults some
  patients may have a ratio less than 0.2 but the ratio is increased
  in most cases in children. The ratio is most helpful if it is more
  than 0.4 when it is most indicative of carcinoma.
Unless the total 17-KS are increased, the beta:alpha ratio is not
  likely to be abnormal.

BLOOD AND URINARY CORTICOSTEROIDS
(17-KETOGENIC STEROIDS)

Increased In
Adrenal hyperplasia
Adrenal adenoma
Adrenal carcinoma
ACTH therapy
Stress

Decreased In
Addison's disease
Panhypopituitarism
Cessation of corticosteroid therapy
General wasting disease

URINARY PORTER-SILBER REACTION

This reaction measures only OH at C-17 and C-21 and O= at C-20;
  does not measure pregnanetriol and other C-20 OH compounds.

Increased In
Cushing's syndrome (sometimes markedly)
Severe stress (e.g., eclampsia, pancreatitis [may be marked], infec-
  tion, burns, surgery)

Third trimester of pregnancy (moderately)
Early pregnancy (slightly)
Severe hypertension (slightly)
Virilism (slightly)

Decreased or Normal In
Addison's disease
Hypopituitarism

Certain drugs (e.g., paraldehyde) interfere with determination.

URINARY DEHYDROISOANDROSTERONE (ALLEN BLUE TEST)

Increased In
Adrenal carcinoma

URINARY PREGNANEDIOL

Increased In
Luteal cysts of ovary
Arrhenoblastoma
Hyperadrenocorticism

Decreased In
Toxemia of pregnancy
Fetal death
Threatened abortion (sometimes)
Amenorrhea

URINARY PREGNANETRIOL

Increased In
Adrenogenital syndrome (congenital adrenal hyperplasia)

URINARY ESTROGENS

Increased In
Granulosa cell tumor of ovary
Theca cell tumor of ovary
Luteoma of ovary
Interstitial cell tumor of testis
Pregnancy
Hyperadrenalism
Liver disease

Decreased In
Primary hypofunction of ovary
Secondary hypofunction of ovary

URINARY CHORIONIC GONADOTROPINS
(see also "Pregnancy" Test, p. 99)

Increased In
Normal pregnancy
Hydatidiform mole (sometimes markedly)

Chorionepithelioma (sometimes markedly)
    Of uterus
    Of testicle

Normal In
Nonpregnant state
Fetal death

URINARY PITUITARY GONADOTROPINS

This is a practical assay only for combined follicle-stimulating hormone and interstitial cell–stimulating hormone.

Increased In
Menopause
Primary hypogonadism
Hyperpituitarism, early

Decreased In
Secondary hypogonadism
Simmonds' disease
Hyperpituitarism, late

Because of small amounts present in 24-hour urine, a 5–10 day continuous collection must be concentrated.

OTHER PROCEDURES
(see also "Pregnancy" Test, p. 99)

Other functional tests on urine (see pp. 76-80)
Urine findings in various diseases (see Table 54, pp. 353-355)
Urine amylase (p. 196)
See also specific tests on urine in various chapters (e.g., Endocrine Diseases, Metabolic and Hereditary Diseases, Gastrointestinal Diseases, Hematologic Diseases).

17

OCCULT BLOOD IN STOOL

Chief usefulness is for screening for asymptomatic ulcerated lesions of gastrointestinal tract, especially carcinoma of the colon that is beyond the reach of routine sigmoidoscopy.

QUALITATIVE SCREENING TEST FOR STOOL FAT

Microscopical examination for neutral fat (ethyl alcohol + Sudan III) and free fatty acids (acetic acid + Sudan III + heat) is made.
Random specimen is taken, on diet of > 60 gm of fat daily.
4+ fat in stool means excessive fecal fat loss.

Increased neutral fat
    Mineral and castor oil ingestion
    Dietetic low-calorie mayonnaise ingestion
    Rectal suppository usage
    Steatorrhea

CHEMICAL DETERMINATION OF FECAL FAT

A 3-day stool sample is taken, on diet of 100 gm of fat daily.
Determination parallels but is more sensitive than triolein ^{131}I test in chronic pancreatic disease.
Normal is less than 6 gm/24 hours.
In chronic pancreatic disease fecal fat is more than 10 gm/24 hours.

UROBILINOGEN IN STOOL

Increased In
Hemolytic anemias

Decreased In
Complete biliary obstruction
Severe liver disease
Oral antibiotic therapy altering intestinal bacterial flora
Decreased hemoglobin turnover (e.g., aplastic anemia, cachexia)

MICROSCOPICAL EXAMINATION OF DIARRHEAL STOOLS FOR FECAL LEUKOCYTES

Primarily polynuclear leukocytes in
    Shigellosis
    Salmonellosis
    Invasive *E. coli* colitis
    Ulcerative colitis
Primarily mononuclear leukocytes in
    Typhoid
Leukocytes absent in
    Cholera
    Viral diarrheas
    Noninvasive *E. coli* diarrhea
    "Nonspecific" diarrheas
    Normal healthy individuals

OTHER PROCEDURES

Examination for ova and parasites
Isotopic studies (pp. 129 ff.)
Trypsin digestion (see Cystic Fibrosis of Pancreas, p. 198)
Microscopical examination (see Laboratory Diagnosis of Malabsorption, p. 170)
Etc.

18

Gastric and Duodenal Fluids

GASTRIC ANALYSIS

One-hour basal acid

Less than 2 mEq	Normal, gastric ulcer, or carcinoma
2–5 mEq	Normal, gastric or duodenal ulcer
More than 5 mEq	Duodenal ulcer
More than 20 mEq	Zollinger-Ellison syndrome

One hour after stimulation (histamine or betazole hydrochloride)

0 mEq	Achlorhydria, gastritis, gastric carcinoma
1–20 mEq	Normal, gastric ulcer, or carcinoma
20–35 mEq	Duodenal ulcer
35–60 mEq	Duodenal ulcer, high normal, Zollinger-Ellison syndrome
More than 60 mEq	Zollinger-Ellison syndrome

Ratio of basal acid to poststimulation outputs

20%	Normal, gastric ulcer, or carcinoma
20–40%	Gastric or duodenal ulcer
40–60%	Duodenal ulcer, Zollinger-Ellison syndrome
More than 60%	Zollinger-Ellison syndrome

Achlorhydria

Gastric carcinoma (50% of patients) even following histamine or betazole stimulation. Hypochlorhydria occurs in 25% of patients with gastric carcinoma; hydrochloric acid is normal in 25% of patients with gastric carcinoma; hyperchlorhydria is rare in gastric carcinoma.

Pernicious anemia (virtually all patients)

Adenomatous polyps of stomach (85% of patients)

Gastric atrophy

Achlorhydria occurs in normal individuals: in 4% of children, increasing to 30% of adults over age 60.

True achlorhydria excludes duodenal ulcer.

Tubeless gastric analysis (Diagnex Blue) is useful to rule out achlorhydria as in pregnant patients with macrocytic anemia or in screening for gastric carcinoma.

If no free acid is demonstrated with Diagnex Blue test or examination of gastric juice, further examination (e.g., stimulation with histamine or betazole) is required to prove the absence of free HCl.

Measure acid output after IV insulin to demonstrate adequacy of vagotomy (see below, Insulin Test Meal).

Hyperchlorhydria and hypersecretion
> Duodenal ulcer
>> Zollinger-Ellison syndrome (see p. 329). Twelve-hour night secretion shows acid of more than 100 mEq/L and volume of more than 1500 ml. Basal secretion is more than 60% of secretion caused by histamine or betazole stimulation.

INSULIN TEST MEAL

Aspirate gastric fluid every 15 minutes for 2 hours after IV administration of sufficient insulin (usually 15–20 units) to produce blood sugar less than 50 mg/100 ml.

Normal: Hypoglycemia increases free HCl.

Successful vagotomy produces achlorhydria.

PANCREOZYMIN-SECRETIN TEST

The test measures the effect of IV administration of pancreozymin and secretin on (1) volume, bicarbonate concentration, and amylase output of duodenal contents; and (2) increase in serum lipase and amylase

Normal duodenal contents
> Volume of 95–235 ml/hour
> Bicarbonate concentration of 74–121 mEq/L
> Amylase output of 87,000–267,000 mg

This is the most sensitive and reliable test of chronic pancreatic disease; avoid gastric contamination (pH 7.5).

Normally, serum lipase and amylase do not rise above normal limits.

19

Serous Fluids
(Pleural, Pericardial, and Ascitic)

Table 13. Comparison of " Typical"* Findings in Transudates and Exudates

Finding	Transudates (e.g., heart failure, nephrosis, cirrhosis)	Exudates (e.g., neoplasm, tuberculosis, infection)
Specific gravity	< 1.016	> 1.016
Protein (gm/100 ml)	< 3.0	> 3.0
Clot (fibrinogen)	Absent	Present
Cells		
WBC	Few lymphocytes	Many WBCs; may be grossly purulent
RBC	Few	Variable; few or may be grossly bloody
Glucose	Equivalent to serum	May be decreased because of bacteria or many WBC

* "Typical" means two-thirds to three-quarters of the cases.
Culture is positive in two-thirds of cases due to tuberculosis.
Cytology is positive in more than 50% of cases due to neoplasm. Pleural or ascitic effusion occurs in 20–30% of patients with malignant lymphoma; cytology establishes the diagnosis in about 50% of the cases.
LDH in nonpurulent, nonhemolyzed, and nonbloody effusions is generally low in cirrhosis and heart failure but increased in malignancy.
Increased amylase level in ascitic fluid occurs in acute pancreatitis, perforated peptic ulcer, necrosis of small intestine (e.g., mesenteric vascular occlusion), and in some cases of pleural and peritoneal metastases (including those originating from nonpancreatic primary sites).
See also Rheumatoid Pleurisy with Effusion, p. 162.

20

Sweat

SWEAT ELECTROLYTES

Increased In

Cystic fibrosis of pancreas
    Chloride: 50–120 mEq/L (mean = 97); normal: 4–60 mEq/L
        (mean = 18)
    Sodium: 50–140 mEq/L (mean = 103); normal: 0–40 mEq/L
        in children and 0–60 mEq/L in adults
    Potassium (mean = 15); normal (mean = 9)
Untreated adrenal insufficiency (Addison's disease)
Some unusual disease syndromes (e.g., glucose-6-phosphatase defi-
    ciency, glycogen-storage disease, vasopressin-resistant diabetes
    insipidus)

*Sweat sodium is reduced by aldosterone administration in both normal
    subjects and cystic fibrosis patients.*

21

Bacteria Commonly Cultured from Various Sites

Table 14. Most Common Bacteria Isolated in Cultures from Various Sites

Site	Normal Flora	Pathogens
External ear	*Staphylococcus epidermis* Alpha-hemolytic streptococcus Coliform bacilli Aerobic corynebacteria *Corynebacterium acnes* *Candida* species *Bacillus* species	*Pseudomonas* species *Staphylococcus aureus* Coliform bacilli Alpha-hemolytic streptococci *Proteus* species *Streptococcus (Diplococcus) pneumoniae* *Corynebacterium diphtheriae*
Middle ear	Sterile	*Acute Otitis Media* *Haemophilus influenzae* Beta-hemolytic streptococci Pneumococci *Chronic Otitis Media* *Staphylococcus aureus* *Proteus* species *Pseudomonas* species Other gram-negative bacilli Alpha-hemolytic streptococci Beta-hemolytic streptococci
Nasal passages	*Staphylococcus epidermis* *Staphylococcus aureus* Diphtheroids Pneumococci Alpha-hemolytic streptococci Nonpathogenic *Neisseria* species Aerobic corynebacteria	*Acute Sinusitis* *Staphylococcus aureus* Pneumococci *Klebsiella-Enterobacter* species Alpha-hemolytic streptococci Beta-hemolytic streptococci *Chronic Sinusitis* *Staphylococcus aureus* Alpha-hemolytic streptococci Pneumococci Beta-hemolytic streptococci

Site	Normal Flora	Pathogens
Pharynx and tonsils	Alpha-hemolytic streptococci *Neisseria* species *Staphylococcus epidermis* *Staphylococcus aureus* (small numbers) Pneumococci Nonhemolytic (gamma) streptococci Diphtheroids Coliforms Beta-hemolytic streptococci (not Group A) *Actinomyces israeli* *Haemophilus* species *Marked predominance of one organism may be clinically significant even if it is a normal inhabitant.*	Beta-hemolytic streptococci *Corynebacterium diphtheriae* *Bordetella pertussis* *Neisseria meningitidis* *Haemophilus influenzae* Group B *Staphylococcus aureus* *Candida albicans*
Gastrointestinal tract		
Mouth	Alpha-hemolytic streptococci Enterococci Lactobacilli Staphylococci Fusobacteria *Bacteroides* species Diphtheroids	*Candida albicans* *Borrelia vincentii* with *Fusobacterium fusiforme*
Stomach	Sterile	
Small intestine	Sterile in one-third Scant bacteria in others *Escherichia coli* *Klebsiella-Enterobacter* Enterococci Alpha-hemolytic streptococci *Staphylococcus epidermis* Diphtheroids	
Colon	Abundant bacteria *Bacteroides* species *Escherichia coli* *Klebsiella-Enterobacter* Paracolons *Proteus* species Enterococci (Group D streptococci) Yeasts	Enteropathogenic *Escherichia coli* *Candida albicans* Various amebae and parasites *Aeromonas* species *Salmonella* species *Shigella* species

Table 14   *(continued)*

Site	Normal Flora	Pathogens
Gall-bladder	Sterile	*Escherichia coli*
		Enterococci
		Klebsiella-Enterobacter-Serratia
		Occasionally
		Coliforms
		Proteus species
		Pseudomonas species
		Salmonella species
Blood	Sterile	Staphylococci (coagulase positive and negative)
		Coliform and related bacilli
		Alpha- and beta-hemolytic streptococci
		Pneumococci
		Enterococci
		Haemophilus influenzae
		Clostridium perfringens
		Pseudomonas species
		Proteus species
		Bacteroides and related anaerobes
		Neisseria meningitidis
		Brucella species
		Pasteurella tularensis
		Listeria monocytogenes
		Achromobacter (Herellea) species
		Streptobacillus moniliformis
		Leptospira species
		Vibrio fetus
		Opportunistic fungi (e.g., *Candida* species, *Nocardia* species, *Blastomyces dermatitidis, Histoplasma capsulatum*)
		Salmonella species
Eye	Usually sterile	*Staphylococcus aureus*
	Occasionally small numbers of diphtheroids and coagulase-negative staphylococci	*Haemophilus* species
		Streptococcus (Diplococcus) pneumoniae
		Neisseria gonorrhoeae
		Alpha- and beta-hemolytic streptococci
		Achromobacter (Herellea) species
		Coliform bacilli
		Pseudomonas aeruginosa
		Other enteric bacilli
		Morax-Axenfeld bacillus
		Bacillus subtilis (occasionally)

Site	Normal Flora	Pathogens
Spinal fluid	Sterile	*Haemophilus influenzae*
		Neisseria meningitidis
		Streptococcus pneumoniae
		Mycobacterium tuberculosis
		Staphylococci, streptococci
		Cryptococcus neoformans
		Coliform bacilli
		Pseudomonas and *Proteus* species
		Bacteroides species
Urethra, male	*Staphylococcus aureus*	*Neisseria gonorrhoeae*
	Staphylococcus epidermis	Enterococci
	Enterococci	Beta-hemolytic streptococci (usually Group B)
	Diphtheroids	Anaerobic and microaerophilic streptococci
	Achromobacter wolffi (Mima)	
	Haemophilus vaginalis	*Bacteroides* species
	Bacillus subtilis	*Escherichia* and *Klebsiella-Enterobacter*
		Staphylococcus aureus
Urethra, female, and vagina	*Lactobacillus* (large numbers)	Yeasts and *Candida albicans*
	Coli-aerogenes	*Clostridium perfringens*
	Staphylococci	*Listeria monocytogenes*
	Streptococci (aerobic and anaerobic)	*Haemophilus vaginalis*
		Trichomonas vaginalis
	Candida albicans	
	Bacteroides species	
	Achromobacter wolffi (Mima)	
	Haemophilus vaginalis	
Prostate	Sterile	*Streptococcus faecalis*
		Staphylococcus epidermis
		Escherichia coli
		Proteus mirabilis
		Pseudomonas species
		Klebsiella species
Uterus		Anaerobic and micro-anaerophilic streptococci (alpha, beta, and gamma types)
		Bacteroides species
		Enterococci
		Beta-hemolytic streptococci (usually Group B)
		Staphylococci
		Proteus species
		Clostridium perfringens
		Escherichia and *Klebsiella-Enterobacter-Serratia*
		Listeria monocytogenes

Table 14 *(continued)*

Site	Normal Flora	Pathogens
Urine	Staphylococci, coagulase negative	*Escherichia coli, Klebsiella-Enterobacter-Serratia*
	Diphtheroids	*Proteus* species
	Coliform bacilli	*Pseudomonas* species
	Enterococci	Enterococci
	Proteus species	Staphylococci, coagulase positive and negative
	Lactobacilli	*Alcaligenes* species
	Alpha- and beta-hemolytic streptococci	*Achromobacter (Herellea)* species
		Candida albicans
		Beta-hemolytic streptococci
		Neisseria gonorrhoeae
		Mycobacterium tuberculosis
		Salmonella and *Shigella* species
Wound		*Staphylococcus aureus*
		Streptococcus pyogenes
		Coliform bacilli
		Bacteroides species; other gram-negative rods
		Proteus species
		Pseudomonas species
		Clostridium species
		Enterococci
		Achromobacter (Herellea) species
		Serratia species

22

Radioisotope Studies

SCHILLING TEST

The fasting patient is given 0.5 µc of ^{60}Co B_{12} (or ^{57}Co) as radiocyanocobalamin orally followed in 1 hour by a "flushing dose" of 1000 µg of intramuscular B_{12} (nonradioactive). Radioactivity is measured in total urine collection for the next 24 hours and compared to the amount of radioactivity ingested.

Normal is 7% or more of ingested radioactivity.
In pernicious anemia, 0–3% of the administered radioactivity appears in 24-hour urine.

If less than 7% appears in the urine, the test is repeated with the addition of 60 µg of intrinsic factor orally.

In pernicious anemia, 24-hour urine radioactivity becomes normal.
In malabsorption, 24-hour urine radioactivity remains low.

BLOOD VOLUME

Blood volume determination is usually done using albumin tagged with ^{125}I or ^{131}I; red cell mass may be measured by labeling RBCs with ^{51}Cr.

May Be Useful To

Determine the most appropriate blood component (whole blood, plasma, or packed cells) for replacement therapy. E.g., normal total blood volume and decreased red cell mass indicate the need for packed red cell transfusion.

Follow the clinical course. E.g., immediately after acute severe hemorrhage, the hemoglobin concentration, hematocrit value, and RBC may be normal and not indicate the severity of blood loss whereas appropriate measurements will show decreased blood volume, plasma volume, and red cell mass. After hemorrhage, the subsequent fluid shift from extravascular to intravascular space may produce a "falling" value for hemoglobin concentration, hematocrit, and RBC and falsely suggest continuing hemorrhage.

Assess the real degree of anemia in chronic conditions in which other mechanisms may disguise or accentuate the extent of RBC deficiency. E.g., anemia and hemoconcentration together may produce an apparently normal hemoglobin concentration, hematocrit reading, and RBC. Hemodilution in uremia may make the anemia more marked and apparently more severe.

Alert the surgeon who compares preoperative and postoperative values in surgical patients to

   Unexpected blood loss

   Need for replacement of the appropriate blood component, which may vary with the surgical procedure (e.g., in thoracoplasty the blood loss may be 900 ml, representing approximately equal red cell and plasma losses; in gastrectomy the blood loss may be 1800 ml, representing a red cell loss of 400 ml and a plasma loss of 1400 ml)

Differentiate polycythemia vera (increased total blood volume, plasma volume, red cell mass) and secondary polycythemia (normal or decreased total blood volume and plasma volume) in most cases.

Radioisotopes should not be administered to children or pregnant women. In the presence of active hemorrhage, the isotope is lost via the bleeding site, and a false value will be produced.

THYROID UPTAKE OF RADIOACTIVE IODINE (^{131}I OR ^{125}I)

A tracer dose of radioactive iodine is administered (usually orally), and the radioactivity over the thyroid is measured at specific intervals (e.g., 1, 2, 6, or 24 hours). The test may also measure radioactivity in urine, saliva, etc.

The test is contraindicated in pregnant or lactating women, infants, and children. It is invalidated for 2–4 weeks after administration of antithyroid drugs, thyroid, or iodides; the effect of organic iodine (e.g., x-ray contrast media) may persist for a much longer time.

	Thyroid Uptake of ^{131}I			24-Hour Excretion of ^{131}I in Urine
	1 hour	6 hours	24 hours	
Normal	9–19%	7–25%	10–50%	40–70%
Hyperthyroid	>20%	>25%	>50%	5–40%
Hypothyroid	<9%	<7%	<15%	70–90%

The test is considered most valuable in the diagnosis of hyperthyroidism. Uptake is usually greater in diffuse toxic goiter than in toxic nodules or recurrent hyperthyroidism following surgery or radioactive iodine treatment.

Administration of triiodothyronine (75 µg/day for 1 week) causes less suppression in the hyperthyroid patient than in the normal person. Failure to suppress uptake to less than 65% after antithyroid drug treatment often means the patient will relapse.

Very low uptake associated with a very high serum PBI probably means ingestion of iodine. Low uptake associated with a moderately high serum PBI suggests thyroiditis.

TRIOLEIN ^{131}I ABSORPTION TEST

The patient fasts overnight after taking 30 drops of Lugol's iodine solution on the previous day.

Administer 15–20 μc of triolein ^{131}I. Collect blood every 1–2 hours for the next 6–8 hours.

Collect stools for 48–72 hours until radioactivity disappears.

Normal: 10% or more of administered radioactivity appears in the blood within 6 hours; less than 5% appears in the feces.

The test is useful for screening patients with steatorrhea. Normal values indicate that digestion of fat in the small bowel and absorption of fat in the small bowel are normal.

If results are abnormal, do an oleic acid ^{131}I absorption test.

OLEIC ACID ^{131}I ABSORPTION TEST

Methodology and normal values are the same as for the triolein absorption test.

An abnormal result indicates a defect in small bowel mucosal absorption function (e.g., sprue, Whipple's disease, regional enteritis, tuberculous enteritis, collagen diseases involving the small bowel, extensive resection). Abnormal pancreatic function does not affect the test.

POLYVINYLPYRROLIDONE (PVP)- ^{131}I

Give 15–25 μc of PVP-^{131}I intravenously and collect all stools for 4–5 days.

Normal: Less than 2% is excreted in feces when the mucosa of the GI tract is intact.

In protein-losing enteropathy more than 2% of administered radioactivity appears in the stool.

^{51}Cr TEST FOR GASTROINTESTINAL BLEEDING

Tag 10 ml of the patient's blood with 200 μc of ^{51}Cr and administer it intravenously. Collect daily stools for radioactivity measurement and also measure simultaneous blood samples.

Radioactivity in the stool establishes GI blood loss. Comparison with radioactivity measurements of 1 ml of blood indicates the amount of blood loss.

The test is useful in ulcerative diseases (e.g., ulcerative colitis, regional enteritis, peptic ulcer).

RBC UPTAKE OF RADIOACTIVE IRON (^{59}Fe)

^{59}Fe is injected intravenously, and blood samples are drawn in 3, 7, and 14 days for measurement of radioactivity.

In pure red cell anemia the rate of uptake of ^{59}Fe is markedly decreased.

PLASMA IRON ^{59}Fe CLEARANCE

^{59}Fe is injected intravenously, and blood samples are drawn in 5, 15, 30, 60, and 120 minutes for measurement of radioactivity.

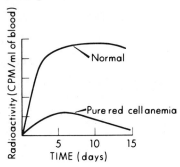

Fig. 2. RBC Uptake of Radioactive Iron (^{59}Fe)

In the normal person, half the radioactivity of plasma disappears in 1–2 hours.

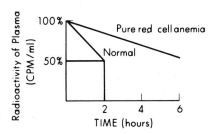

Fig. 3. Plasma Iron (^{59}Fe) Clearance

In pure red cell anemia, half of the plasma radioactivity may not disappear for 7–8 hours.

ERYTHROCYTE SURVIVAL IN HEMOLYTIC DISEASES
^{51}Cr

Increased In
Thalassemia minor

Decreased In
Idiopathic acquired hemolytic anemia
Paroxysmal nocturnal hemoglobinuria
Association with chronic lymphatic leukemia
Association with uremia
Congenital nonspherocytic hemolytic anemia
Hereditary spherocytosis
Elliptocytosis with hemolysis
Hemoglobin C disease
Sickle cell–hemoglobin C disease
Sickle cell anemia
Pernicious anemia
Megaloblastic anemia of pregnancy

Normal In
Sickle cell trait
Hemoglobin C trait
Elliptocytosis without hemolysis or anemia

EVALUATION OF RENAL TRANSPLANT FUNCTION BY SODIUM IODOHIPPURATE ^{131}I CLEARANCE

Blood samples taken 20 and 30 minutes after IV hippuran [131]I
This test is useful for early detection of renal function impairment due to rejection of renal transplant, especially in the first 24 hours when other tests of renal function are less useful.

THYROID SCAN WITH RADIOACTIVE IODINE

Useful To
Differentiate "hot" nodule from "cold" nodule
Detect presence and localization of functioning metastases
Differentiate mediastinal tumors from substernal thyroid (use ^{131}I rather than ^{125}I); first stimulate uptake with TSH
Differentiate tongue mass from lingual thyroid
Diagnose subacute thyroiditis
　　Differentiates inflammatory transient cold nodules from cancer since inflammatory nodule may disappear after prednisone treatment
　　Shows migration of focal thyroiditis
　　Differentiates diffuse and focal types of thyroiditis

LIVER SCANNING
(radioactive technetium-^{99m}Tc)

Indications
Assess hepatic size, shape, location in abdomen
Differentiation of abdominal mass as being part of liver or extrahepatic
Focal lesions (primary or secondary tumors, abscess, cyst, hematoma)—minimal size to be visualized = 1 inch; must be located within range of instrument focus (30% of patients with metastatic carcinoma of liver have lesions too small to visualize)
Location of focal lesions prior to needle biopsy
Subphrenic abscess (combine with lung scan or chest x-ray to locate diaphragm)
Cirrhosis of liver—mottled appearance of small liver and isotope uptake in reticuloendothelial system of vertebrae; enlarged spleen that may have a density equal to or greater than that of liver

Beware of variability in porta hepatis region.
A diffuse pattern may occur with hepatitis or diffuse metastases.
False negative diagnosis is made in up to 12% of patients; false positive in up to 5%.

LUNG SCANNING
(macroaggregates of radioactive iodinated serum albumin (RISA); 150–300 μc ^{131}I and 0.6 mg albumin—after first blocking thyroid gland)

Useful In

Demonstration of pulmonary blood flow; i.e., detects regional pulmonary ischemia. Down to vessels 1–2 mm in size. May demonstrate emboli too small for angiographic demonstration.

Evaluation of pulmonary function of individual lungs (instead of bronchospirometry) in preoperative evaluation of candidates for pulmonary resection

BRAIN SCANNING

^{99m}Tc has wider application and repeatability than ^{197}Hg or ^{203}Hg.

The scan is safe, nontoxic, easy to administer intravenously or orally, and painless; patient must remain quiet.

It is most accurate with meningiomas and malignant glioblastomas; least accurate with slow-growing astrocytomas. At present, it is more accurate in scanning cerebral hemispheres than midline or posterior fossa and more accurate for supratentorial (80%) than infratentorial lesions (70%)—somewhat less precise, that is, than angiography or positive contrast ventriculography.

A positive scan is not specific for tumor (scan may also be positive in infarct, contusion, abscess, subdural hematoma, granuloma, arteriovenous malformation, scalp hematomas, and fluid accumulations, etc.).

A negative scan does not rule out tumor or other structural lesions.

The scan does not reveal type of tumor, blood supply, or ventricular system.

RENAL SCANNING

Use of ^{99m}Tc-iron complex may be the best at present.

Useful To

Detect renal masses (not as useful as renal arteriogram, which provides higher resolution and distinguishes benign from malignant lesions by vascular patterns)

Localize kidney prior to needle biopsy in children (permits greater frequency of successful biopsy)

Localize functioning renal parenchyma (e.g., extent of the bridge in horseshoe kidney)

The scan represents renal plasma flow in each kidney. If total renal plasma flow is measured by PAH clearance, individual renal plasma flow can be determined without ureteral catheterization.

CARDIAC BLOOD POOL SCANNING (^{99m}Tc)

Useful In

Pericardial effusion or tumor (halo area around heart)

Ventricular aneurysm (tumor in vicinity of left ventricle that contains tracer isotope)

Aortic aneurysm (differentiated from mediastinal tumors)

Localization of other aneurysms in body

Localization of placenta

Demonstration of cardiac dilation

SPLEEN SCANNING

Method 1

Use patient's RBCs which have been damaged (by heat or chemicals) after tagging with isotope such as ^{51}Cr, ^{197}Hg, or ^{81}Rb; these damaged RBCs are preferentially sequestered in splenic sinusoids. This method is indicated for

Demonstration of ectopic spleen location

Demonstration that functional splenic tissue is absent

Demonstration of accessory spleens after splenectomy

Detecting rejection of splenic transplant

Demonstrating spleen size quantitatively or detecting some cases of minimal splenomegaly

Method 2

Use radioactive colloids such as ^{198}Au, ^{99m}Tc, or ^{113m}In which are phagocytosed by the reticuloendothelial cells in the spleen (and other organs). This method is preferred (because of lower radiation dose) in the differential diagnosis of left upper quadrant abdominal masses or delineation of space-occupying lesions of the spleen. This is the only method that visualizes spleen and liver simultaneously in cases of diffuse hepatic disease and splenomegaly.

BONE SCANNING

Sodium fluoride ^{18}F is superior to previously used ^{47}Ca and ^{85}Sr.

The scan is used for detection of bone metastases (both osteolytic and osteoblastic). Diagnosis prior to definite x-ray evidence of these lesions is its chief clinical usefulness.

It may also be positive in primary bone tumors (e.g., Ewing's sarcoma, osteogenic sarcoma).

It is not useful in soft-tissue sarcomas.

Since ^{18}F is indicator of increased bone metabolism, nonneoplastic reparative bone activity may cause positive scan in patients with Paget's disease, osteomyelitis, fractures, healing postoperative areas, osteoarthritis, rheumatoid spondylitis, and osteoporosis. For these cases, roentgenograms are essential to establish diagnosis and rule out tumor.

PAROTID GLAND SCANNING
(using ^{99}Tc)

Preliminary Findings

"Hot" nodule in Warthin's tumor (papillary cystadenoma lymphomatosum); probably will also be found in other ductal tumors (oncocytoma, mucoepidermoid tumor)

"Cold" nodules (more than 2 cm in size)

Benign tumors or cysts—smooth, sharply defined outlines

Adenocarcinoma—ragged irregular outlines

SCANNING OF THE PANCREAS
(using Selenomethionine—^{75}Se)

The liver may also be scanned with ^{198}Au to delineate the medial border of the liver.

Inability to demonstrate the pancreas is the most reliable sign of pancreatic disease. Distortion of pancreatic shape is not always indicative of abnormality.

Radioactivity in the upper jejunum is a sign of pancreatic normality.

Diagnosis of normal pancreas is correct in 90% of cases.

Diagnosis of abnormal pancreas is correct in less than 60% of cases.

SCANNING OF THE PARATHYROID GLANDS
(using ^{75}Se)

Useful in consistently visualizing adenomas larger than 2 gm

Not useful for detecting adenomas smaller than 1 gm or mediastinal lesions or parathyroid hyperplasia

SCANNING OF THE ADRENAL GLANDS
(using ^{131}I-19-iodocholesterol)

In Cushing's syndrome that persists or recurs after total adrenalectomy, photoscanning demonstrates residual adrenal tissue.

In primary aldosteronism, localizes site of adrenal adenoma and distinguishes unilateral from bilateral tumor. May become useful to distinguish adenoma from bilateral hyperplasia (photoscanning before and after administration of dexamethasone shows suppression of adrenal uptake in hyperplasia but no suppression in adenoma).

23

Nuclear Sex Chromatin and Karyotyping

NUCLEAR SEXING

Epithelial cells from buccal smear (or vaginal smear, etc.) are stained with cresyl violet and examined microscopically.

A dense body (Barr body) on the nuclear membrane represents one of the X chromosomes and occurs in 30–60% of female somatic cells. The maximum number of Barr bodies is one less than the number of X chromosomes.

If there are < 10% of the cells containing Barr bodies in a patient with female genitalia, karyotyping should be done to delineate probable chromosomal abnormalities.

A normal count does not rule out chromosomal abnormalities.

Two Barr bodies may be found in
  47 XXX female
  48 XXXY male (Klinefelter's syndrome)
  49 XXXYY male (Klinefelter's syndrome)

Three Barr bodies may be found in
  49 XXXXY male (Klinefelter's syndrome)

EVALUATION OF SEX CHROMOSOME IN LEUKOCYTES

Presence of a "drumstick" nuclear appendage in approximately 3% of leukocytes in normal females indicates the presence of 2 X chromosomes in the karyotype, It is not found in males.

It is absent in the XO type of Turner's syndrome.

There is a lower incidence of drumsticks in Klinefelter's syndrome (XXY) as opposed to the extra Barr body. (*Mean lobe counts of neutrophils are also decreased.*)

Incidence of drumsticks is decreased and mean lobe counts are lower also in mongolism.

Double drumsticks are exceedingly rare and diagnostically impractical.

SOME CLINICAL INDICATIONS FOR SEX CHROMATIN STUDIES

Klinefelter's syndrome
Turner's syndrome

Primary amenorrhea or oligomemorrhea
Mental retardation with sex anomalies
Ambiguous genitalia
Hypogonadism
Delayed puberty
Abnormal development at puberty
Disturbance of somatic growth

SOME CLINICAL INDICATIONS FOR KARYOTYPING

Chromatin-negative females
Chromatin-positive males
Multiple Barr bodies
Decreased number of Barr bodies (*suspect mosaicism, e.g., XO/XX in females, XY/XXY in males*)
Ambiguous genitalia (some patients)
Chromatin-negative males with hypogonadism (some patients)

SEX CHROMATIN NUMBER AND KARYOTYPE

Normal male	46 XY
Normal female	46 XX
Turner's syndrome	45 XO
Testicular feminization (normal external female genitalia and secondary sex characteristics, sterility, amenorrhea; biopsy of gonads shows testes)	46 XY
"Normal" male (children potentially mentally defective)	47 XYY
"Normal" female (may be mentally defective, sterile)	47 XXX
Trisomy 21 (mongolism [Down's syndrome]) in female	47 XX, G+
Klinefelter's syndrome	47 XXY
	48 XXYY
	48 XXXY
	49 XXXYY
	49 XXXXY
Mosaicism (more than one karyotype present in different cells)	E.g., 45 XO/46 XX

III

Diseases of Organ Systems

24
Cardiovascular Diseases

HYPERTENSION

Laboratory findings due to the primary disease. *These conditions are often occult or unsuspected and should always be carefully ruled out since many of them represent curable causes of hypertension.*

Systolic hypertension
   Hyperthyroidism
   Chronic anemia with hemoglobin less than 7 gm/100 ml
   Arteriovenous fistulas—advanced Paget's disease of bone; pulmonary arteriovenous varix
   Beriberi
Systolic and diastolic hypertension
   Essential (primary) hypertension (causes 80% of cases of hypertension)
   Secondary hypertension (causes 20% of cases of hypertension)
      Endocrine diseases
         Adrenal
            Pheochromocytoma (0.5% of cases of hypertension)
            Aldosteronism (5–15% of cases of hypertension)
            Cushing's syndrome
         Pituitary disease
            Signs of hyperadrenal function
            Acromegaly
         Hyperthyroidism
         Hyperparathyroidism
      Renal diseases
         Vascular (5–15% of cases of hypertension)
            Renal artery stenosis
            Nephrosclerosis
            Embolism
            Arteriovenous fistula
         Parenchymal
            Glomerulonephritis
            Pyelonephritis
            Polycystic kidneys

              Kimmelstiel-Wilson syndrome
              Amyloidosis
              Collagen diseases
              Renin-producing renal tumor
              Miscellaneous
        Urinary tract obstructions
      Central nervous system diseases
              Cerebrovascular accident
              Brain tumors
              Poliomyelitis
      Others
              Toxemia of pregnancy
              Polycythemia

Laboratory findings indicating the functional renal status, e.g., urinalysis, BUN, creatinine, uric acid, serum electrolytes, PSP, creatinine clearance, Addis count, radioisotope scan of kidneys, renal biopsy

Laboratory findings due to complications of hypertension, e.g., congestive heart failure, uremia, cerebral hemorrhage, myocardial infarction

Laboratory findings due to administration of some antihypertensive drugs

    Oral diuretics (e.g., benzothiadiazines)

        Increased incidence of hyperuricemia (to 65–75% of hypertensive patients from incidence of 25–35% in untreated hypertensive patients)

        Hypokalemia

        Hyperglycemia or aggravation of preexisting diabetes mellitus

        Less common: bone marrow depression, aggravation of renal or hepatic insufficiency by electrolyte imbalance, cholestatic hepatitis, toxic pancreatitis

    Hydralazine

        Long-term dosage of more than 200 mg/day may produce syndrome not distinguishable from systemic lupus erythematosus (SLE). Usually regresses after drug is discontinued. Antinuclear antibody may be found in up to 50% of asymptomatic patients.

    Methyldopa

        Up to 20% of patients may have positive direct Coombs' test, but relatively few have hemolytic anemia. When drug is discontinued, Coombs' test may remain positive for months but anemia usually reverses promptly.

        Abnormal liver function tests indicate hepatocellular damage without jaundice associated with febrile influenza-like syndrome.

        RA and LE tests may occasionally be postive.

        Rarely, granulocytopenia or thrombocytopenia may occur.

    Monamine oxidase inhibitors (e.g., pargyline hydrochloride)

        Wide range of toxic reactions, most serious of which are

            Blood dyscrasias

            Hepatocellular necrosis

    Diazoxide

        Sodium and fluid retention

        Hyperglycemia (usually mild and manageable by insulin or oral hypoglycemic agents)

When hypertension is associated with decreased serum potassium, rule out
>   Primary aldosteronism
>   Pseudo-aldosteronism (due to excessive ingestion of licorice)
>   Secondary aldosteronism (e.g., malignant hypertension)
>   Hypokalemia due to diuretic administration
>   Potassium loss due to renal disease
>   Cushing's syndrome

Approximately 8% of patients with hypertension have primary aldoster-onism and show increased aldosterone in urine and decreased plasma renin activity. An additional 15% of patients show a normal urine aldosterone level with decreased plasma renin activity.

CORONARY HEART DISEASE

Beware of coronary heart disease in presence of
>   Increased serum cholesterol (over 260 mg/100 ml)
>   Increased serum triglyceride (over 250 mg/100 ml)
>   Abnormal lipoprotein electrophoresis (see pp. 295–297).
>   Hyperglycemia (fasting blood sugar over 120 mg/100 ml; postprandial blood sugar over 180 mg/100 ml)
>   Decreased glucose tolerance
>   Significant glycosuria
>   Increased serum uric acid (over 8.5 mg/100 ml)
>   Laboratory findings due to hypertension (see preceding section)

ACUTE MYOCARDIAL INFARCTION

Laboratory Determinations Required
Because ECG changes may be inconclusive (e.g., masked by bundle-branch block or Wolff-Parkinson-White syndrome or may not reveal intramural or diaphragmatic infarcts)

For differential diagnosis (e.g., angina pectoris, pulmonary infarction). Normal serum enzyme levels during 48 hours after onset of clinical symptoms indicate no myocardial infarction.

To follow the course of the patient with acute myocardial infarction

To estimate prognosis (e.g., marked elevation of serum enzymes [4–5 times normal] correlates with increased incidence of ventricular arrhythmia, shock, heart failure, and with higher mortality)

Blood should be drawn promptly after onset of symptoms. Repeat determinations should be performed at appropriate intervals (see Fig. 4, p. 147) and also if symptoms recur or new signs or symptoms develop. Changes may indicate additional myocardial infarction or other complications (e.g., pulmonary infarction).

Specific Findings
Serum creatine phosphokinase (CPK) is particularly valuable for the following reasons
>   Increased levels occur in more than 90% of the patients when blood is drawn at the appropriate time.
>   It allows early diagnosis because increased levels appear within 3–6 hours after onset and peak levels in 24–36 hours.

It is a more sensitive indicator because increased CPK level shows a larger amplitude of change (6–12 times normal) than that of other enzymes.

Less diagnostic confusion occurs because CPK is not increased by many diseases that may be associated with myocardial infarction (e.g., liver damage due to congestion, drug therapy, etc., may increase SGOT) or that may be difficult to distinguish from myocardial infarction (e.g., pulmonary infarction may increase LDH).

It returns to normal by third day; a poorer prognosis is suggested if the increase lasts more than 3–4 days. Reinfarction is indicated by an elevated level after the fifth day that has previously returned to normal.

It is useful in differential diagnosis of diseases with normal enzyme level (e.g., angina pectoris) or with increased levels of other enzymes (e.g., increased LDH in pulmonary infarction).

Serum SGOT is useful for the following reasons.

It is increased in more than 95% of the patients when blood is drawn at the appropriate time.

It allows early diagnosis because increased levels appear within 6–8 hours and peak levels in 24 hours. Usually returns to normal in 4–6 days.

Peak level is usually about 200 units (5 times normal). A higher level (more than 300 units), along with a more prolonged increase, suggests a poorer prognosis.

Reinfarction is indicated by a rise following a return to normal.

Serum SGPT is usually not increased unless there is liver damage due to congestive heart failure, drug therapy, etc.

Serum LDH is almost always increased, beginning in 10–12 hours and reaching a peak in 48–72 hours (of about 3 times normal). The prolonged rise (average 11 days) is particularly useful for late diagnosis in cases in which earlier blood samples were not studied. Levels of more than 2000 units suggest a poorer prognosis. Because many other diseases may increase the LDH level, isoenzyme studies may be useful. In myocardial infarction, the heat-stable fast-moving fractions (LDH_1 and LDH_2) are increased.

Serum α-HBD parallels increase of fast-moving LDH with peak (3–4 times normal) in 48 hours and persistent elevation for up to 2 weeks.

Serum MDH is useful because an early increase (4–6 hours) parallels changes in CPK.

Serum ICD is normal.

Leukocytosis is almost invariable; commonly detected by second day but may occur as early as 2 hours. Usually the WBC count is 12,000 to 15,000; up to 20,000 is not rare; sometimes it is very high. Usually there are 75–90% neutrophilic leukocytes with only a slight shift to the left. Leukocytosis is likely to develop before fever.

Sedimentation rate (ESR) is increased, usually by second or third day (may begin within a few hours); peak rate is in 4–5 days; persists for 2–6 months. Increased ESR is sometimes more sensitive than WBC as it may occur before fever and it persists after temperature and WBC have returned to normal. Degree of increase of ESR does not correlate with severity or prognosis.

Glycosuria and hyperglycemia occur in up to 50% of patients.

Glucose tolerance is decreased.

Table 15. Summary of Increased Serum Enzyme Levels After Acute Myocardial Infarction

Serum Enzymes	Earliest Increase (hours)	Maximum Level (hours)	Return to Normal By (days)	Amplitude of Increase X Normal	Comment
CPK	3–6	24–36	3	7	Recommended for early diagnosis
MDH	4–6	24–48	5	4	Early use parallels CPK; no advantage over other enzymes; technically difficult to do
SGOT	6–8	24–48	4–6	5	Most commonly used
LDH	10–12	48–72	11	3	See α-HBD; isoenzyme determination to differentiate pulmonary infarction, congestive heart failure, etc.
α-HBD	10–12	48–72	13	3–4	Particularly useful for later diagnosis (in 2d week) when other enzymes have returned to normal, because of longer duration of increased activity; more specific than LDH
ALD	6–8	24–48	4	4	
SGPT	Usually normal unless liver damage due to congestive heart failure, shock, drug therapy (e.g., Coumadin)				
ICD	Usually normal				

The time periods all represent average values.
Least number of false positive results occur with CPK, α-HBD, heat-stable LDH.

Table 16. Some Laboratory Tests in Differential Diagnosis of Acute Myocardial Infarction*

Serial Tests Done Within 2 Days of Onset	Acute Myocardial Infarction	Angina Pectoris	Pulmonary Embolism or Infarction†	Pneumonia or Atelectasis	Congestive Heart Failure	Pulmonary Embolism and Myocardial Infarction
SGOT	I	N	Usually N	N	N	I
LDH	I	N	I	N	N	I
Serum bilirubin	N	N	I in about 20% of cases	N	May be slightly I	I

I = increased; N = normal.
* Not useful in presence of severe liver disease.
† "Triad" of increased LDH and serum bilirubin associated with normal SGOT is found in about 15% of these cases.

Differential Diagnosis

Serum enzymes not elevated in angina pectoris; increased levels
mean myocardial infarction or other condition.

Serum enzymes usually show little or no increase in inflammatory
myocardial lesions (e.g., rheumatic fever) unless disease is severe.
(Salicylates may cause some increase of SGOT and SGPT due to
liver damage.)

Little or no change occurs in chronic heart failure.

Some increase of SGOT and SGPT may occur in acute heart failure
due to liver congestion; it is quickly reversed with appropriate
therapy. There may be marked increase in cardiac tamponade due
to pericardial effusion.

SGPT is higher than SGOT (which is only slightly increased) in
pulmonary infarction and upper abdominal disease (e.g., liver
injury).

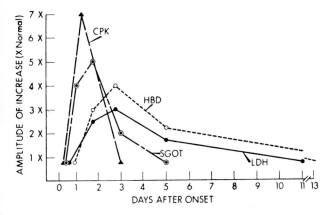

Fig. 4. Sequential Changes in Serum Enzymes After Acute Myocardial Infarction. Source: J. H. Wilkinson, "The Diagnostic Value
of LDH Isoenzymes in Clinical Medicine," *Clinical Profile* 1 (1968):
1–12.

CONGESTIVE HEART FAILURE

Renal changes. Urine—slight albuminuria (less than 1 gm/day) is
common. There are isolated RBC and WBC, hyaline and sometimes granular casts. Urine is concentrated, with specific gravity
more than 1.020. Oliguria is a characteristic feature of right-sided
failure. PSP excretion and urea clearance are usually depressed.
Moderate azotemia (BUN usually less than 60 mg/100 ml) is
evident with severe oliguria; may increase with vigorous diuresis.
(*Primary renal disease is indicated by proportionate increase in serum
creatinine and low specific gravity of urine despite oliguria.*)

ESR may be decreased because of decreased serum fibrinogen.

Plasma volume is increased. Serum albumin and total protein are
decreased, with increased gamma globulin. Hematocrit reading is
slightly decreased but red cell mass may be increased.

Liver function changes. See pp. 188–189.

Fluid and electrolytes

Urine sodium is decreased. Plasma sodium and chloride tend to fall but may be normal before treatment. Total body sodium is markedly increased. Plasma potassium is usually normal or slightly increased (because of shift from intracellular location); may be somewhat reduced with hypochloremic alkalosis due to some diuretics. Total body potassium is decreased. Saliva sodium and chloride is decreased and potassium is increased.

Acidosis (reduced blood pH) occurs when renal insufficiency is associated or there is CO_2 retention due to pulmonary insufficiency, low plasma sodium, or ammomium chloride toxicity.

Alkalosis (increased blood pH) occurs in uncomplicated heart failure itself, hyperventilation, alveolar-capillary block due to associated pulmonary fibrosis, after mercurial diuresis that causes hypochloremic alkalosis, because of potassium depletion.

Alkalosis (with normal or increased blood pH) showing increased plasma bicarbonate and moderately increased pCO_2 after acute correction of respiratory acidosis is due to CO_2 retention when there is chloride deficit and usually decreased potassium.

ACUTE RHEUMATIC FEVER

Antistreptolysin O titer increase indicates recent hemolytic streptococcus infection and indirectly corroborates clinical findings of rheumatic fever. Increased titer develops only after second week and reaches a peak in 4–6 weeks. Increasing titer is more significant than a single determination. Titer is usually more than 250 units; more significant if over 400–500 units. A normal titer helps to rule out clinically doubtful rheumatic fever. Sometimes ASO is not increased even when other titers (antifibrinolysin, antihyaluronidase) are increased. Increased titer is found in 80% of patients within the first 2 months. Height of titer is not related to severity; rate of fall is not related to course of disease.

Antihyaluronidase titer of 1000–1500 follows recent streptococcus A disease and up to 4000 with rheumatic fever. Average titer is higher in early rheumatic activity than in subsiding or inactive rheumatic fever or nonrheumatic streptococcal disease or nonstreptococcal infections. Antihyaluronidase titer is increased as often as ASO and antifibrinolysin titers.

Antifibrinolysin (antistreptokinase) titer is increased in rheumatic fever and in recent hemolytic streptococcus infections.

One of the above three titers is elevated in 95% of cases of acute rheumatic fever; if all are normal, a diagnosis of rheumatic fever is less likely.

Sedimentation rate (ESR) increase is a sensitive test of rheumatic activity; returns to normal with adequate treatment with ACTH or salicylates. It may remain increased after WBC becomes normal. It is said to become normal with onset of congestive heart failure even in the presence of rheumatic activity. It is normal in uncomplicated chorea alone.

C-reactive protein (CRP) parallels ESR.

Serum proteins are altered, with decreased serum albumin and increased alpha$_2$ and gamma globulins. (*Streptococcus A infections do not increase alpha$_2$ globulin.*) Fibrinogen is increased.

White blood count may be normal but usually is increased (10,000–16,000/cu mm) with shift to the left; increase may persist for weeks after fever subsides. Count may decrease with salicylate and ACTH therapy.

Anemia (hemoglobin usually 8–12 gm/100 ml) is common; gradually improves as activity subsides; microcytic type. Anemia may be related to increased plasma volume that occurs in early phase of acute rheumatic fever.

Urine. There is a slight febrile albuminuria. Often mild abnormality of Addis count (protein, casts, RBC, WBC) indicates mild focal nephritis. Concomitant glomerulonephritis appears in up to 2.5% of cases.

Blood cultures are usually negative. Occasional positive culture is found in 5% of cases (bacteria usually grow only in fluid media, not on solid media), in contrast to bacterial endocarditis.

SGOT may be increased, but SGPT is normal unless the patient has cardiac failure with liver damage.

Determine clinical activity: follow ESR, CRP, and WBC. Return to normal should be seen in 6–12 weeks in 80–90% of patients; it may take up to 6 months. Normal findings do not prove inactivity if patient is receiving hormone therapy. When therapy is stopped after findings have been suppressed for 6–8 weeks, there may be a mild rebound for 2–3 days and then a return to normal. Relapse after cessation of therapy occurs within 1–8 weeks.

CHRONIC RHEUMATIC VALVULAR HEART DISEASE

Laboratory findings due to complications
    Congestive heart failure
    Rheumatic activity
    Bacterial endocarditis
    Embolic phenomena

CHRONIC NONRHEUMATIC VALVULAR HEART DISEASE

Laboratory findings due to associated or underlying disease
    Syphilis
    Carcinoid syndrome
    Marfan's syndrome
    Genetic disease of mucopolysaccharide metabolism (Hurler's syndrome, Schei's syndrome, Morquio-Ulrich syndrome)
    Rheumatoid arthritis
    Congenital defect (e.g., Ebstein's abnormality of tricuspid valve, bicuspid aortic valve)
    Calcific aortic stenosis
    Endocardial fibroelastosis
    Nonbacterial thrombotic endocarditis (see next section)
Laboratory findings due to complications
    Heart failure
    Bacterial endocarditis
    Embolic phenomena

NONBACTERIAL THROMBOTIC ENDOCARDITIS
(TERMINAL ENDOCARDITIS, MARANTIC ENDOCARDITIS)

Laboratory findings due to underlying or predisposing conditions
    Rheumatic valvular disease
    Congenital valvular heart disease
    Terminal systemic neoplasms
    Etc.
Laboratory findings due to complications
    Systemic emboli (e.g., cerebral, renal)
    Bacterial endocarditis

BACTERIAL ENDOCARDITIS

Blood culture is positive in 80–90% of patients. Streptococcus viridans, enterococcus, or staphylococcus causes 95% of cases. Others may be: gram-negative bacteria (e.g., *Haemophilus influenzae*), gram-positive bacteria (e.g., hemolytic streptococcus), fungi (e.g., *Candida, Histoplasma, Cryptococcus*).

Progressive normochromic normocytic anemia is a characteristic feature; in 10% of cases hemoglobin is less than 7 gm/100 ml. Rarely there is a hemolytic anemia with a positive Coombs' test. Serum iron is decreased. Bone marrow contains abundant hemosiderin. White blood count is normal in about half of the patients and elevated up to about 15,000/cu mm in the rest, with 65–85% neutrophils. Higher WBC indicates presence of a complication (e.g., cerebral, pulmonary). Occasionally there is leukopenia. Monocytosis may be pronounced. Large macrophages may occur in peripheral blood.

Platelet count is usually normal but occasionally it is decreased; rarely purpura occurs.

Serum proteins are altered, with an increase in gamma globulin; therefore positive cephalin flocculation, thymol turbidity, ESR, cryoglobulins, rheumatoid factor (RA test), etc., are found.

Hematuria (usually microscopic) occurs at some stage in many cases due to glomerulitis or renal infarct or focal embolic glomerulonephritis. Albuminuria is almost invariable even without these complications. Renal insufficiency with azotemia and fixed specific gravity is infrequent now. Nephrotic syndrome is rare.

Cerebrospinal fluid findings in various complications. See sections on meningitis, brain abscess, mycotic aneurysm.

Proper blood cultures require: adequate volume of blood (20–25 ml), cultures taken daily for 5 days with temperature 101°F or more (preferably when highest), anaerobic as well as aerobic growth, variety of enriched media, prompt incubation, prolonged observation (growth is usual in 1–4 days but may require 2–3 weeks). Beware of negative culture due to recent antibiotic therapy. Beware of transient bacteremia following dental procedures, tonsillectomy, etc., which does not represent bacterial endocarditis (in these cases, streptococci usually grow only in fluid media; in bacterial endocarditis, many colonies also occur on solid media). Blood culture is also negative in bacterial endocarditis due to *Rickettsia burnetii*, but Phase 1 complement fixation test is positive.

Laboratory findings due to underlying or predisposing diseases
    Rheumatic heart disease
    Congenital heart disease
    Infection of genitourinary system
    Etc.

MYXOMA OF LEFT ATRIUM OF HEART

Anemia which is hemolytic in type and mechanical in origin (due to local turbulence of blood) is to be looked for and may be severe. Bizarre poikilocytes may be seen in blood smear. Reticulocyte count may be increased. Other findings may reflect effects of hemolysis or compensatory erythroid hyperplasia. The anemia is recognized in about half of the patients with this tumor. Increased serum LDH reflects hemolysis.

Serum gamma globulin is recognized to be increased in about half the patients.

Increased ESR is a reflection of abnormal serum proteins.

Platelet count may be decreased (possibly the cause here also is mechanical) with resultant findings due to thrombocytopenia.

Negative blood cultures differentiate this tumor from bacterial endocarditis.

Occasionally WBC is increased, and CRP may be positive.

Laboratory findings due to complications
    Emboli to various organs (*Increased SGOT may reflect many small emboli to striated muscle.*) (see next section)
    Congestive heart failure

These findings are reported much less frequently in myxoma of the right atrium, which is more likely to be accompanied by secondary polycythemia than anemia.

EMBOLIC LESIONS

See separate sections for laboratory findings due to infarction of kidney, intestine, brain, etc.

Laboratory findings due to underlying causative disease
    Bacterial endocarditis
    Nonbacterial thrombotic vegetations on heart valves
    Chronic rheumatic mitral stenosis with mural thrombi
    Chronic atrial fibrillation (*Rule out underlying hyperthyroidism.*)
    Mural thrombus due to underlying myocardial infarction
    Myxoma of left atrium (see preceding section)

POSTCOMMISSUROTOMY SYNDROME

This condition occurs after cardiac surgery (e.g., commissurotomy, correction of pulmonary stenosis with atrial septal defect); it is the same as the postcardiac injury syndrome.

WBC is increased.

ESR is increased.

CRP is present by the second day.

SGOT is increased to 4–7 times normal by the second day.

COR PULMONALE

Secondary polycythemia

Increased blood CO_2 when cor pulmonale is secondary to chest deformities or pulmonary emphysema

Laboratory findings of the primary lung disease (e.g., chronic bronchitis and emphysema, multiple small pulmonary emboli, pulmonary schistosomiasis)

TETRALOGY OF FALLOT

Secondary polycythemia is present. Mortality for complete surgical correction is higher in cases with Hb over 18 gm/100 ml than in those with Hb less than 18 gm/100 ml. Surgical risk is decreased if polycythemia is first reduced by a preliminary systemic-pulmonary anastomosis.

Laboratory findings due to complications (see below)

COMPLICATIONS OF CONGENITAL HEART DISEASE

Laboratory findings due to
    Congestive heart failure
    Bacterial endocarditis
    Pulmonary tuberculosis, especially with pulmonary stenosis
    Paradoxical embolism—with right-to-left communication, especially patent foramen ovale
    Brain abscess, especially with interventricular septal defect, particularly in tetralogy of Fallot; also in atrial septal defect
    Rupture of aorta
    Secondary polycythemia

COBALT-BEER CARDIOMYOPATHY
(bizarre syndrome of fulminating heart failure in drinkers of large amounts of beer of a brand that contains cobalt)

Polycythemia

Lactic acidosis and shock

Increased SGOT, CPK, and LDH, often to extremely high levels; these may rise even further after recovery from shock

Laboratory findings due to pericardial effusion and, less frequently, pleural effusion

ACUTE PERICARDITIS

Due To

Active rheumatic fever (40% of cases)

Bacterial infection (20% of cases)

Uremia (11% of cases)

Benign nonspecific pericarditis (10% of cases)

Neoplasms (3.5% of cases)

Collagen disease (e.g., disseminated lupus erythematosus, polyarteritis nodosa) (2% of cases)

Also acute myocardial infarction, postcardiac injury syndrome

Findings

See appropriate sections above for laboratory findings of primary disease.

Radioisotope scan of cardiac pool
WBC—usually increased in proportion to fever; normal or low in viral disease and tuberculous pericarditis; markedly increased in suppurative bacterial pericarditis
Examination of aspirated pericardial fluid (see Table 13, p. 122)
    Smears and cultures for pyogenic bacteria and tubercle bacilli
    Cytologic examination for LE cells and neoplastic cells

CHRONIC PERICARDIAL EFFUSION
(see appropriate sections listed below for primary diseases and section on body fluids)

Due To
Tuberculosis
Myxedema
Metastatic tumor
Disseminated lupus erythematosus

Rarely Due To
Severe anemia
Scleroderma
Polyarteritis nodosa
Rheumatoid arthritis
Radiation therapy
Mycotic infections
Endomyocardial fibrosis of Africa
"Idiopathic" causes

CHRONIC CONSTRICTIVE PERICARDITIS

Altered liver function tests
    BSP retention increased
    Thymol turbidity increased (some cases)
    Other abnormalities as occur in congestive heart failure
Decreased serum albumin with normal total protein

LOEFFLER'S PARIETAL FIBROPLASTIC ENDOCARDITIS

Eosinophilia up to 70%; may be absent at first but appears sooner or later
WBC frequently increased
Laboratory findings due to frequently occurring
    Mural thrombi in heart and embolization of spleen and lung
    Mitral and tricuspid regurgitation

AORTIC ARCH SYNDROME (TAKAYASU'S SYNDROME; PULSELESS DISEASE)

WBC usually normal
Serum proteins abnormal with increased gamma globulins (mostly composed of IgM)
Increased ESR

Women have a continuous high level of urinary total estrogens (rather than the usual rise during luteal phase after a low excretion during follicular phase)

SYPHILITIC AORTITIS

Laboratory findings due to associated lesions
    Syphilitic aortic insufficiency, with congestive heart failure
    Myocardial infarction due to coronary ostial stenosis
Laboratory findings due to complications
    Hemorrhage (into pericardium, esophagus, bronchial tree, etc.)
    Pressure or erosion or obstruction of adjacent structures in
        mediastinum
Laboratory evidence of syphilis (see Serologic Tests for Syphilis, p.
    101)
    Serologic tests for syphilis (e.g., VDRL, Kolmer complement-
        fixation) are negative in more than one-quarter of patients
        with syphilitic aortitis at autopsy.

DISSECTING ANEURYSM OF AORTA

If patient survives the immediate episode
    Increased WBC
    Increased ESR
    Laboratory findings due to hemorrhage
    Normal serum CPK, SGOT, SGPT, LDH, α-HBD unless
        complications occur (see below)
Laboratory findings due to complications
    Hemopericardium
    Interference with blood supply to heart, brain, kidney, intestine,
        etc.
Laboratory findings due to underlying disease
    Marfan's disease

ARTERIOSCLEROTIC ANEURYSM OF ABDOMINAL AORTA

Laboratory findings due to complications
    Hemorrhage, especially retroperitoneal; rarely into duodenum,
        etc.
    Obstruction of branches (e.g., renal arteries)

MYOCARDIAL DISEASE ASSOCIATED WITH MARKED EOSINOPHILIA

Due To
Trichinosis
Polyarteritis nodosa
Eosinophilic leukemia with infiltration of heart
Loeffler's fibroplastic endocarditis

MYOCARDIAL INVOLVEMENT IN SYSTEMIC DISEASES

Laboratory findings due to primary disease
    Infections (viral; rickettsial, e.g., scrub typhus; bacterial, e.g.,
        diphtheria; protozoan, e.g., trypanosomiasis; parasitic, e.g.,
        trichinosis)
    Hyperthyroidism
    Myxedema
    Chronic anemias (with Hg $<$ 7 gm/100 ml)

Beriberi (alcoholism)
Arteriovenous fistulas (e.g., Paget's disease of bone, pulmonary arteriovenous fistula)
Acute glomerulonephritis
Collagen diseases (polyarteritis nodosa, SLE, scleroderma, rheumatoid arthritis)
Hypokalemia
Sarcoidosis
Amyloidosis
Muscular dystrophy
Mucopolysaccharidoses
Glycogen-storage disease
Leukemia and metastatic tumor
Idiopathic causes (e.g., hypertrophic subaortic stenosis)
Others
Laboratory findings due to complications
    Systemic emboli
    Pulmonary emboli
    Heart failure
    Pericardial effusion

Serum LDH, SGOT, SGPT, etc., show variable mild increase.

SHOCK

Leukocytosis is common, especially with hemorrhage. There may be leukopenia when shock is severe as in gram-negative bacteremia. Circulating eosinophils are decreased.

Hemoconcentration (e.g., dehydration, burns) or hemodilution (e.g., hemorrhage, crush injuries, and skeletal trauma) takes place.

Hyperglycemia occurs early.

Acidosis appears when shock is well developed, with increased blood lactate, low serum sodium, low CO_2 —combining power with decreased alkaline reserve. Serum potassium may be increased. Blood pH is usually relatively normal but may be decreased. BUN may be increased.

Oliguria with low specific gravity (unless due to dehydration) or anuria is seen, as are decreased renal blood flow and glomerular filtration.

THROMBOPHLEBITIS OF DEEP VEINS OF LEG

Laboratory findings of pulmonary infarction (see p. 162) should be sought as evidence of embolization.

RECURRENT THROMBOPHLEBITIS

Laboratory findings will be due to the underlying disease, which is often occult and may be without other manifestations.

Due To
Carcinoma, especially of pancreas; also bronchus, ovary, others
Kaposi's disease
Polycythemia
Vibrio fetus infection

CONGENITAL ANGIOMATOUS ARTERIOVENOUS FISTULAS

Platelet count may be decreased.

RAYNAUD'S PHENOMENON

May Occur With
High titer of cold agglutinins
Presence of cryoglobulins (e.g., in multiple myeloma, leukemia)
Scleroderma (CREST)
Other diseases without specific laboratory findings

LABORATORY FINDINGS OF HEART TRANSPLANT REJECTION AS GUIDE TO IMMUNOSUPPRESSIVE TREATMENT

Increasing ESR
Increasing WBC
Increasing LDH isoenzyme-1 as amount ($>$ 100 I.U.) and percent (35%) of total LDH during first 4 weeks after surgery

These findings are reversed with effective immunosuppressive therapy. Total LDH continues to be increased even when LDH_1 becomes normal.

25

Respiratory Diseases

DISEASES OF LARYNX

Culture and smears for specific organisms (e.g., tubercle bacilli, fungi)

Biopsy for diagnosis of visible lesions (e.g., leukoplakia, carcinoma)

CHRONIC BRONCHITIS

WBC normal or increased

Eosinophil count increased if there is allergic basis or component

ESR normal or increased

Sputum bacterial smears and cultures (most common pathogens: pneumococcus, *Haemophilus influenzae*; occasionally *Staphylococcus aureus* or gram-negative rods)

Smears and cultures of bronchoscopic secretions

Laboratory findings due to associated or coexisting diseases (e.g., emphysema, bronchiectasis)

BRONCHIAL ASTHMA

Sputum is white and mucoid without blood or pus (unless infection is present). Eosinophils, crystals (Curschmann's spirals), and mucus casts of bronchioles may be found.

Eosinophilia may be present.

Blood CO_2 may be decreased in early stages and may be increased in later stages.

Laboratory findings due to underlying diseases that may be primary and that should be ruled out, especially

    Polyarteritis nodosa

    Parasitic infestation

    Bronchial carcinoid

    Drug reaction (especially aspirin)

    Poisoning (especially cholinergic drugs and pesticides)

BRONCHIECTASIS

WBC usually normal unless pneumonitis is present

Mild to moderate normocytic normochromic anemia with chronic severe infection

[*157*]

Sputum abundant, and mucopurulent (often contains blood); sweet-ish smell
Sputum bacterial smears and cultures
Laboratory findings due to complications (pneumonia, pulmonary hemorrhage, brain abscess, sepsis, cor pulmonale)

Rule out cystic fibrosis of the pancreas and hypogammaglobulinemia or agammaglobulinemia.

OBSTRUCTIVE PULMONARY EMPHYSEMA

Laboratory findings of underlying disease that may be primary (e.g., pneumoconiosis, tuberculosis, sarcoidosis, kyphoscoliosis, marked obesity, fibrocystic disease of pancreas)
Laboratory findings of associated conditions, especially duodenal ulcer
Laboratory findings due to decreased lung ventilation
    Arterial blood oxygen decreased and CO_2 increased
    Ultimate development of respiratory acidosis
    Secondary polycythemia
    Cor pulmonale

ATELECTASIS

No specific laboratory findings

Rule out underlying lesions (e.g., tumor, tuberculosis, cystic fibrosis of pancreas).

PNEUMONIA

Due To
Bacteria—pneumococcus, staphylococcus, *Klebsiella pneumoniae, Haemophilus influenzae,* streptococcus, enterobacteria, tularemia, plague, tubercle bacilli

	Isolated in % of Cases	*Mortality**
Diplococcus	62%	19%
Gram-negative bacilli	20%	79%
(e.g., *K. pneumoniae*		
Enterobacteria		
Escherichia coli		
Proteus mirabilis		
Pseudomonas aerugi-		
nosa)		
Staphylococcus	10%	41%
Haemophilus influenzae	8%	14%

---

* *Mortality is much greater over the age of 40 years.*

Mycoplasma pneumoniae
Viruses—influenza, parainfluenza, adenoviruses, respiratory syncy-
tial virus, ECHO, Coxsackie, reovirus, cytomegalic inclusion
virus, viruses of exanthems, herpes simplex
Rickettsiae—Q fever, typhus
Fungi— *Histoplasma* and *Coccidioides* in particular
Protozoans— *Toxoplasma*, pneumocystis carinii

Laboratory Findings
WBC is frequently normal or slightly increased in nonbacterial
pneumonias; considerable increase in WBC is more common in
bacterial pneumonia. *In severe bacterial pneumonia, WBC may be
very high or low or normal. Since individual variation is considerable,
there is limited value in distinguishing bacterial and nonbacterial
pneumonia.*
In the urine, protein, WBC, hyaline and granular casts in small
amounts are common. Ketones may occur with severe infection.
Check for glucose to rule out underlying diabetes mellitus.
A blood culture should be taken before antibiotic therapy is started.
Sputum reveals abundant WBC in bacterial pneumonias. Gram
stain shows abundant organisms in bacterial pneumonias (e.g.,
pneumococcus, staphylococcus). Culture sputum for appropriate
bacteria.
Acute-phase serum should be stored at onset. If etiologic diagnosis
is not established, a convalescent-phase serum should be taken. A
fourfold increase in antibody titer establishes the etiologic diagnosis.
Serologic tests determine whether pneumonia is due to *Histoplasma*,
Coccidioides, etc.

LIPID PNEUMONIA

Sputum shows fat-containing macrophages that stain with Sudan.
They may be present only intermittently; *therefore examine sputum
more than once.*

DIFFUSE INTERSTITIAL PNEUMONITIS

Serum LDH is increased.

LUNG ABSCESS

Sputum
    Abundant, foul
    Purulent; may be bloody; contains elastic fibers
    Bacterial cultures (including tubercle bacilli)—anaerobic as well
        as aerobic (*Rule out amebas, parasites.*)
    Cytologic examination for malignant cells
Blood culture—may be positive in acute stage
Increased WBC in acute stages (15,000—30,000/cu mm)
Increased ESR
Normochromic normocytic anemia in chronic stage
Albuminuria frequent
Findings of underlying disease—especially bronchogenic carci-
noma; also drug addiction, postabortal state, coccidioidomycosis,
amebic abscess, tuberculosis, alcoholism

BRONCHOGENIC CARCINOMA

Cytologic examination of sputum for malignant cells—positive in 60–70% of patients; false positive rare

Biopsy of scalene lymph nodes for metastases to indicate inoperable status—positive in 15% of patients

Findings of complicating conditions (e.g., pneumonitis, atelectasis, lung abscess)

Findings due to metastases (e.g., Addison's disease, diabetes insipidus, liver metastases with functional hepatic changes, malignant cells in pleural fluid)

Findings due to secretion of active hormone substances (e.g., Cushing's syndrome, hypercalcemia, serotonin production by carcinoid of bronchus) (See pp. 349, 351.)

Biopsy of bronchus, pleura, lung, metastatic sites in appropriate cases

Cancer cells in bone marrow and rarely in peripheral blood

PULMONARY ALVEOLAR PROTEINOSIS

Serum LDH increases when protein accumulates in lungs and drops to normal when infiltrate resolves.

PAS-positive material appears in sputum.

PSP dye injected intravenously is excreted in sputum for long periods of time.

Biopsy of lung for histologic examination is in order.

HYALINE MEMBRANE SYNDROME

Laboratory findings of
    Increased catabolism: increased BUN and serum potassium
    Impaired ventilation: increased CO_2 and decreased O_2 tension; decreased blood pH (to 7.3 or less) (Acidosis is first respiratory, later also metabolic.)

PULMONARY INFILTRATIONS ASSOCIATED WITH EOSINOPHILIA

Due To

Allergic conditions (e.g., asthma, serum sickness, drug reaction, farmer's lung)

Collagen disorders (e.g., polyarteritis nodosa, Wegener's granulomatosis, SLE)

Neoplasms (e.g., malignant lymphoma, eosinophilic leukemia)

Infections (e.g., fungus, tuberculosis, brucellosis)

Infestations (e.g., trichinosis, ascariasis, tropical eosinophilia due to *Dirofilaria immitis*)

Idiopathic causes, including Loeffler's syndrome of recurrent transient pulmonary infiltration

PNEUMOCONIOSIS

Biopsy of lung, scalene lymph node—histologic, chemical, spectrographic, and x-ray diffraction studies (e.g., silicosis, berylliosis; also metastatic tumor, sarcoidosis, tuberculosis, fungus infection)

Increased WBC if associated infection

Secondary polycythemia or anemia

Bacterial smears and cultures of sputum (*especially for tubercle bacilli*)

Cytologic examination of sputum and bronchoscopic secretions for malignant cells

Asbestosis
> Asbestos bodies sometimes in sputum after exposure to asbestos dust even without clinical disease
> Associated malignancy, especially mesothelioma of pleura and squamous cell carcinoma of bronchus

Acute beryllium disease
> Occasional transient hypergammaglobulinemia

Chronic beryllium disease
> Secondary polycythemia
> Increased serum gamma globulin
> Increased urine calcium
> *Increased beryllium in urine for long time after beryllium exposure has ended*

Coal worker's pneumoconiosis

Diatomaceous earth pneumoconiosis

Talcosis

Bauxite fume fibrosis (shaver's disease)

Siderosis

Byssinosis (dust from carding and spinning of cotton contains fibers, mold, fungi, etc.)

Bagassosis (dust from sugar cane fibers)

FARMER'S LUNG (BAGASSOSIS, THRESHER'S LUNG, RESPIRATORY DISEASE OF MUSHROOM WORKERS, ETC.)

Due To
Hypersensitivity to inhaled organic dusts (e.g., sugar cane, wheat, corn, oats, straw, hay, barley, tobacco)

Laboratory Findings
Normal WBC; increased in presence of infection
Eosinophilia up to 45%
Increased ESR
Sputum smear and culture nonspecific
Lung biopsy—acute granulomatous interstitial pneumonitis

IDIOPATHIC PULMONARY HEMOSIDEROSIS

Hemosiderin-laden macrophages in sputum
Hypochromic microcytic anemia due to pulmonary hemorrhages with normal serum iron and iron-binding capacity; sometimes findings of hemolytic type of anemia (increased indirect serum bilirubin and urine urobilinogen)
Eosinophilia in up to 20% of patients

GOODPASTURE'S SYNDROME

Malignant hypertension associated with malignant nephrosclerosis
Pulmonary hemorrhages
Eosinophilia absent and anemia more marked than in idiopathic pulmonary hemosiderosis

PULMONARY HEMOSIDEROSIS SECONDARY TO MITRAL STENOSIS

Hemosiderin-laden macrophages in sputum

PULMONARY EMBOLISM AND INFARCTION

Serum LDH increased (isozymes LD_2 and LD_3) (may be useful as screening test); rises on first day, peaks on second day, normal by tenth day; increased in more than 80% of patients

Lung scan (radioactive isotope scans) (see p. 133)

Serum bilirubin increased (as early as fourth day up to 5+ mg/100 ml) in about 20% of cases

Urine urobilinogen increased

Serum SGOT usually normal or only slightly increased

Serum aldolase slightly increased

Leukocytosis up to 15,000/cu mm in about 50% of patients

ESR increased

"Triad" of increased LDH and bilirubin with normal SGOT found in about 15% of cases

See Table 16, p. 146.

These laboratory findings depend on the size and duration of the infarction, and the tests must be performed at the appropriate time to detect abnormalities.

CAVERNOUS HEMANGIOMA (CONGENITAL ARTERIOVENOUS ANEURYSM OR VARIX) OF LUNG

Polycythemia

PULMONARY SEQUESTRATION

The only laboratory findings are due to associated localized chronic bronchitis and bronchiectasis.

TUMORS (PRIMARY OR SECONDARY) OF PLEURA

Examination of pleural fluid (see Table 13, p. 122)

Biopsy of pleura

RHEUMATOID PLEURISY WITH EFFUSION

Decreased glucose level (less than 30 mg/100 ml in three-fourths of cases) is the most useful finding clinically. Nonpurulent nonmalignant effusions other than those due to tuberculosis or rheumatoid arthritis almost always have glucose levels higher than 70 mg/100 ml.

Exudate is frequently turbid and may be milky.

Smears and cultures for bacteria, tubercle bacilli, and fungi are negative.

Cytologic examination for malignant cells is negative. RA cells may be found.

Protein level is more than 3 gm/100 ml.

Increased LDH (usually higher than in serum) is commonly found in other chronic pleural effusions and is not useful in differential diagnosis.

Rheumatoid factor may be present but may also be found in other types of pleural effusions (e.g., with carcinoma, tuberculosis, bacterial pneumonia).

Needle biopsy of pleura usually shows nonspecific chronic inflammation, but characteristic changes of rheumatoid pleuritis may be found histologically.

Other laboratory findings of rheumatoid arthritis are found (see p. 234).

PNEUMOTHORAX

No abnormal laboratory findings

Laboratory findings *if* underlying disease is present (e.g., tuberculosis, sarcoidosis, lung abscess, silicosis, carcinoma)

PNEUMOMEDIASTINUM

Leukocytosis—variable, nonspecific

MEDIASTINAL NEOPLASMS

See
Thymoma
Malignant lymphoma
Ganglioneuroma
Neuroblastoma
Pheochromocytoma
Substernal goiter
Parathyroid adenoma
Metastatic tumors
Sarcoidosis
Tuberculosis
Etc.

DERMOID CYST OF MEDIASTINUM

Hair in sputum may occur with rupture into bronchus.

DIAPHRAGMATIC HERNIA

Microcytic anemia (due to blood loss) may be present.
Stool may be positive for blood.

TIETZE'S SYNDROME (COSTOCHONDRITIS, COSTOCHONDRALGIA, RIB SYNDROME, ETC.)

No abnormal laboratory findings

26

Gastrointestinal Diseases

LABORATORY FINDINGS IN ORAL MANIFESTATIONS OF SOME SYSTEMIC DISEASES

Infections
    Bacterial (e.g., diphtheria, scarlet fever, syphilis, Vincent's angina)
    Viral (e.g., herpes simplex, herpangina, measles, infectious mononucleosis)
    Fungal (e.g., actinomycosis, histoplasmosis, mucormycosis, moniliasis)
Hematologic diseases
    Pernicious anemia—glossitis
    Iron-deficiency anemia—atrophy
    Polycythemia—erosions
    Granulocytopenia—ulceration and inflammation
    Acute leukemia—edema and hemorrhage
Vitamin deficiencies
    Pellagra
    Riboflavin deficiency
    Scurvy
Systemic diseases
    Systemic lupus erythematosus
    Primary amyloidosis
    Hereditary hemorrhagic telangiectasia (Osler-Weber-Rendu disease)

GASTROINTESTINAL MANIFESTATIONS OF SOME SYSTEMIC DISEASES

Lymphoma and leukemia
Metastatic carcinoma
Collagen diseases (e.g., scleroderma, polyarteritis nodosa, SLE)
Amyloidosis
Parasitic infestation (schistosomiasis)
Bacterial infection (lymphogranuloma venereum)
Osler-Weber-Rendu disease
Henoch's purpura

Hemolytic crises (e.g., sickle cell disease)
Porphyria
Lead poisoning
Embolic accidents in rheumatic heart disease, bacterial endocarditis
Ischemic vascular disease
Uremia
Allergy
Cystic fibrosis of pancreas
Hirschsprung's disease
Cirrhosis (esophageal varices, hemorrhoids, peptic ulcer)
Zollinger-Ellison syndrome (peptic ulcer)
Peptic ulcer associated with other diseases (in 8–22% of patients with hyperparathyroidism, 10% of patients with pituitary tumor, etc.)
Others

SYSTEMIC MANIFESTATIONS OCCURRING IN SOME GASTROINTESTINAL DISEASES

Carcinoid syndrome
Anemia (e.g., due to bleeding occult neoplasm)
Arthritis, uveitis, etc., in ulcerative colitis
Vitamin deficiency (e.g., sprue, malabsorption)
Endocrine manifestations due to replacement by metastatic tumors of GI tract

MALLORY-WEISS SYNDROME
(spontaneous cardioesophageal laceration following retching)

Laboratory findings due to hemorrhage from cardioesophageal laceration

SPONTANEOUS PERFORATION OF ESOPHAGUS

Gastric contents in thoracocentesis fluid

PLUMMER-VINSON SYNDROME

Hypochromic anemia associated with dysphagia and cardiospasm in women

CARCINOMA OF ESOPHAGUS

Cytologic examination of esophageal washings is positive for malignant cells in three-quarters of the patients. It is falsely positive in less than 2% of the patients.

DIAPHRAGMATIC HERNIA

Microcytic anemia (due to blood loss) may be present.
Stool may be positive for blood.

ESOPHAGEAL INVOLVEMENT DUE TO PRIMARY DISEASES ELSEWHERE

Scleroderma (*esophageal involvement in more than half of patients with scleroderma*)

Esophageal varices (see Cirrhosis of Liver)
Malignant lymphoma

SOME CONDITIONS OF GASTROINTESTINAL TRACT IN WHICH NO USEFUL ABNORMAL LABORATORY FINDINGS OCCUR

Acute esophagitis
Chronic esophagitis
Diverticula of esophagus and stomach
Esophageal spasm
Prolapse of gastric mucosa
Foreign bodies in stomach

PEPTIC ULCER OF STOMACH

Laboratory findings due to underlying conditions
    Administration of ACTH and adrenal steroids
    Acute burns (Curling's ulcer)
    Cerebrovascular accidents and trauma and inflammation (Cushing's ulcer)
    Various drugs (e.g., salicylates)
    Uremia
    Cirrhosis
Laboratory findings due to complications
    Gastric retention—dehydration, hypokalemic alkalosis
    Perforation—increased WBC with shift to the left, dehydration, increased serum amylase, increased amylase in peritoneal fluid
    Hemorrhage

Curling's ulcer—hemorrhage 8–10 days and perforation 30 days after burn, causes death in 15% of fatal burn cases
See Chronic Duodenal Ulcer, p. 167.

NONSPECIFIC GASTRITIS

Hypochromic microcytic anemia due to blood loss
Occult blood in stool
Gastric analysis
    Hypochlorhydria in early cases
    Achlorhydria with complete atrophy
Hypoalbuminemia possible

BENIGN GIANT HYPERTROPHIC GASTRITIS (MENETRIER'S DISEASE)

See Protein-Losing Enteropathy, p. 172.

ADENOMATOUS POLYP OF STOMACH

Gastric analysis—achlorhydria in 85% of patients
Sometimes evidence of bleeding

Polyps occur in 5% of patients with pernicious anemia and 2% of patients with achlorhydria.

CARCINOMA OF STOMACH

Anemia due to chronic blood loss
Occult blood in stool
Gastric analysis
  Achlorhydria following histamine or betazole in 50% of patients
  Hypochlorhydria in 25% of patients
  Normal in 25% of patients
  Hyperchlorhydria rare
Exfoliative cytology positive in 80% of patients; false positive in less than 2%
Lymph node biopsy for metastases; needle biopsy of liver, bone marrow, etc.

Carcinoma of the stomach should always be searched for by periodic prophylactic screening in high-risk patients, especially those with pernicious anemia, gastric atrophy, gastric polyps.

LEIOMYOMA, LEIOMYOSARCOMA, MALIGNANT LYMPHOMA OF STOMACH

May show evidence of bleeding

CHRONIC DUODENAL ULCER

Laboratory findings due to associated conditions
  Zollinger-Ellison syndrome (ulcerogenic tumor of pancreas) (see p. 329)
  Chronic pancreatitis
  Mucoviscidosis
  Rheumatoid arthritis
  Chronic pulmonary disease (e.g., pulmonary emphysema)
  Cirrhosis
  Certain drugs (e.g., ACTH)
  Hyperparathyroidism
  Polycythemia vera
Laboratory findings due to treatment
  Milk-alkali (Burnett's) syndrome—alkalosis, hypercalcemia, azotemia, renal calculi or nephrocalcinosis
  Inadequate vagotomy: insulin test (see p. 121)
    Gastric acidity shows late response of more than 4.5 mEq total free acid in 30 minutes or any early response.

  (*To obtain valid collection, Levin tube must be correctly placed fluoroscopically.*)

  Dumping syndrome (occurs in up to 70% of post–subtotal gastrectomy patients)—during symptoms may have
    Rapid prolonged alimentary hyperglycemia
    Decreased plasma volume
    Decreased serum potassium
    Increased blood and urine serotonin
  Hypoglycemic syndrome (occurs in less than 5% of post–subtotal gastrectomy patients)
    Prolonged alimentary hyperglycemia followed after 2 hours by precipitous hypoglycemia
    Late hypoglycemia shown by 6-hour oral GTT

Stomal gastritis—anemia due to chronic bleeding
Postgastrectomy malabsorption
Postgastrectomy anemia (due to chronic blood loss, malabsorption, vitamin B_{12} deficiency, etc.)
Afferent-loop obstruction—marked increase in serum amylase to more than 1000 units
Laboratory findings due to complications of gastric or duodenal ulcer
Hemorrhage
Perforation
Obstruction
Etc.
Gastric analysis
True achlorhydria following maximum stimulation rules out duodenal ulcer. Normal secretion or hypersecretion does not prove the presence of an ulcer.

Duodenal ulcer is absent in patients with ulcerative colitis (unless under steroid therapy), carcinoma of stomach, pernicious anemia, pregnancy.

REGIONAL ENTERITIS (CROHN'S DISEASE)

Inflammation—increased WBC and ESR
Iron-deficiency type of anemia due to blood loss
Malabsorption
Laboratory findings due to complications
Perforation and peritonitis
Hemorrhage
Arthritis
Secondary amyloidosis

ACUTE APPENDICITIS

Increased WBC (12,000–14,000/cu mm) with shift to the left in acute catarrhal stage; higher and more rapid rise with suppuration or perforation
ESR—may be normal during first 24 hours
Later: Laboratory findings due to complications (e.g., dehydration, abscess formation, perforation with peritonitis)

ACUTE DIVERTICULITIS

Increased WBC and ESR
Hypochromic microcytic anemia (some cases)
Occult blood in stool
Cytologic examination of stool—negative for malignant cells
Laboratory findings due to complications
Hemorrhage
Perforation
Obstruction

ACUTE MEMBRANOUS ENTEROCOLITIS

Laboratory findings due to antecedent condition
Disease for which antibiotics are administered

Myocardial infarction
Surgical procedure
Etc.
Laboratory findings due to shock, dehydration
Culture of staphylococci from stool or rectal swab

WHIPPLE'S DISEASE (INTESTINAL LIPODYSTROPHY)

Characteristic biopsy of intestine and mesenteric lymph nodes
Malabsorption syndrome (see p. 170)
Arthritis

CELIAC DISEASE (GLUTEN-SENSITIVE ENTEROPATHY, NONTROPICAL SPRUE, IDIOPATHIC STEATORRHEA)

Malabsorption syndrome (see p. 170); return to normal on gluten-free diet
Biopsy of small intestine

TUMORS OF SMALL INTESTINE

Laboratory findings due to complications
Hemorrhage
Obstruction
Intussusception
Malabsorption
Laboratory findings due to underlying condition
Peutz-Jeghers syndrome
Malignant lymphoma
Carcinoid syndrome

MULTIPLE DIVERTICULA OF JEJUNUM

Laboratory findings due to malabsorption syndrome

MECKEL'S DIVERTICULUM

Laboratory findings due only to complications
Gastrointestinal hemorrhage
Intestinal obstruction
Perforation or intussusception (about 20% of cases; the other 80% of patients are asymptomatic)

CLASSIFICATION OF MALABSORPTION

Inadequate mixing of food with bile salts and lipase (e.g., pyloroplasty, subtotal or total gastrectomy, gastrojejunostomy)
Inadequate lipolysis due to lack of lipase (e.g., cystic fibrosis of the pancreas, chronic pancreatitis, cancer of the pancreas or ampulla of Vater, pancreatic fistula, vagotomy)
Inadequate emulsification of fat due to lack of bile salts (e.g., obstructive jaundice, severe liver disease)
Primary absorptive defect in small bowel
Inadequate absorptive surface due to extensive mucosal disease (e.g., regional enteritis, tumors, amyloid disease, scleroderma, radiation)

Biochemical dysfunction of mucosal cells (e.g., celiac-sprue
syndrome, severe starvation, intestinal infections, infestations, or administration of drugs such as neomycin sulfate,
colchicine, or PAS)

Obstruction of mesenteric lymphatics (e.g., by lymphoma, carcinoma, Whipple's disease, intestinal tuberculosis)

Inadequate length of normal absorptive surface (e.g., surgical
resection, fistula, shunt)

Miscellaneous (e.g., "blind loops" of intestine, diverticula,
Zollinger-Ellison syndrome, agammaglobulinemia, endocrine
and metabolic disorders)

LABORATORY DIAGNOSIS OF MALABSORPTION

Direct stool examination
Gross—oil droplets, egg particles, buttery materials
Sudan III stain—more than 3 globules/microscopical hpf or
globules larger than 75 μ
Weight—much heavier than normal (normal weight is less than
200 gm/24 hours or normal fecal solids of 25–30 gm/24
hours)

Chemical analysis of fecal fat
Normal—less than 6 gm of fat/24 hours as average of 3-day
collection when diet includes 100 gm of fat/day
Chronic pancreatic disease—more than 10 gm/24 hours

Indirect indices of fat absorption
Serum carotene (for screening purposes) is always abnormal in
steatorrhea unless therapy is successful.
Normal is 70–290 μg/100 ml.
30–70 μg/100 ml indicates mild depletion; less than 30
indicates severe depletion.
May also be low in liver disease and diets low in carotene-
containing foods

Vitamin A tolerance test (for screening steatorrhea)
Measure plasma vitamin A level 5 hours after ingestion.
Normal rise is 9 times fasting level.
Flat curve in liver disease
Not useful after gastrectomy

Triolein ^{131}I absorption with measurement of blood and fecal
radioactivity (see p. 131)
Oleic acid ^{131}I (see p. 131)

Carbohydrate absorption indices
Oral glucose tolerance test—limited value
Flat curve or delayed peak occurs in celiac disease and
nontropical sprue.
Curve is normal in pancreatic insufficiency.

D-xylose tolerance test—useful test of carbohydrate absorption
Measure total 5-hour urine excretion; perhaps also measure blood levels at $\frac{1}{2}$, 1, and 2 hours (almost no
absorption from ileum). Accuracy is 90% in distinguishing pancreatic disease from intestinal mucosal disease.
Absorption is normal, but urinary excretion is decreased in
renal disease and myxedema; also decreased in the
elderly.

Na_2CO_3 and Nile blue dye give blue color to stool proportional
to the concentration of oleates.

Protein absorption indices
> Normal fecal nitrogen is less than 2 gm/day. There is marked increase in sprue and severe pancreatic deficiency.
>
> Measure plasma glycine or urinary excretion of hydroxyproline after gelatin meal. Plasma glycine increases 5 times in 2½ hours in normal persons. In those with cystic fibrosis of the pancreas, the increase is less than 2½ times.

Schilling test (using ^{60}Co- or ^{58}Co-labeled vitamin B_{12}) shows poor absorption of vitamin B_{12} that is not improved by the addition of intrinsic factor.

^{131}I PVP test is indicated (see p. 131).

^{51}Cr albumin test (IV dose of 30–50 μc) shows increased excretion in 4-day stool collection due to protein-losing enteropathy.

Biopsy of small intestine mucosa is excellent for verification of sprue, celiac disease, and Whipple's disease.

Anemia is due to deficiency of iron, folic acid, vitamin B_{12}, or various combinations, depending on their decreased absorption.

DISACCHARIDE MALABSORPTION

Due To
Primary malabsorption (congenital or acquired) due to absence of specific disaccharidase in brush border of small intestine mucosa
> Sucrose-isomaltose malabsorption (inherited recessive defect)
>> Oral sucrose tolerance is flat, but glucose plus fructose tolerance test is normal. Occasionally there is an associated malabsorption with increased stool fat and abnormal D-xylose tolerance test although intestinal biopsy is normal.
>
> Isolated lactase deficiency (most common defect; occurs in more than 10% of whites and 60% of Negroes; congenital or acquired)
>> Oral lactose tolerance is flat, but glucose plus galactose tolerance test is normal. Intestinal biopsy shows normal histology but decreased lactose activity.

Secondary malabsorption
> Resection of more than half of disaccharidase activity
>> Lactose is most marked, but there may also be sucrose.
>>> Oral disaccharide tolerance (especially lactose) is abnormal, but intestinal histology and enzyme activity are normal.
>
> Diffuse intestinal disease—especially celiac disease in which activity of all disaccharidases may be decreased, with later increase as intestine becomes normal on gluten-free diet
>> Oral tolerance tests (especially lactose) are frequently abnormal, with later return to normal with gluten-free diet. Tolerance tests with monosaccharides may also be abnormal because of defect in absorption as well as digestion.

Laboratory Findings
Oral carbohydrate (disaccharide) tolerance test is abnormal (blood glucose rises 0–21 mg/100 ml above fasting level).

Oral tolerance test using constituent monosaccharides. Normal result demonstrates normal absorption of monosaccharides.
Examine stool during disaccharide tolerance test.
  pH of 5 or less is abnormal.
    Measure disaccharide (Clinitest tablet).
      More than 0.5% is abnormal.
      0.25–0.5% is suspicious.
      Less than 0.25% is normal.
Biopsy of small intestine mucosa will reveal activity of specific disaccharidase.

PROTEIN-LOSING ENTEROPATHY

Secondary (i.e., disease states in which clinically significant protein-losing enteropathy may occur as a manifestation)
    Giant hypertrophy of gastric rugae
    Gastric neoplasms
    Regional enteritis
    Whipple's disease
    Nontropical sprue
    Inflammatory and neoplastic diseases of small and large intestine
    Ulcerative colitis
    Constrictive pericarditis
Primary (i.e., hypoproteinemia is the major clinical feature)
    Intestinal lymphangiectasia
    Nonspecific inflammatory or granulomatous disease of small intestine
Serum albumin and gamma globulin decreased
Serum alpha and beta globulins normal
Serum cholesterol usually normal
Mild anemia
Eosinophilia (occasionally)
Serum calcium decreased
Steatorrhea with abnormal tests of lipid absorption
Increased permeability of GI tract to large molecular substances shown by IV ^{131}I PVP test (see p. 131)

PERORAL BIOPSY OF THE PROXIMAL SMALL INTESTINE*

For differential diagnosis of malabsorption, diarrhea, and associated nutritional deficiencies

Biopsy is always useful in
    Celiac sprue
    Whipple's disease
    Agammaglobulinemia
    A-beta-lipoproteinemia (see p. 59: acanthocytic RBCs, steatorrhea, failure of beta lipoprotein manufacture, neurologic findings)
Biopsy may or may not be of specific diagnostic value in
    Amyloidosis
    Intestinal lymphangiectasia

---

* J. S. Trier, "Diagnostic Value of Peroral Biopsy of the Proximal Small Intestine," *New Eng. J. Med.* 285 (Dec. 23, 1971): 1470–1473.

      Malignant lymphoma of small bowel
      Eosinophilic gastroenteritis
      Regional enteritis
      Hypogammaglobulinemia and dysgammaglobulinemia
      Systemic mastocytosis
      Parasitic infestations (giardiasis, coccidiosis, strongyloidiasis, capillariasis)
Biopsy may be abnormal but not diagnostic in
      Tropical sprue
      Folate deficiency
      Vitamin B_{12} deficiency
      Radiation enteritis
      Zollinger-Ellison syndrome
      Stasis with intraluminal bacterial overgrowth
      Drug-induced lesions (neomycin, antimetabolites)
      Malnutrition
Biopsy is normal in
      Cirrhosis
      Pancreatic exocrine insufficiency
      Postgastrectomy malabsorption without intestinal mucosal disease
      Functional bowel disease (irritable colon, nonspecific diarrhea)

(*Biopsy taken at duodenojejunal junction by x-ray localization, prompt fixation of tissue, proper orientation of tissue for histologic sectioning, and serial sectioning of specimen are all necessary for proper interpretation.*)

RECTAL BIOPSY

Rectal biopsy is particularly useful in diagnosis of
      Cancer of rectosigmoid
      Polyps of rectosigmoid
      Secondary amyloidosis
      Amebic ulceration
      Schistosomiasis (even when no lesions are visible)
      Hirschsprung's disease

HIRSCHSPRUNG'S DISEASE (AGANGLIONIC MEGACOLON)

Rectal biopsy to include muscle layers shows absence of myenteric plexus ganglia in muscle layers.

CHRONIC NONSPECIFIC ULCERATIVE COLITIS

Parallels severity of the disease
      Anemia due to blood loss (frequently Hb = 6 gm/100 ml)
      WBC usually normal unless complication occurs (e.g., abscess)
      ESR often normal or only slightly increased
Stools
      Positive for blood (gross and/or occult)
      Negative for usual enteric bacterial pathogens and parasites; high total bacterial count
Changes in liver function
      Microscopic changes in needle biopsy of liver
      BSP test sometimes abnormal

Serum alkaline phosphatase often increased slightly
Other liver function tests usually normal
Changes in serum electrolytes due to diarrhea or to therapy with
adrenal steroids or ACTH
Laboratory changes due to complications or sequelae
Malabsorption due to involvement of small intestine
Perforation
Abscess formation
Hemorrhage
Carcinoma
Arthritis
Etc.
Rectal biopsy

GONOCOCCAL PROCTITIS
(See pp. 378–379)

HEREDITARY GASTROINTESTINAL POLYPOSIS

Laboratory findings due to intestinal polyps and due to associated
lesions
Familial polyposis of colon
Occasional discrete polyps of colon and rectum
Peutz-Jeghers syndrome
Gardner's syndrome (see following section)
Turcot syndrome
Zollinger-Ellison syndrome

GARDNER'S SYNDROME
(multiple osteomas, fibrous and fatty tumors of skin and mesentery,
epidermoid inclusion cysts of skin, multiple polyposis)

Polyposis of the colon and rectum may develop before puberty and
show great tendency to become malignant.

CARCINOMA OF COLON

Blood in stool (occult or gross)
Evidence of inflammation
Increased WBC and ESR
Anemia
May be the only symptom of carcinoma of right side of colon
(present in more than 50% of these patients)
Usually hypochromic
Stools sometimes negative for occult blood
Evidence of metastases (see p. 188, on metastatic lesions of liver)
Biopsy of colon lesion

*Villous tumor of rectum may cause potassium depletion with decreased
serum potassium.*
Carcinoid tumors may cause increased 5-HIAA in urine.

Laboratory findings due to complications
Hemorrhage
Perforation
Obstruction

VILLOUS ADENOMA OF RECTUM

Stool
    Large amount of mucus tinged with blood; frequent watery
        diarrhea
Serum potassium sometimes decreased
Biopsy of lesion

MESENTERIC VASCULAR OCCLUSION

Chronic (mesenteric arterial insufficiency)
    Laboratory findings due to malabsorption and starvation
Acute
    Marked increase in WBC (15,000–25,000/cu mm or more) with
        shift to the left
    Laboratory findings due to intestinal hemorrhage, intestinal
        obstruction, metabolic acidosis, shock

INTESTINAL OBSTRUCTION

WBC is normal early. Later it tends to rise, with increase in
    polynuclear leukocytes; 15,000–25,000/cu mm suggests strangula-
    tion; more than 30,000/cu mm suggests mesenteric thrombosis.
Hemoglobin and hematocrit levels are normal early but later
    increase, with dehydration.
Urine
    Specific gravity increases, with deficit of water and electrolytes
        unless preexisting renal disease is present. Urinalysis helps
        rule out renal colic, diabetic acidosis, etc.
Gastric contents
    Positive guaiac test suggests strangulation; there may be gross
        blood if strangulated segment is high in jejunum.
Rectal contents
    Gross rectal blood suggests carcinoma of colon or intussuscep-
        tion.
Decreased serum sodium, potassium, chloride, and pH, and in-
    creased CO_2 are helpful indications for following the course of the
    patient and to guide therapy.
Increased BUN suggests blood in intestine or renal damage.
Serum amylase may be moderately increased in absence of pancrea-
    titis.
Increased serum LDH may indicate strangulation (infarction) of
    small intestine.

GALLSTONE ILEUS

Laboratory findings due to preceding chronic cholecystitis and
    cholelithiasis
Laboratory findings due to acute obstruction of terminal ileum
    (*accounts for 1–2% of these cases*)

GASTROINTESTINAL COMPLICATIONS OF
ANTICOAGULANT THERAPY

Hemorrhage into gastrointestinal tract occurs in 3–4% of patients on
    anticoagulant therapy; may be spontaneous or secondary to
    unsuspected disease (e.g., peptic ulcer, carcinoma, diverticula,

hemorrhoids). Occasionally there is hemorrhage into the wall of the intestine with secondary ileus. Prothrombin time may be in the therapeutic range or, more commonly, is increased. *Coumarin drug action is potentiated by administration of aspirin, antibiotics, phenylbutazone, and thyroxine and T tube drainage of the common bile duct, especially if pancreatic disease is present.*
Hypersensitivity to phenindione may cause hepatitis or steatorrhea.

GASTROINTESTINAL HEMORRHAGE

Due To
Duodenal ulcer (25% of patients)
Esophageal varices (18%)
Gastric ulcer (12%)
Gastritis (12%)
Esophagitis (6%)
Mallory-Weiss syndrome (5%)
Others (22%)

With previously known GI tract lesions, 40% of patients bled from a different lesion.

In addition to the main cause of bleeding, 50% of patients have an additional lesion that could cause hemorrhage (especially duodenal ulcer, esophageal varices, hiatus hernia).

27

Hepatobiliary Diseases and Disorders of the Pancreas

HEPATIC INVOLVEMENT IN SYSTEMIC DISEASES

Infections (e.g., infectious mononucleosis, cytomegalic inclusion disease, Q fever, leptospirosis, lobar pneumonia, typhoid, granulomas such as those with tuberculosis and brucellosis)

Infestations (e.g., schistosomiasis, echinococciasis, ascariasis, infection with *Toxocara canis*, amebiasis, toxoplasmosis)

Intoxications (e.g., alcohol)

Vascular diseases (e.g., congestive heart failure)

Hematologic diseases (e.g., leukemias, lymphomas, hemolytic anemias, polycythemia)

Endocrine diseases (e.g., hyperthyroidism, diabetes mellitus, pregnancy)

Hereditary and metabolic diseases (e.g., mucopolysaccharidoses, glycogen-storage diseases, sickle cell disease, histiocytoses, Wilson's disease, mucoviscidosis, fatty liver, ulcerative colitis)

Collagen diseases (e.g., SLE, polyarteritis)

ACUTE VIRAL HEPATITIS

Prodromal period
> BSP retention is the earliest abnormality, followed by bilirubinuria before serum bilirubin increases.
>
> Cephalin flocculation becomes positive at the same time that direct serum bilirubin increases.
>
> There is an increase in urinary urobilinogen and total serum bilirubin just before clinical jaundice occurs.
>
> Serum SGOT and SGPT both rise during the preicteric phase and show very high peaks (more than 500 units) by the time jaundice appears.
>
> ESR is normal.
>
> Leukopenia (lymphopenia and neutropenia) is noted with onset of fever, followed by relative lymphocytosis and monocytosis; atypical lymphocytes and plasma cells may be found.

Acute icteric period (tests show parenchymal cell damage)
> Serum bilirubin is one-half to three-quarters direct in the early stage; later, indirect bilirubin is proportionately more.

Serum SGOT and SGPT fall rapidly in the several days after jaundice appears and become normal 2–5 weeks later.

In hepatitis associated with infectious mononucleosis, peak levels are usually less than 200 units and peak occurs 2–3 weeks after onset, becoming normal by the fifth week. *In toxic hepatitis*, levels depend upon severity; slight elevations may be associated with therapy with anticoagulants, anovulatory drugs, etc.; poisoning (e.g., carbon tetrachloride) may cause levels up to 300 units. *In severe toxic hepatitis* (*especially carbon tetrachloride poisoning*), serum enzymes may be 10–20 times higher than in acute hepatitis and show a different pattern, i.e., increase in LDH > SGOT > SGPT. *In acute hepatitis*, SGPT > SGOT > LDH.

Serum aldolase is increased in 90% of patients, up to 10 times normal. It parallels transaminase with a sharp rise before serum bilirubin rises and a return to normal 2–3 weeks after jaundice begins.

Serum isocitric dehydrogenase (ICD) is usually elevated in the early stage (5–10 times normal) but returns to normal in 2–3 weeks; increase persists in chronic hepatitis.

Abnormal thymol turbidity and cephalin flocculation occur frequently; changes in toxic hepatitis are less striking.

Other liver function tests are often abnormal, depending on severity of the disease—bilirubinuria, abnormal serum protein electrophoresis, alkaline phosphatase, etc.

Serum cholesterol : ester ratio is usually depressed early; total serum cholesterol is decreased only in severe disease. Serum phospholipids are increased in mild but decreased in severe hepatitis. Plasma vitamin A is decreased in severe hepatitis.

Urine urobilinogen is increased in the early icteric period; at peak of the disease it disappears for days or weeks; urobilinogen simultaneously disappears from stool.

ESR is increased; falls during convalescence.

Serum iron is often increased.

Urine. Cylindruria is common; albuminuria occurs occasionally; concentrating ability is sometimes decreased.

Defervescent period

Diuresis occurs at onset of convalescence.

Bilirubinuria disappears while serum bilirubin is still increased. Urine urobilinogen increases.

Serum bilirubin becomes normal after 3–6 weeks.

Later, cephalin flocculation becomes normal. Still later, thymol turbidity is normal.

ESR falls.

Anicteric Hepatitis

Laboratory findings are the same as in the icteric type, but abnormalities are usually less marked and there is slight or no increase of serum bilirubin.

Acute Fulminant Hepatitis with Hepatic Failure

Findings are the same as in acute hepatitis but more severe.

There are findings of hepatic failure.

Serum bilirubin is very high unless death occurs in the prodromal period.

Serum cholesterol and esters are markedly decreased.
Aminoaciduria occurs.
Patient may show anemia, leukocytosis, thrombocytopenia, etc.

Cholangiolitic Hepatitis
Same as acute hepatitis but evidence of obstruction is more prominent (e.g., increased serum alkaline phosphatase and direct serum
bilirubin) and tests of parenchymal damage are less marked (e.g.,
thymol turbidity is frequently normal; SGOT increase may be 3–6
times normal).

Viral Hepatitis Carrier State
Usually liver function tests and needle biopsy are normal.

Table 17. Comparison of Infectious Hepatitis and Serum Hepatitis

	Infectious Hepatitis	Serum Hepatitis
Incubation period	15–40 days	50–160 days
Abnormal SGOT	Transient 1–3 weeks	More prolonged 1–8+ months
Thymol turbidity	Usually increased during acute phase	Usually normal
Serum IgM levels	Usually increased above 400 mg/100 ml during acute phase	Usually normal
Australia antigen in blood	Not present	Present during incubation period and acute phase; occasionally may persist

Chronic Active Hepatitis
This is a nonalcoholic chronic liver disease of uncertain cause. Most
often is subacute form of viral hepatitis that progresses to
postnecrotic cirrhosis. Clinical course is variable and diagnosis
requires histologic confirmation. Includes some diseases labeled
autoimmune hepatitis, plasma cell hepatitis, chronic progressive
hepatitis, lupoid hepatitis, postnecrotic cirrhosis, juvenile cirrhosis, etc.

Serum SGOT and SGPT are usually increased (up to 10 times
normal range).
Serum bilirubin is increased (1–30 mg/100 ml).
Serum albumin may be decreased.
Serum gamma globulin may be increased.
LE preparation is positive in 10–20% of patients.
Hepatitis-associated antigen (HAA) is found in 25% of patients.
Anemia, leukopenia, and thrombocytopenia occur in 40–60% of
patients.

Laboratory findings due to associated conditions
(see appropriate separate sections)
    Ulcerative colitis
    Thyroiditis

Rheumatoid arthritis
SLE
After renal transplantation

"LUPOID" HEPATITIS

This is a severe active hepatitis with liver autoantibodies particularly in young adult females but is not part of systemic lupus erythematosus.

Liver function tests of severe hepatitis (increased transaminases, bilirubin, etc.)
Characteristic marked increase of serum gamma globulin
LE cells present in circulating blood
Positive Coombs' test, hemolytic anemia, etc., sometimes present
Positive autoimmune complement fixation tests in about half of patients
Increased plasma cells in bone marrow which may appear in peripheral blood
Decreased serum haptoglobins
Abnormal laboratory tests reversed by steroid therapy

SERUM ENZYME DETERMINATIONS IN LIVER DISEASES

Useful In
Diagnosis of asymptomatic, prodromal, or anicteric hepatitis (e.g., in infectious mononucleosis). Occurs earlier than other chemical abnormalities (e.g., thymol turbidity, increased serum bilirubin)
Following the course of hepatitis. Determine return to physical activity (if enzymes increase in response to activity, return to bed rest). Determine prognosis by recurring acute episodes or prolonged course with increased serum enzymes levels.
Differential diagnosis of diseases of liver, biliary tract, etc.
Screening prior to surgery for carcinoma (e.g., sudden rise in SGOT may indicate early liver metastases)
Screening of all blood donors

FATTY LIVER

Laboratory findings are due to underlying conditions (most commonly alcoholism; also diabetes mellitus, poor nutritional state, toxic chemicals, etc.).
Needle biopsy of liver establishes the diagnosis.
Liver function tests are normal in at least half the patients; others may show abnormalities of 1 or several tests including clinical jaundice.
Mild anemia and increased WBC may occur.

Not infrequently, fatty liver is the only postmortem finding in cases of sudden, unexpected death.

Table 18. Increased Serum Enzyme Levels in Liver Diseases

Serum Enzyme	Acute Viral Hepatitis		Obstructive Jaundice		Cirrhosis		Liver Metastases*	
	Frequency	Amplitude	Frequency	Amplitude	Frequency	Amplitude	Frequency	Amplitude
SGOT	>95%	14	>95%	3	75%	2	50%	1–2
SGPT	>95%	17	>95%	4	50%	1	25%	1–2
Alkaline phosphatase	60%	1–2	>95%	4–5	55%	1–2	50%	2
LAP	80%	1–2	85%	3	30%	1	70%	2–3
ICD	>95%	6	10%	1	20%	1	40%	2
5'-Nucleotidase	70%	1–2	>95%	6	50%	1–2	65%	3–4
Aldolase	90%	10		N		N	20%	

Frequency = average % frequency of cases with increased serum enzyme level when blood taken at optimal time.
Amplitude = average number of times normal that serum level is increased.
*E.g., tumor, tuberculosis, sarcoid, amyloid.

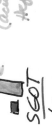

Alk Phos

Obstructive → Hepatitis

LDH

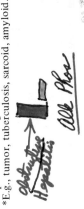

SGOT

Hepatocellular (acute Viral) Hepatitis

(SGPT even more marked, as more specific to liver)

Table 19. Serum Enzymes in Differential Diagnosis of Various Liver Diseases

Disease	Alkaline Phosphatase	SGOT	SGPT	ICD
Hepatitis	5–15 BU in over 80% of cases; 15–70 BU in 100% of cases during obstructive phase	Both rise during preicteric phase to peaks (more than 500 U) by the time jaundice appears; then rapid fall in several days; become normal 2–5 weeks after onset of jaundice		500–2000 in first week; less than 800 after 2 weeks; slightly elevated in 3rd week
Cirrhosis	5–15 BU in 40–55% of cases	Up to 300 U in 65–75% of cases	Up to 200 U in 50% of cases; wide fluctuation reflects activity of disease	Less than 500; poor prognosis if higher
Metastatic disease		Up to 300 U in 50% of cases	40–150 U	250–1000
Metastatic cancer	Up to 70 BU in 80% of cases			
Tuberculosis	Up to 50 BU in 50% of cases			
Sarcoidosis	Up to 18 BU in 40% of cases			
Amyloidosis	Up to 100 BU frequently			
Biliary obstruction Complete	Up to 70 BU in 100% of cases	Up to 300 U — Both return to normal within 1 week after obstruction is relieved	20–200 U	100–500
Incomplete (occlusion of 1 duct or incomplete occlusion of bile ducts)	Frequently 10–14 BU			
Congenital intrahepatic atresia	50–70 BU in 100% of cases			
Congenital extrahepatic atresia	Normal unless rickets is present			

U = units; BU = Bodansky units.

[182]

Table 20. Liver Function Tests in Differential Diagnosis of Jaundice

Disease	Urine		Stool		Serum Bilirubin		Serum Cholesterol		Cephalin Flocculation and Thymol Turbidity
	Bilirubin	Urobilinogen	Bilirubin	Urobilinogen	Direct	Indirect	Total	Esters	
Viral hepatitis	I	N or I	D	D	I early	I predom.	N or D	Mild to marked D	I
Hepatitis due to drugs Hepatitic type	I	N or I	D	D	I early	I predom.	N		I
Cholestatic type	I	N or D	D	D	I	Slight I	I		N or slight I
Cirrhosis	I	N or I			I < indirect	I > direct	N or D	Mild to marked D	I
Extrahepatic biliary obstruction	I	D	D	Marked D	I	N or slight I	Mild to marked I		N or slight I

I = increase; D = decrease; N = normal.

[183]

Table 21. Comparison of Three Main Types of Liver Disease Due to Drugs

	Predominantly Cholestatic	Predominantly Hepatitic	Mixed Biochemical Pattern
Laboratory findings	Obstructive type of jaundice (See p. 189)		Some aspects of each type, but one may be more marked
	Average duration of jaundice = 2 weeks; may last for years		
	Serum bilirubin may be > 30 mg/100 ml		
	Alkaline phosphatase and LAP are markedly increased; may remain increased for years after jaundice has disappeared	Less markedly increased	
	SGOT, SGPT, LDH show mild to moderate increase	More markedly increased	
Some causative drugs	Organic arsenicals	Cinchophen	PAS and other antituberculosis agents
	Anabolic steroids	Monamine oxidase inhibitors (particularly iproniazid) *(MAO)*	
	Sulfonyl urea derivatives (including sulfonamides, phenothiazine tranquilizers, antidiabetic drugs, oral diuretics)	Isonicotinic acid hydrazide *(INH)*	
	Chlorpromazine		
	PAS (usually this type but may be mixed)		
	Erythromycin		
Pathology	Centrilobular bile stasis	Same as acute viral hepatitis	
	Low incidence		
	High mortality rate (20%)		

CIRRHOSIS OF LIVER

Serum bilirubin is often increased; may be present for years. Fluctuations may reflect liver status due to insults to the liver (e.g., alcoholic debauches). Most bilirubin is of the indirect type unless cirrhosis is of the cholangiolitic type. Higher and more stable levels occur in postnecrotic cirrhosis; lower and more fluctuating levels occur in Laennec's cirrhosis. Terminal icterus may be constant and severe.

Serum SGOT is increased (up to 300 units) in 65–75% of patients. Serum SGPT is increased (up to 200 units) in 50% of patients. Transaminases vary widely and reflect activity or progression of the process (i.e., hepatic parenchymal cell necrosis).

Serum ICD is normal or only slightly increased (less than 500 units) in 20% of patients. A large increase suggests a poorer prognosis.

Serum 5′-nucleotidase is increased in 50% of patients.

Serum alkaline phosphatase is increased (up to 15 Bodansky units) in 40–50% of patients. Serum LAP is slightly increased in 30% of patients.

Total serum protein is usually normal or decreased. Serum albumin parallels functional status of parenchymal cells and may be useful for following progress of liver disease; but it may be normal in the presence of considerable liver cell damage. Lowering of serum albumin may reflect development of ascites or hemorrhage. Serum globulin level is usually increased; it reflects inflammation and parallels the severity of the inflammation. Increased serum globulin may cause increased total protein especially in chronic (viral) hepatitis and posthepatitis cirrhosis. Increased globulin is usually gamma. (See Table 4, p. 56.)

Cephalin flocculation and thymol turbidity are usually abnormal and remain so for long periods. Therefore they are useful for differentiating parenchymal cell disease from obstructive or hemolytic jaundice but are not helpful guides for following the course of cirrhosis.

Total serum cholesterol is normal or decreased. Decreased esters reflect more severe parenchymal cell damage.

BSP retention is a rather sensitive index of liver function and is most useful in the absence of jaundice to follow the course of disease when the other liver function tests are normal.

Urine bilirubin is increased; urobilinogen is normal or increased.

Laboratory findings due to complications or sequelae
>   Ascites
>   Bleeding esophageal varices
>   Hypersplenism
>   Hepatoma
>   Portal vein thrombosis
>   Hepatic coma
>   Etc.

BUN is often decreased (less than 10 mg/100 ml); increased with gastrointestinal hemorrhage.

Serum uric acid is often increased.

Electrolytes and acid-base balance are often abnormal and reflect various combinations of circumstances at the time, such as malnutrition, dehydration, hemorrhage, metabolic acidosis, respiratory alkalosis. In cirrhosis with ascites, the kidney retains increased sodium and excessive water causing dilutional hyponatremia.

Anemia reflects increased plasma volume and some increased destruction of RBCs. If more severe, rule out hemorrhage in gastrointestinal tract, folic acid deficiency, excessive hemolysis, etc.

WBC is usually normal with active cirrhosis; increased (up to 50,000/cu mm) with massive necrosis, hemorrhage, etc.; decreased with hypersplenism.

Blood ammonia level is increased in liver coma and cirrhosis and with portacaval shunting of blood.

Abnormalities of coagulation mechanisms

> Prolonged prothrombin time (does not respond to parenteral vitamin K as frequently as in patients with obstructive jaundice)

> Abnormal TGT reflecting various abnormalities

Biopsy of liver is valuable.

Laboratory findings due to associated diseases or conditions (see appropriate separate sections)

> Alcoholism
> Wilson's disease
> Hemochromatosis
> Mucoviscidosis
> Glycogen-storage diseases
> Porphyria
> Fanconi syndrome
> Schistosomiasis
> Gaucher's disease
> Ulcerative colitis
> Osler-Weber-Rendu disease

CHOLANGIOLITIC CIRRHOSIS (HANOT'S HYPERTROPHIC CIRRHOSIS, PRIMARY INTRAHEPATIC BILIARY CIRRHOSIS, ETC.)

Laboratory findings of complete biliary obstruction (see p. 189) of long duration (may last for years) but often of fluctuating intensity are noted.

Laboratory findings show relatively little evidence of parenchymal damage.

Marked increase in total cholesterol and phospholipids takes place, with normal triglycerides; serum is not lipemic. The increase is associated with xanthomas and xanthelasmas.

Serum globulins (especially beta and alpha$_2$) are increased. Albumin is normal or slightly decreased early; later decreased.

Thymol turbidity is usually increased; cephalin flocculation is negative or positive.

There are laboratory findings of steatorrhea, but prothrombin time is normal or restored to normal by parenteral vitamin K.

Urine contains urobilinogen and bilirubin.

WILSON'S DISEASE

Serum ceruloplasmin is decreased (less than 20 mg/100 ml). (*It is normal in 5% of patients with overt Wilson's disease.*)

Total serum copper is decreased.

Nonceruloplasmin copper is increased.

Urinary copper is increased (more than 100 μg/24 hours).

Liver biopsy shows high copper concentration (more than 250 μg/gm of dry liver).

Liver biopsy may show no abnormalities, moderate to marked fatty changes with or without fibrosis, or active or inactive cirrhosis.
Liver function tests are abnormal depending on the type and severity of disease (e.g., transaminase).
Aminoaciduria, especially cystine and threonine, may be found.
Decreased serum uric acid may occur.

Decreased serum ceruloplasmin (less than 20 mg/100 ml) with increased hepatic copper (more than 250 µg/gm) occurs only in Wilson's disease or normal infants less than 6 months of age.
Heterozygous gene for Wilson's disease occurs in 1 in 200 in the general population; 10% of these have decreased serum ceruloplasmin.
Homozygous gene (clinical Wilson's disease) occurs in 1 in 200,000 in the general population.

PORTAL HYPERTENSION (WITH SHUNT FROM PORTAL SYSTEM VIA COLLATERAL CIRCULATION)

Increased blood ammonia
Increased postprandial blood glucose
Increased urine urobilinogen
Laboratory findings due to underlying disease
    Posthepatic obstruction (e.g., constrictive pericarditis, obstruction of hepatic veins, obstruction of inferior vena cava, cirrhosis)
    Intrahepatic obstruction (e.g., sickle cell disease)
    Prehepatic obstruction (e.g., occlusion of portal vein by thrombus or tumor, tumors, scars—as from schistosomiasis)
    Shunts (e.g., arteriovenous fistulas, hamartomas of liver)
Laboratory findings due to complications and sequelae
    Hypersplenism
    Intestinal malabsorption or protein loss
    Bleeding from esophageal varices

SURGICAL PORTACAVAL ANASTOMOSIS

In cirrhosis
    Operative mortality is less than 5% if
        Serum bilirubin is less than 3.0 mg/100 ml.
        Serum albumin is at least 3.5 gm/100 ml.
    Operative mortality is about 50% if
        Serum bilirubin is more than 8.0 mg/100 ml.
        Serum albumin is about 2.5 gm/100 ml.
Following surgery
    Serum indirect bilirubin is slightly increased.
    Blood ammonia is increased.
    Laboratory findings of hypersplenism decrease.

PORTAL VEIN THROMBOSIS

Laboratory findings due to underlying conditions (e.g., polycythemia, cirrhosis, neoplastic invasion of portal vein)
Laboratory findings due to infarction of intestine

HEPATOMA

Serum alpha-fetoprotein present in 50% of white and 75–90% of nonwhite patients
Laboratory findings associated with metastatic lesions of liver

Laboratory findings associated with underlying disease (more than 60% occur with preexisting cirrhosis)

    Hemochromatosis (up to 20% of patients die of hepatoma)

    More frequent in postnecrotic than in alcoholic cirrhosis

Sudden progressive worsening of laboratory findings of underlying disease

Hemoperitoneum—ascites in about 50% of patients but tumor cells found irregularly

Laboratory findings due to obstruction of hepatic or portal veins or inferior vena cava

Occasional marked hypoglycemia unresponsive to adrenalin injection

ESR and WBC sometimes increased

Anemia uncommon unless hemorrhage occurs

METASTATIC OR INFILTRATIVE DISEASE OF LIVER

Increased serum alkaline phosphatase is the most useful index of *partial obstruction of the biliary tree* when serum bilirubin is usually normal and urine bilirubin is increased.

    Increased in 80% of patients with metastatic carcinoma (up to 70 Bodansky units)

    Increased in 50% of patients with tuberculosis (up to 50 Bodansky units)

    Increased in 40% of patients with sarcoidosis (up to 18 Bodansky units)

    Increased frequently in patients with amyloidosis (up to 100 Bodansky units)

Increased serum LAP parallels alkaline phosphatase but is not affected by bone disease.

Whenever the alkaline phosphatase is increased, a simultaneous increase of 5'-N establishes biliary disease as the cause of the elevated alkaline phosphatase.

SGOT is increased in 50% of patients (up to 300 units).

SGPT is increased less frequently (up to 150 units).

ICD may show a moderate increase.

Increased serum alkaline phosphatase and increased BSP retention is 65% reliable to establish this diagnosis.

Radioactive scanning of the liver is 80% reliable.

Blind needle biopsy of the liver is positive in 65–75% of the patients.

Laboratory findings due to primary disease are noted. See also

    Carcinoid syndrome

    Pyogenic liver abscess

    Etc.

LIVER FUNCTION ABNORMALITIES IN CONGESTIVE HEART FAILURE

BSP retention is the most frequently abnormal test. It may indicate circulatory stasis as well as cellular damage.

Serum bilirubin is frequently increased (indirect more than direct); usually 1–5 mg/100 ml. It usually represents combined right- and left-sided failure with hepatic engorgement and pulmonary infarcts. Serum bilirubin may suddenly rise rapidly if superimposed myocardial infarction occurs.

Urine urobilinogen is increased. Urine bilirubin is increased in the presence of jaundice.

Thymol turbidity is abnormal in about 30% and cephalin flocculation test is positive in about 20% of cases.

SGOT and SGPT are increased in about 12% of patients.

Serum LDH is increased in about 40% of patients.

Serum alkaline phosphatase shows mild to moderate increase (6–25 Bodansky units) in 45% of cases.

Hypoalbuminemia is common with cardiac fibrosis of liver.

Prothrombin time may be slightly increased, with increased sensitivity to anticoagulant drugs.

Serum cholesterol and esters may be decreased.

These findings may occur with marked liver congestion due to other conditions, e.g., Chiari's syndrome (occlusion of hepatic veins) and constrictive pericarditis.

COMPLETE BILIARY OBSTRUCTION (INTRAHEPATIC OR EXTRAHEPATIC)

Direct serum bilirubin is increased; indirect serum bilirubin is normal or slightly increased.

Urine bilirubin is increased; urine urobilinogen, decreased.

There is decreased stool bilirubin and urobilinogen (clay-colored stools).

Serum alkaline phosphatase is markedly increased (15–70 Bodansky units). In extrahepatic type, the increase is related to the completeness of obstruction.

Serum LAP parallels alkaline phosphatase.

SGOT is increased (up to 300 units) and SGPT is increased (up to 200 units); they usually return to normal in 1 week after relief of obstruction.

Thymol turbidity, cephalin flocculation, and BSP test are normal or may later become only slightly increased.

Serum cholesterol is increased (acute, 300–400 mg/100 ml; chronic, up to 1000 mg/100 ml).

Serum phospholipids are increased.

Prothrombin time is prolonged, with response to parenteral vitamin K more frequent than in hepatic parenchymal cell disease.

Laboratory findings due to underlying causative disease are noted (e.g., stones, carcinoma of duct, metastatic carcinoma to periductal lymph nodes).

OBSTRUCTION OF ONE HEPATIC BILE DUCT

Serum bilirubin remains normal in the presence of serum alkaline phosphatase that is markedly increased.

DUBIN-JOHNSON SYNDROME (SPRINZ-NELSON DISEASE)

The disease resembles mild viral hepatitis. It is characterized by mild recurrent jaundice with hepatomegaly and right upper quadrant abdominal pain. It is due to inability to transport bilirubin-glucuronide through the parenchymal hepatic cell into the canaliculi; however, conjugation of bilirubin-glucuronide is normal. Usually it is compensated except in periods of stress. Jaundice (innocuous and reversible) may be produced by estrogens, last trimester of pregnancy, or oral contraceptives.

Serum bilirubin is increased (3–10 mg/100 ml; approximately 50% is indirect) in the chronic or intermittent form; usually familial.

Urine contains bile and urobilinogen.
Thymol turbidity may be increased.
Cephalin flocculation may be positive.
BSP excretion is impaired with *late* (1½- and 2-hour) rise.
Serum alkaline phosphatase is normal.
Liver biopsy shows large amounts of yellow brown or slate black
pigment in hepatic cells in centrilobular location; small amounts
in Kupffer's cells.

GILBERT'S DISEASE (CONSTITUTIONAL HEPATIC DYSFUNCTION)

Mild asymptomatic benign cases have an evanescent increase of
indirect serum bilirubin that is usually discovered on routine
laboratory examinations. The disease is due to inadequacy of
glucuronyl-transferase and probably represents a heterogeneous
group (e.g., late infectious hepatitis, mild familial congenital
disease) or may be a congenital defect that is aggravated by other
medical conditions. Jaundice is usually accentuated by pregnancy, fever, exercise, and various drugs including alcohol and oral
contraceptives.
Indirect serum bilirubin is increased. It may rise to 18 mg/100 ml
but usually is less than 4 mg/100 ml.
Fecal urobilinogen is decreased.
Urine shows no bilirubin.
BSP retention may be slightly increased.
Liver function tests are usually normal.

CRIGLER-NAJJAR SYNDROME

This rare familial autosomal recessive disease is due to marked
congenital deficiency or absence of glucuronyl-transferase that
conjugates bilirubin to bilirubin-glucuronide in hepatic cells
(counterpart is the homozygous Gunn rat).
Indirect serum bilirubin is increased; it appears on first or second
day of life, rises to 12–45 mg/100 ml, and persists for life.
Fecal urobilinogen is very low.
Liver function tests are normal.
Liver biopsy is normal.
There is no evidence of hemolysis.
Nonjaundiced parents have diminished capacity to form glucuron-
ide conjugates with menthol, salicylates, and tetrahydrocortisone.
This syndrome has been divided into two groups:

	Group I	Group II
Transmission	Autosomal recessive	Autosomal dominant
Hyperbilirubinemia	More severe	Less severe
Kernicterus	Frequent	Absent
Bile	Essentially colorless	Normal color
	Only traces of unconjugated bilirubin	Contains bilirubin glucuronide
Phenobarbital administration	Hyperbilirubine-mia unaffected	Jaundice disappears

Table 22. Liver Function Tests in Differential Diagnosis of Additional Causes of Jaundice

Disease	Urine		Stool		Serum Bilirubin		Liver Function Tests for	
	Bilirubin	Urobilinogen	Bilirubin	Urobilinogen	Direct	Indirect	Obstruction	Parenchymal Damage
Hemolytic jaundice	O	I	I	I	N or slight I ($<15\%$ of total)	I	N	N
Jaundice of the newborn	N	N	N or D	N or D	N or slight I	I		
Crigler-Najjar syndrome	N	N or D	D	N or D		I	N	N
Dubin-Johnson syndrome	I	I			I		N	N; late BSP excretion impaired
Rotor syndrome	N or I	N or I			I			Late BSP excretion impaired
Gilbert's disease	N	N or D	D	N or D		I	N	N

I = increase; D = decrease; N = normal; O = absent.

LUCEY-DRISCOLL SYNDROME
(transient familial neonatal hyperbilirubinemia)

Newborn infants have severe nonhemolytic unconjugated hyperbilirubinemia with high risk of kernicterus.

Syndrome is due to unidentified substance in mother's serum only
during last trimester of pregnancy that inhibits glucuronyl transferase activity.

NEONATAL PHYSIOLOGIC HYPERBILIRUBINEMIA

This is a transient unconjugated hyperbilirubinemia ("physiologic
jaundice") that occurs in most newborns.

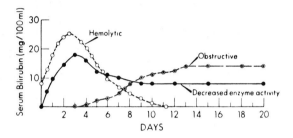

Fig. 5. Comparison of Progressive Changes in Serum Bilirubin
Levels During Prolonged Jaundice in Infancy Due to Hemolytic
Jaundice, Obstruction (e.g., biliary atresia, cystic fibrosis, "inspissat-
ed bile syndrome," neonatal hepatitis, galactosemia), Decreased
Liver Enzyme Activity (e.g., prematurity, Gilbert's disease, Crigler-
Najjar syndrome, breast feeding, infections such as cytomegalic
inclusion disease and toxoplasmosis, "physiologic" disorders)

HEPATIC CHOLESTEROL ESTER STORAGE DISEASE

In this inherited familial disorder an enlarged liver contains excessive deposition of cholesterol esters and serum bile acid levels are
increased.

Liver chemical function tests are normal.

Other blood chemistries are normal (including carotene, vitamin A,
ceruloplasmin).

Serum lipid profiles may show a moderate increase in esterified
cholesterol, phospholipid, triglyceride.

Lipoprotein electrophoresis may show slight decrease in alpha or
slight increase in beta and prebeta.

Biopsy of liver reveals brilliant orange yellow color. Polarized light
shows crystalline material in parenchymal cells. There is chemical
and histochemical confirmation of cholesterol esters. Septate
cirrhosis may be present histologically.

LIVER TRAUMA

Serum LDH is frequently increased (more than 1400 units) 8-12
hours after major injury. *Shock due to any injury may also increase
LDH.*

Other serum enzymes and liver function tests are not generally helpful.

Findings of abdominal paracentesis

Bloody fluid (in about three-quarters of the patients) confirming traumatic hemoperitoneum and indicating exploratory laparotomy

Nonbloody fluid (especially if injury occurred more than 24 hours earlier)

Microscopic—some red and white blood cells

Determine amylase, protein, pH, presence of bile.

SUPPURATIVE CHOLANGITIS

Marked increase in WBC (up to 30,000/cu mm) with increase in granulocytes

Blood culture often positive

Laboratory findings of incomplete duct obstruction due to inflammation or of preceding complete duct obstruction that caused the cholangitis (e.g., stone, tumor, scar)

Laboratory findings of parenchymal cell necrosis and malfunction

Increased serum SGOT, SGPT, etc.

Increased urine urobilinogen

SUPPURATIVE PYLEPHLEBITIS

Polynuclear leukocytosis in more than 90% of patients; usually over 20,000/cu mm

Anemia of varying severity

Moderate increase in serum bilirubin in about 33% of patients

Other liver function tests positive in about 25% of patients

Needle biopsy of liver not helpful; contraindicated

Blood culture sometimes positive

Laboratory findings due to preceding disease (e.g., acute appendicitis, diverticulitis, ulcerative colitis)

PYOGENIC LIVER ABSCESS

Increase in WBC due to increase in granulocytes

Abnormalities of liver function tests

BSP retention

Decreased serum albumin, increased serum globulin

Positive cephalin flocculation

Increased serum alkaline phosphatase

Increased serum bilirubin ($>$ 10 mg/100 ml usually indicates pyogenic rather than amebic and suggests poorer prognosis because of more tissue destruction)

Other laboratory findings (see Metastatic or Infiltrative Disease of Liver, p. 188)

Anemia frequent

Laboratory findings due to complications (e.g., subphrenic abscess, pneumonia, empyema, bronchopleural fistula)

Patients with amebic abscess of liver due to *Entamoeba histolytica* also show positive serologic tests for ameba (see p. 419).

Stools may be negative for cysts and trophozoites.

Needle aspiration of abscess may show *E. histolytica* in 50% of the cases. (*Characteristic brown or anchovy-sauce color may be absent; secondary bacterial infection may be superimposed.*)

ACUTE CHOLECYSTITIS

Increased ESR, WBC (up to 20,000/cu mm) and other evidences of acute inflammatory process

Increased BSP retention (some cases) even if serum bilirubin is normal

Increased serum alkaline phosphatase (some cases) even if serum bilirubin is normal

Increased serum amylase and lipase in some cases

Laboratory findings of associated biliary obstruction if such obstruction is present

Laboratory findings of preexisting cholelithiasis (sometimes)

Laboratory findings of complications (e.g., empyema of gallbladder, perforation, cholangitis, liver abscess, pylephlebitis, pancreatitis, gallstone ileus)

Serum SGOT may be increased in 75% of patients.

CHRONIC CHOLECYSTITIS

May be mild laboratory findings of acute cholecystitis or no abnormal laboratory findings

May be laboratory findings of associated cholelithiasis

CHOLELITHIASIS

Laboratory findings of underlying conditions causing hypercholesterolemia (e.g., diabetes mellitus)

Laboratory findings of causative chronic hemolytic disease (e.g., hereditary spherocytosis)

Laboratory findings of resultant cholecystitis or choledocholithiasis, etc.

CHOLEDOCHOLITHIASIS

During or soon after an attack of biliary colic
    Increased WBC
    Increased serum bilirubin in about one-third of patients
    Increased urine bilirubin in about one-third of patients
    Increased serum and urine amylase

Fluctuating laboratory evidence of biliary obstruction (see p. 189)

Laboratory findings due to secondary cholangitis

In duodenal drainage, crystals of both calcium bilirubinate and cholesterin (some cases); 50% accurate (only useful in nonicteric patients)

BILIARY DYSKINESIA

Normal laboratory tests of biliary, hepatic, and pancreatic function
Normal WBC

CANCER OF GALLBLADDER AND BILE DUCTS

Laboratory findings reflect varying location and extent of tumor infiltration that may cause partial intrahepatic duct obstruction or obstruction of hepatic or common bile duct, metastases in liver, or associated cholangitis (see pp. 189, 188, 193); 50% of patients have jaundice at the time of hospitalization.

Laboratory findings of duct obstruction are of progressively increasing severity in contrast to the intermittent or fluctuating changes due to duct obstruction caused by stones. A papillary intraluminal duct carcinoma may undergo periods of sloughing, producing the findings of intermittent duct obstruction.

Stool is frequently positive for occult blood.

Anemia is present.

Cytologic examination of aspirated duodenal fluid may demonstrate malignant cells.

Laboratory findings of the preceding cholelithiasis are present (gallbladder cancer occurs in about 3% of patients with gallstones).

PARASITIC INFESTATION OF BILIARY SYSTEM

Laboratory findings due to biliary obstruction and to cholangitis
Infestation due to echinococcus, ascaris, liver flukes

POSTOPERATIVE JAUNDICE

This is usually due to a combination of factors.

Overproduction of bilirubin
Resorption of blood (e.g., hematoma, hemoperitoneum)
G-6-PD deficiency (see p. 259)
Sickle cell disease (see p. 254)
Hemolysis of transfused RBCs. The amount of hemoglobin produced is insufficient to cause jaundice unless other conditions (e.g., sepsis, hypoxemia, anesthesia) are present.
Impaired hepatocellular function
Halothane toxicity. Occurs 1 in 10,000 cases. WBC is increased in 2 days. Jaundice may not appear for several weeks but may occur earlier if there has been previous exposure. Laboratory findings of severe liver necrosis are present (e.g., marked increase of SGOT, prolonged prothrombin time), and there is 20% fatality.
Shock. Severe jaundice in 2% of these patients is due to trauma. (*Multiple factors are usually present, e.g., drugs, infection, transfusions.*) Serum bilirubin reaches 5–20 mg/100 ml 2–10 days after surgery; SGOT is 100–500 units; serum alkaline phosphatase is 2–3 times normal. *Clinical jaundice is found in only 20% of these patients with massive liver necrosis.*
Syndrome of benign postoperative intrahepatic cholestasis. Occurs in patients with difficult prolonged surgery, multiple transfusions, postoperative complications (e.g., hemorrhage, sepsis, kidney failure, heart failure). Serum bilirubin reaches 15–40 mg/100 ml 2–10 days after surgery; SGOT is usually less than 200 units; serum alkaline phosphatase shows marked but variable increase. Liver biopsy reveals dilated

bile canaliculi with bile casts, and minimal necrosis or infiltration of lymphocytes.

Bacterial infections, especially gram-negative septicemia and pneumococcal pneumonia. Occurs 5–12 days after onset of infection. Increased serum bilirubin is mild; there is variable increase in SGOT and serum alkaline phosphatase. Liver biopsy reveals intrahepatic cholestasis with mild periportal infiltration of leukocytes; there is little or no hepatic cell necrosis.

Preexisting anicteric hepatitis or cirrhosis

Drugs (see Table 21, p. 184)

Extrahepatic bile duct obstruction

Injury to bile duct. Jaundice usually occurs within 1 week. See also Cholangitis, p. 193; Subphrenic Abscess

See also Cholecystitis; Choledocholithiasis, p. 194.

ACUTE PANCREATITIS

Serum amylase increase begins in 3–6 hours, rises to over 250 Somogyi units within 8 hours in three-quarters of the patients, reaches maximum in 20–30 hours, and may persist for 48–72 hours. The increase may be up to 40 times normal, but the height of the increase does not correlate with the severity of the disease. The level should be at least 500 Somogyi units/100 ml to be significant of acute pancreatitis. *More than 10% of patients with acute pancreatitis may have normal values even when dying of acute pancreatitis. Similar high values may occur in obstruction of pancreatic duct which tend to fall after several days.*

Serum lipase increases in half of the patients and may remain elevated for as long as 14 days after amylase returns to normal. (*Lipase should always be determined whenever amylase is determined since the amylase may have already returned to normal values.*) Urinary lipase is not clinically useful.

Serum calcium is decreased in severe cases 1–9 days after onset (due to binding to soaps in fat necrosis). The decrease usually occurs after amylase and lipase levels have become normal. Tetany may occur. (*Rule out hyperparathyroidism if serum calcium is high or fails to fall in hyperamylasemia of acute pancreatitis.*)

Increased urinary amylase tends to reflect serum changes by a time lag of 6–10 hours, but sometimes increased urine levels are higher and of longer duration than serum levels. The 24-hour level may be normal even when some of the 1-hour specimens show increased values. Amylase levels in hourly samples of urine may be useful.

Serum bilirubin may be increased when pancreatitis is of biliary tract origin but is usually normal in alcoholic pancreatitis.

Other nonspecific serum enzymes may also be increased (e.g., LDH, MDH, LAP, ALD, SGOT). Serum SGOT may correlate with serum bilirubin rather than with amylase, lipase, or calcium levels. Serum alkaline phosphatase is increased when serum bilirubin is elevated and parallels serum bilirubin.

Serum trypsin is increased.

WBC is slightly to moderately increased (10,000–20,000/cu mm).

Hemoconcentration occurs (increased hematocrit).

Mild increase of blood sugar is common.

Glycosuria appears in one-quarter of the patients.

Ascites may develop, cloudy or bloody or "prune juice" fluid, one-half liter to 2 liters in volume, containing increased amylase with a level higher than that of serum amylase. No bile is evident (unlike the situation in perforated ulcer). Gram stain shows no bacteria (unlike the situation in infarct of intestine).

CHRONIC PANCREATIC DISEASE (CHRONIC PANCREATITIS; CARCINOMA OF PANCREAS)

Examine duodenal contents (volume, bicarbonate concentration, amylase output) after IV administration of pancreozymin and secretin. Some abnormality occurs in more than 85% of patients with chronic pancreatitis. Amylase output is the most frequent abnormality. When all three are abnormal, there is a greater frequency of abnormality in the tests listed below.

Serum amylase and lipase increase after administration of pancreozymin and secretin in almost 20% of patients with chronic pancreatitis. They are more often abnormal when duodenal contents are normal.

Fasting serum amylase and lipase increase in 10% of patients with chronic pancreatitis.

There will be a diabetic oral glucose tolerance test (GTT) in 65% of patients with chronic pancreatitis and frank diabetes in more than 10% of patients with chronic relapsing pancreatitis. When GTT is normal in the presence of steatorrhea, the cause should be sought elsewhere than in the pancreas.

Chemical determination of fecal fat demonstrates steatorrhea. It is more sensitive than tests using triolein ^{131}I.

Triolein ^{131}I is abnormal in 33% of patients with chronic pancreatitis.

Starch tolerance test is abnormal in 25% of patients with chronic pancreatitis.

Radioactive scanning of pancreas (selenium) yields variable findings in different clinics.

See Laboratory Diagnosis of Malabsorption, p. 170.

Laboratory findings due to underlying conditions are noted (e.g., alcoholism, trauma, duodenal ulcer, cholelithiasis).

PSEUDOCYST OF PANCREAS

Serum direct bilirubin is increased (more than 2 mg/100 ml) in 10% of patients.

Serum alkaline phosphatase is increased (more than 5 Bodansky units) in 10% of patients.

Fasting blood sugar is increased in less than 10% of patients.

Laboratory findings of preceding acute pancreatitis are present (this is mild and unrecognized in one-third of the cases). Persistent increase of serum amylase and lipase after an acute episode may indicate formation of a pseudocyst.

Duodenal contents after secretin-pancreozymin stimulation usually show decreased bicarbonate content (less than 70 mEq/L) but normal volume and normal content of amylase, lipase, and trypsin.

Laboratory findings due to conditions preceding acute pancreatitis are noted (e.g., alcoholism, trauma, duodenal ulcer, cholelithiasis).

CYSTIC FIBROSIS OF PANCREAS (MUCOVISCIDOSIS)

Striking increase in sweat sodium and chloride (more than 60 mEq/L) and to a lesser extent potassium is present in virtually all homozygous patients. It is present throughout life from time of birth and is not related to severity of disease or organ involvement. There is a broad range of values in this disease and in normal but minimal overlap (see Sweat Electrolytes, p. 123). (*Sweat chloride is somewhat more reliable than sodium for diagnostic purposes.*) Sweat sodium and chloride increase is not useful for determination of heterozygosity or genetic counseling.

Serum chloride, sodium, potassium, calcium, and phosphorus are normal unless complications occur (e.g., chronic pulmonary disease with accumulation of CO_2, massive salt loss due to sweating).

Urine electrolytes are normal.

Submaxillary saliva has slightly increased chloride and sodium but not potassium; however, considerable overlap with normal individuals prevents diagnostic usage. Submaxillary saliva also is more turbid, with increased calcium, total protein, and amylase. These changes are not generally found in parotid saliva.

Serum protein electrophoresis shows increasing gamma globulin with progressive pulmonary disease, mainly due to immunoglobulin G and A; M and D are not appreciably increased.

Serum albumin is often decreased (because of hemodilution due to cor pulmonale; may be found before cardiac involvement is clinically apparent). In late stages of chronic lung disease, decreased serum electrolytes, hemoglobin, hematocrit level, etc., may also reflect hemodilution.

Bacteriology. Hemolytic *Staphylococcus aureus* is the most frequent and important organism in the respiratory tract; *Pseudomonas aeruginosa* has recently been found increasingly often.

Adrenal and pituitary function tests are normal.

Laboratory changes secondary to complications (e.g., pancreatic deficiency, chronic pulmonary disease, excessive loss of electrolytes in sweat, cirrhosis of liver, intestinal obstruction)

> Pancreas
>> 80% of patients show loss of all pancreatic enzyme activity
>> 10% of patients show decrease of pancreatic enzyme activity
>> 10% of patients show normal pancreatic enzyme activity
> Cirrhosis (infrequent)
> Chronic lung disease (*especially upper lobes*) with laboratory changes due to accumulation of CO_2, severe recurrent infection, secondary cor pulmonale, etc.
> Meconium ileus during early infancy

Stool shows lack of trypsin digestion of x-ray film gelatin; this is a useful screening test up to the age of 4 years.

CARCINOMA OF BODY OR TAIL OF PANCREAS

Laboratory tests are often normal.

Serum amylase and lipase may be slightly increased in early stages (less than 10% of cases); with later destruction of pancreas, they are normal or decreased. They may increase following secretin-pancreozymin stimulation before destruction is extensive; therefore, the increase is less marked with a diabetic glucose tolerance curve. Serum amylase response is less reliable.

Glucose tolerance curve is of the diabetic type in one-half of the patients. Flat blood sugar curve with IV tolbutamide tolerance test indicates destruction of islet cell tissue. Unstable, insulin-sensitive diabetes that develops in an older man should arouse suspicion of carcinoma of the pancreas.

Secretin-pancreozymin stimulation evidences duct obstruction when duodenal intubation shows decreased volume of duodenal contents (less than 10 cc/10-minute collection period) with usually normal bicarbonate and enzyme levels in duodenal contents. Acinar destruction (as in pancreatitis) shows normal volume (20–30 cc/10-minute collection period), but bicarbonate and enzyme levels may be decreased. In carcinoma, the test result depends on the relative extent and combination of acinar destruction and of duct obstruction. Cytologic examination of duodenal contents shows malignant cells in 40% of cases.

Serum leucine amino peptidase (LAP) is increased (over 300 units) in 60% of patients with carcinoma of pancreas due to liver metastases or biliary tract obstruction. *It may also be increased in chronic liver disease.*

Triolein ^{131}I test demonstrates pancreatic duct obstruction with absence of lipase in the intestine causing flat blood curves and increased stool excretion.

Radioisotope scanning of pancreas may be done (^{75}Se) for lesions > 2 cm.

CARCINOMA OF HEAD OF PANCREAS

The abnormal pancreatic function tests that occur with carcinoma of the body of the pancreas (see above) may be evident.

Laboratory findings due to complete obstruction of common bile duct

> Serum bilirubin increased (12–25 mg/100 ml), mostly direct. (Increase is persistent and nonfluctuating.)
>
> Serum alkaline phosphatase increased (usually 12–30 Bodansky units)
>
> Urine and stool urobilinogen absent
>
> Increased prothrombin time; normal after IV vitamin K administration
>
> Increased serum cholesterol (usually more than 300 mg/100 ml) with esters not decreased
>
> Other liver function tests (e.g., thymol turbidity, cephalin flocculation) usually normal

See tests listed in sections on other diseases of pancreas, pp. 196–199.

MACROAMYLASEMIA

Serum amylase persistently increased
Urine amylase normal or low

28

Diseases of the Central and Peripheral Nervous System

METABOLIC CAUSES OF COMA

Hypoglycemia (due to insulin, liver diseases, etc.)
Metabolic deficiencies (e.g., vitamin B_{12}, thiamine, niacin, pyridoxine)
Diseases of other organs
  Hepatic coma
  Uremia
  Lung (CO_2 narcosis)
  Pancreas (diabetic coma, hypoglycemia)
  Thyroid (myxedema, thyrotoxicosis)
  Parathyroid (hypoparathyroidism, hyperparathyroidism)
  Adrenal (Addison's disease; pheochromocytoma; Cushing's disease)
  Pituitary
  Porphyria
  Aminoacidurias
  Also leukodystrophies, lipid storage diseases, Bassen-Kornzweig syndrome, etc.
Abnormalities of electrolytes and acid-base balance
  Acidosis (metabolic, respiratory)
  Alkalosis (metabolic, respiratory)
  Water and sodium (hypernatremia, hyponatremia)
  Serum potassium (increased, decreased)
  Serum calcium (increased, decreased)
  Serum magnesium (increased, decreased)
Poisons
  Sedatives (especially alcohol, barbiturates)
  Enzyme inhibitors (especially salicylates, heavy metals, organic phosphates, cyanide)
  Others (e.g., methyl alcohol, paraldehyde, ethylene glycol)
Cerebral hypoxia
  Decreased blood O_2 content with normal tension (e.g., anemia, carbon monoxide poisoning, methemoglobinemia)
  Decreased blood O_2 tension and content (e.g., decreased atmos-

pheric O_2 tension [high altitude], lung disease, alveolar hypoventilation)

Cerebral ischemia

Decreased cardiac output (e.g., cardiac arrhythmias and Adams-Stokes disease, congestive heart failure, myocardial infarction, aortic stenosis)

Decreased peripheral resistance in systemic circulation (e.g., low blood volume, syncope, carotid sinus hypersensitivity)

Increased cerebral vascular resistance (e.g., increased blood viscosity as in polycythemia, hypertensive encephalopathy, hyperventilation syndrome)

NORMAL CSF

Found in

Korsakoff's syndrome

Wernicke's encephalopathy

Alzheimer's disease (diffuse cerebral atrophy)

Jakob-Creutzfeld disease

Tuberous sclerosis (protein rarely increased)

Idiopathic epilepsy (*If protein is increased, rule out neoplasm; if cell count is increased, rule out neoplasm or inflammation.*)

Narcolepsy, cataplexy, etc.

Parkinson's disease

Hereditary cerebellar degenerations

Migraine

Ménière's syndrome

Psychiatric conditions (e.g., neurocirculatory asthenia, hysteria, depression, anxiety, schizophrenia) (*Rule out psychiatric condition as a manifestation of primary disease, e.g., drugs, porphyria, primary endocrine diseases.*)

Transient cerebral ischemia

Amyotrophic lateral sclerosis

Muscular dystrophy

Progressive muscular atrophy

Syringomyelia

Vitamin B_{12} deficiency with subacute combined degeneration of spinal cord

Pellagra

Beriberi

Subacute myelo-optico-neuropathy (SMON)

Table 23. Cerebrospinal Fluid Findings in Various Diseases

Disease	Appearance	Initial Pressure (mm of water)	Protein (mg/100 ml)	Fasting Sugar (mg/100 ml)	WBC/cu mm
Normal	Clear, colorless, no clot	70–180		45–80	0–10
Ventricular			5–15		
Cisternal			10–25		
Lumbar			15–45		
Tuberculous meningitis	O, slightly yellow, delicate clot	Usually I	45–500	10–45	25–1000, chiefly L
Acute pyogenic meningitis	O to Pu, slightly yellow, coarse clot	Usually I	50–1500	0–45	25–10,000, chiefly P
Aseptic meningeal reaction	C or T or X	Often N	20–200+	N	Up to 500, occasionally 2000
Syphilis					
Tabes dorsalis	N	N	25–100	N	10–80
General paresis	N	N	50–300	N	10–150
Meningovascular syphilis	N	N	45–150, N in 30%	N	10–100, N in 45%
Acute anterior poliomyelitis	C or slightly O, may be slightly yellow, may be delicate clot	Usually N, may be I	20–350	N	10–500+, L P
Other virus					
Mumps	N or O	N or slightly I	20–125	N	0–2000+
Measles	N or O	N or slightly I	Slightly I	N	Up to 500
Herpes zoster	N	N	20–110	N	1 up to 300 in 40% of patients

Equine, St. Louis, choriomeningitis	N or slightly T	N or I	20–200+	N	10–200, occasionally to 3000
Postinfectious encephalitis	N	May be slightly I	15–75	N	5–200, rarely to 1000
Toxoplasmosis (congenital)	X	I	Up to 2000		50–500, chiefly monocytes
Cryptococcal meningitis	N		Up to 500 mg/100 ml in 90% of cases	Moderately decreased in 55% of cases	Up to 800 (more L than P)
Coccidioidomycosis		I	I	Frequently D	Up to 200
Primary amebic meningoencephalitis (due to free-living naegleria)	Sanguinopurulent, may be T or Pu	I	I	Usually D	400–21,000 (predominantly P) Usually RBC are also found. Amebas seen on Wright's stain
Tumor					
Cord	C, occasionally X	N or D	Up to 3500 in 85%, N in 15%	N	Up to 100, chiefly L; N in 60%
Brain	C, occasionally X	I	Up to 500	N	Up to 150, N in 75%
Pseudotumor cerebri	N	I	N	N	N
Cerebral thrombosis	N	25% I, 75% N	Up to 100+, N in 60%	N	Up to 50, N in 75%

Continued on next page

See footnotes on page 205.

Table 23 *(continued)*

Disease	Appearance	Initial Pressure (mm of water)	Protein (mg/100 ml)	Fasting Sugar (mg/100 ml)	WBC/cu mm
Cerebral hemorrhage	N in 15%, X in 10%, B in 75%	80% I, 20% N	Up to 2000, usually I	N	Same as in blood, N in 10%
Subarachnoid hemorrhage (ruptured berry aneurysm)	B, X in 24 hours, no clot	Usually I	Up to 1000+, usually I	N	Same as in blood
Bloody tap (traumatic)	B	N or D	I by blood	N	Same as in blood
Head trauma	N, B, or X	Often I	I if bloody	N	Same as in blood
Subdural hematoma	N, B only with contusion	80% I, 20% N	N or slightly I	N	Same as in blood
Multiple sclerosis	N	N	Up to 130, N in 75%; IgG I in 75%	N	Up to 40, N in 70%
Polyneuritis	N; X if protein is very I	N	Usually N	N	N, but albumino-cytologic dissociation in Guillain-Barré syndrome that may occur in heavy metal poisoning, infection, etc.
Polyarteritis		N	Usually N	N	
Porphyria		N	Usually N	N	
Beriberi		N	Usually N	N	
Alcohol		N	Usually N	N	
Arsenic		N	Usually N	N	
Diabetes mellitus		N	Often up to 300	N	
Acute infections		N	Up to 1500	N	
Lead encephalopathy	N or slightly yellow	I	Up to 100	N	0–100
Alcoholism	N	May be I	N	N	Usually N
Diabetic coma	N	D	N	I	Usually N
Uremia	N	Usually I	N or I	N or I	Usually N
Epilepsy	N	N	N	N	N

C = clear; O = opalescent; T = turbid; N = normal; X = xanthochromic; B = bloody; Pu = purulent; I = increased; D = decreased; P = polynuclear neutrophilic leukocyte; L = lymphocyte.

General comments:

1. Spinal fluid sugar decreased by utilization by bacteria (pyogens or tubercle bacilli) or occasionally cancer cells in spinal fluid. Normally is about 20 mg/100 ml less than blood sugar (40–80% of blood sugar), a determination of which should be performed simultaneously. In pyogenic meningitis, may rapidly become N after antibiotic therapy. May be decreased in 10–20% of cases of lymphocytic choriomeningitis, encephalitis due to mumps, or herpes simplex.

2. Blood and spinal fluid serology positive in case of CNS syphilis; positive in 7–10% of active cases of infectious mononucleosis.

3. Must routinely make smears for gram stain and acid-fast stain since the other findings may be normal in these diseases. Occasionally animal inoculations may be required.

4. Cytology smears may be useful in finding cancer cells in occasional cases.

5. Spinal fluid chloride reflects only blood chloride level although in tuberculous meningitis a decrease of 25% may exceed the decrease of serum chlorides on account of dehydration and electrolyte loss.

6. Colloidal gold test is usually not of diagnostic value. Paretic or luetic colloidal gold curve is strongly suggestive of active multiple sclerosis in the absence of syphilis.

7. Cell counts refer to lymphocytes except for monocytes in toxoplasmosis and polynuclear neutrophils in pyogenic meningitis. *Beware of misinterpreting RBCs as leukocytes.*

8. Toxicology examination for drugs (e.g., alcohol, barbiturates), heavy metals (e.g., lead, arsenic).

9. SGOT and LDH are normal in primary brain tumor but may be increased in malignant tumor (carcinoma, leukemia, lymphoma), meningitis, and subarachnoid hemorrhage.

10. Viral isolation and serologic studies.

DIFFERENTIATION OF BLOODY CSF DUE TO SUBARACHNOID HEMORRHAGE AND TRAUMATIC LUMBAR PUNCTURE

CSF Findings	Subarachnoid Hemorrhage	Traumatic Lumbar Puncture
CSF pressure	Often increased	Low
Blood in tubes for collecting CSF	Mixture with blood is uniform in all tubes	Earlier tubes more bloody than later tubes
CSF clotting	Does not clot	Often clots
Xanthochromia	Present if more than 8–12 hours since cerebral hemorrhage	Absent unless patient is icteric
Immediate repeat of lumbar puncture at higher level	CSF same as initial puncture	CSF clear

TRANSAMINASE (GOT) IN CEREBROSPINAL FLUID

Normal CSF is not permeable to serum enzymes. Changes in GOT are irregular and generally of limited diagnostic value.

Increased In

Large infarcts of brain during first 10 days (In severe cases, serum GOT may also be increased; occurs in approximately 40% of patients.)

Approximately 40% of CNS tumors (various benign, malignant, and metastatic), depending on location, growth rate, etc.; chiefly useful as indicator of organic neurologic disease

Some other conditions (e.g., head injury, subarachnoid hemorrhage)

LACTIC DEHYDROGENASE (LDH) IN CEREBROSPINAL FLUID

Changes are of limited diagnostic value.

Increased In

Cerebrovascular accidents. Increase occurs frequently, reaches maximum level in 1–3 days, and is apparently not related to xanthochromia, RBC, WBC, protein, sugar, or chloride levels.

CNS tumors (primary and metastatic), depending on location, growth rate, etc.

Meningitis—mild increase in viral meningitis due to LDH_1 and LDH_2; more marked increase in bacterial meningitis due to LDH_4 and LDH_5

CREATINE PHOSPHOKINASE (CPK) IN SPINAL FLUID

Test not useful because
> It does not consistently increase in various CNS diseases.
> No relationship to CSF protein, WBC, or RBC values
> No pattern of relationship of LDH and GOT in CSF
> No correlation of serum CPK and cerebrospinal fluid CPK

See Serum Creatine Phosphokinase, p. 53.

HEAD TRAUMA

Laboratory findings due to single or various combinations of brain injuries
> Contusion
> Laceration
> Subdural hemorrhage
> Extradural hemorrhage
> Subarachnoid hemorrhage

Laboratory findings due to complications (e.g., pneumonia, meningitis)

ACUTE EPIDURAL HEMORRHAGE

CSF is usually under increased pressure; clear unless there is associated cerebral contusion, laceration, or subarachnoid hemorrhage.

SUBDURAL HEMATOMA

CSF findings are variable: clear, bloody, or xanthochromic, depending on recent or old associated injuries (e.g., contusion, laceration).

Chronic subdural hematoma fluid is usually xanthochromic; protein content is 300–2000 mg/100 ml.

CEREBROVASCULAR ACCIDENT (NONTRAUMATIC)

Due To
Occlusion (thrombosis, embolism, etc.) in 80% of cases
Hemorrhage
> Ruptured berry aneurysm in 45% of cases
> Hypertension in 15% of cases
> Angiomatous malformations in 8% of cases
> Miscellaneous (e.g., brain tumor, blood dyscrasia)—infrequent
> Undetermined in the rest of the cases

CSF
> *In early subarachnoid hemorrhage* (less than 8 hours after onset of symptoms) the test for occult blood may be positive before xanthochromia develops. After bloody spinal fluid occurs, WBC:RBC ratio may be higher in CSF than in peripheral blood.
> *Bloody CSF* clears by tenth day in 40% of patients. *CSF is persistently abnormal* after 21 days in 15% of patients.
> *About 5% of cerebrovascular episodes due to hemorrhage* are wholly within the parenchyma with normal CSF.

See Serum Creatine Phosphokinase, p. 53.
See Serum Transaminase, p. 50.

CEREBRAL THROMBOSIS

Laboratory findings due to some diseases which may be causative
    Hematologic (e.g., polycythemia, sickle cell disease, thrombotic thrombopenia, macroglobulinemia)
    Arterial (e.g., polyarteritis nodosa, Takayasu's syndrome, dissecting aneurysm of aorta, syphilis, meningitis)
    Hypotension (e.g., myocardial infarction, shock)
CSF
    Protein normal or may be increased up to 100 mg/100 ml
    Cell count normal or up to 10 leukocytes/cu mm during first 48 hours and rarely up to 2000 leukocytes/cu mm transiently on third day
See Serum Creatine Phosphokinase, p. 53.
See Serum Transaminase, p. 50, and Table 23, pp. 202–205.

CEREBRAL EMBOLISM

Laboratory findings due to underlying causative disease
    Bacterial endocarditis
    Nonbacterial thrombotic vegetations on heart valves
    Chronic rheumatic mitral stenosis with mural thrombi
    Chronic atrial fibrillation (*Rule out underlying hyperthyroidism.*)
    Mural thrombus due to underlying myocardial infarctions
    Myxoma of left atrium
    Myocardial infarction
CSF
    Usually findings are the same as in cerebral thrombosis. One-third of patients develop hemorrhagic infarction, usually producing slight xanthochromia several days later; some of these cases may have grossly bloody CSF (10,000 RBC/cu mm). Septic embolism (e.g., bacterial endocarditis) may cause increased WBC (up to 200/cu mm with variable lymphocytes and polynuclear leukocytes), increased RBC (up to 1000/cu mm), slight xanthochromia, increased protein, normal sugar, negative culture.

INTRACEREBRAL HEMORRHAGE

Increased WBC (15,000–20,000/cu mm) (*higher than in cerebral occlusion, e.g., embolism, thrombosis*)
Increased ESR
Urine
    Transient glycosuria
    Laboratory findings of concomitant renal disease
Laboratory findings due to other causes of intracerebral hemorrhage (e.g., leukemia, aplastic anemia, purpuras, hemophilias, anticoagulant therapy, SLE, polyarteritis)
CSF
    See Table 23, pp. 202–205.

See Differentiation of Bloody CSF, p. 206.
See Cerebrovascular Accident (Nontraumatic), p. 207.

Especially if blood pressure is normal, always rule out ruptured berry aneurysm, hemorrhage into tumor, angioma.

RUPTURED BERRY ANEURYSM OF CEREBRAL VESSELS

See preceding section and Cerebrovascular Accident (Nontraumatic) (p. 207).
Laboratory findings due to other diseases which occur with increased frequency in association with berry aneurysm
    Coarctation of the aorta
    Polycystic kidneys
    Hypertension

HYPERTENSIVE ENCEPHALOPATHY

Laboratory findings due to changes in other organ systems
    Cardiac
    Renal
    Endocrine
    Toxemia of pregnancy
Laboratory findings due to progressive changes that may occur (e.g., focal intracerebral hemorrhage)
CSF frequently shows increased pressure and protein (up to 100 mg/100 ml).

PSEUDOTUMOR CEREBRI

CSF normal except for increased pressure
Laboratory findings due to underlying causative condition
    Corticosteroid administration, usually after reduction of dosage or change to different preparation
    Sex hormone administration
    Addison's disease
    Lateral sinus thrombosis (most commonly after otitis media)
    Acute hypocalcemia

BRAIN TUMOR

CSF findings
    CSF is clear, occasionally xanthochromic or bloody if there is hemorrhage into the tumor.
    WBC may be increased up to 150 cells/cu mm in one-quarter of cases; normal in others.
    Protein is usually increased.
    Tumor cells may be demonstrable.
    Glucose may be decreased if cells are present.

    CSF protein is particularly increased with meningioma of the olfactory groove and with acoustic neurinoma.

Laboratory findings due to underlying causative disease
    Primary brain tumors

Metastatic tumors, especially of bronchus, breast, kidney, GI tract (*hemorrhagic tumor particularly with choriocarcinoma and some bronchogenic carcinomas*)

Leukemias and lymphoma

Infections (e.g., tuberculoma, schistosomiasis, torulosis, hydatid cyst, cysticercosis)

Pituitary adenomas—CSF protein and pressure usually normal

See Brain Scanning, p. 134.

ANGIOMAS OF BRAIN (ARTERIAL-VENOUS COMMUNICATIONS)

Laboratory findings due to complications
Subarachnoid hemorrhage in 20%
Intracerebral hemorrhage in 20%
Convulsion in 50%

LEUKEMIC INVOLVEMENT OF CNS

Intracranial hemorrhage—principal cause of death in leukemia (may be intracerebral, subarachnoid, subdural)
More frequent when WBC is more than 100,000/cu mm and with rapid increase in WBC, especially in blastic crises
Platelet count frequently decreased
Evidence of bleeding elsewhere
Cerebrospinal fluid findings of intracranial hemorrhage (see pp. 207, 208)
Meningeal infiltration of leukemic cells
CSF may show
Increased pressure
Increased cells which are not usually recognized as blast cells because of poor preservation
Increased protein
Glucose decreased to less than half of blood level
Complicating meningeal infection (see next two sections)
Various bacteria
Opportunistic fungi (see pp. 409, 413, 416)

BACTERIAL MENINGITIS

CSF
See Table 23, pp. 202-205.

Three-quarters of cases are due to *Neisseria meningitidis*, pneumococcus, *Haemophilus influenzae. Bacteria can be identified in 90% of cases; culture is more reliable than gram stain although the stain offers a more immediate guide to therapy.*

Laboratory findings due to preceding diseases
Pneumonia, otitis media, sinusitis, skull fracture prior to pneumococcus meningitis
Neisseria epidemics prior to this meningitis
Bacterial endocarditis, septicemia, etc.
Laboratory findings due to complications (e.g., Waterhouse-Friderichsen syndrome)

Table 24. Etiology of Bacterial Meningitis by Age

	Newborns	Less Than 1 Year Old	1 to 5 Years Old	5 to 14 Years Old	More Than 15 Years Old
Most frequent	*Escherichia coli*	*Haemophilus influenzae*	*Haemophilus influenzae*	*Neisseria meningitidis*	Pneumococcus
Common	*Klebsiella-Aerobacter* Beta-hemolytic streptococcus *Staphylococcus aureus*	*Neisseria meningitidis* Pneumococcus	*Neisseria meningitidis* Pneumococcus	*Haemophilus influenzae* Pneumococcus	*Neisseria meningitidis* *Staphylococcus aureus*
Uncommon	Paracolon bacilli *Pseudomonas* species *Haemophilus influenzae*	*Pseudomonas* species *Staphylococcus aureus* Beta-hemolytic streptococcus *Escherichia coli*	Beta-hemolytic streptococcus		Beta-hemolytic streptococcus *Escherichia coli* *Pseudomonas* species
Rare	*Neisseria meningitidis*	*Klebsiella-Aerobacter*, paracolons, various other gram-negative organisms			*Haemophilus influenzae*

ASEPTIC MENINGITIS

CSF
> Protein is normal or slightly increased.
> Increased cell count shows predominantly leukocytes at first, later mononuclear cells.
> Glucose is normal.
> Bacterial cultures are negative.

> *If glucose levels are decreased, rule out tuberculosis, cryptococcosis, leukemia, lymphoma, metastatic carcinoma, sarcoid.*

Due To   (clinically most important types)
Viral infections (especially poliomyelitis, Coxsackie, ECHO, lymphocytic choriomeningitis, infectious mononucleosis, and many others)
Leptospirosis, syphilis
Tuberculosis, cryptococcosis (*CSF glucose levels may not be decreased until later stages.*)
Brain abscess, incompletely treated bacterial meningitis
Neoplasm (leukemia, carcinoma)

RECURRENT MENINGITIS

May Be Associated With
Bacterial infections
> Anatomic defects (traumatic or congenital)
> Adjacent foci of infection (e.g., paranasal sinusitis, mastoiditis, brain abscess, epidural abscess, subdural empyema)
> Immunologic deficiencies (e.g., sickle cell anemia, lymphoma, decreased immunoglobulins)
> Various infections (brucellosis, leptospirosis, tuberculosis, idiopathic)
Fungal infections
> Cryptococcosis
> Treatment failure in cases of blastomycosis, coccidioidomycosis, and histoplasmosis
Other infections
> Viral
> Cerebral hydatid cyst
Neoplasms of brain and spinal cord (e.g., hemangioma of third ventricle, ependymoma, craniopharyngioma)
Unknown etiology
> Sarcoidosis
> Mollaret's meningitis
> Behçet's syndrome
> Vogt-Koyanagi syndrome
> Harada's syndrome

PRIMARY AMEBIC MENINGOENCEPHALITIS
(due to free-living amebas—naegleria)

Increased WBC, predominantly neutrophils
CSF findings (see Table 23, pp. 202–205)
> Fluid may be cloudy, purulent, or sanguinopurulent.
> Protein is increased.
> Glucose is usually decreased; may be normal.

Increased WBCs are chiefly polynuclear neutrophilic leukocytes. RBCs are frequently present also. Motile amebas are seen in hemocytometer chamber.

Amebas are seen on Wright's stain. Gram's stain and cultures are negative for bacteria and fungi.

VON ECONOMO'S ENCEPHALITIS LETHARGICA

CSF changes appear in one-half of patients: increase in lymphocytes and variable increase in protein.

ACUTE ENCEPHALOMYELITIS
(postvaccinal, postexanthematous, postinfectious)

CSF shows increased protein and lymphocytes.
Laboratory findings due to preceding condition (e.g., measles) are noted.

MOLLARET'S MENINGITIS

Numerous recurrent episodes (2–7 days each) of aseptic meningitis occur over a period of several years with symptom-free intervals showing mild leukopenia and eosinophilia. Other organ systems are not involved. There is frequently a history of previous severe trauma with fractures and concussions.

CSF during first 12–24 hours may contain up to several thousand cells/cu mm, predominantly polynuclear neutrophils and up to 66% of a large type of mononuclear cell. The mononuclear cells (sometimes called "endothelial" cells) are of unknown origin and significance and are characterized by vague nuclear and cytoplasmic outline with rapid lysis even while being counted in the hemocytometer chamber; they may be seen only as "ghosts" and are usually not detectable after the first day of illness. After the first 24 hours, the polynuclear neutrophils disappear and are replaced by lymphocytes, which, in turn, rapidly disappear when the attack subsides.

CSF protein may be increased up to 100 mg/100 ml. CSF glucose is normal or may be slightly decreased.

GUILLAIN-BARRÉ SYNDROME

CSF shows albuminocytologic dissociation with normal cell count and increased protein (average, 50–100 mg/100 ml). Protein increase parallels increasing clinical severity; increase may be prolonged.

Laboratory findings due to underlying disease are noted (e.g., infectious mononucleosis, Refsum's disease).

MENTAL RETARDATION

Laboratory findings due to underlying causative condition
    Cretinism
    Mongolism
    Aminoacidurias
    Glycogen-storage disease
    Infections (e.g., syphilis, toxoplasmosis, cytomegalic inclusion disease)

Associated diseases (e.g., Turner's syndrome, congenital heart disease, tuberous sclerosis)
Kernicterus (erythroblastosis fetalis)

SENILE DEMENTIA (ALZHEIMER-PICK DISEASE; CEREBRAL ATROPHY)

There are no abnormal laboratory findings, but laboratory findings are useful to rule out other diseases that may resemble these syndromes but are amenable to therapy:
Neurosyphilis
Bromism
Myxedema
Vitamin B_{12} deficiency
Brain tumors
Others (see conditions listed under Metabolic Causes of Coma, pp. 200-201)

REFSUM'S DISEASE

This is a rare hereditary recessive lipidosis of the nervous system with retinitis pigmentosa, peripheral neuropathy, cerebellar ataxia, nerve deafness, and ichthyosis.
CSF shows albuminocytologic dissociation.

LEUKODYSTROPHY (DIFFUSE DEGENERATIVE TYPES OF CEREBRAL SCLEROSIS)

Urine sediment may contain metachromatic lipids (from breakdown of myelin products).

PROGRESSIVE CEREBELLAR ATAXIA WITH SKIN TELANGIECTASIAS

This is an autosomal recessive multisystem disease with cerebellar ataxia and oculocutaneous telangiectasia.
Some patients have
Glucose intolerance
Abnormal liver function tests
Decreased or absent serum IgA and IgE causing recurrent pulmonary infections; IgM present
Increased serum alpha-fetoprotein
See also Table 38, pp. 276-277.

TUBEROUS SCLEROSIS

This is a hereditary, familial, congenital anomaly of adenoma sebaceum, epilepsy, and mental retardation associated with sclerotic areas in the brain.
There are no abnormal laboratory findings.
Rarely, CSF protein is increased.

BASSEN-KORNZWEIG SYNDROME

Abnormal RBCs (acanthocytes) are present in the peripheral blood smear.

There may be
> Marked deficiency of serum beta lipoprotein and cholesterol
> Abnormal pattern of RBC phospholipids
> Marked impairment of GI fat absorption

LINDAU-VON HIPPEL DISEASE (HEMANGIOBLASTOMAS OF RETINA AND CEREBELLUM)

Laboratory findings due to associated conditions
> Polycythemia
> Pheochromocytomas
> Various tumors (e.g., kidney)

MULTIPLE SCLEROSIS

CSF shows a slight increase in mononuclear cells and normal or slightly increased protein (50% of cases). (*Diagnosis is probably multiple sclerosis if more than 20% is gamma globulin.*) The protein increase causes abnormal colloidal gold curves.

CRANIAL ARTERITIS

ESR is markedly increased.

CAVERNOUS SINUS THROMBOPHLEBITIS

CSF is usually normal unless there is associated subdural empyema or meningitis. *In the diabetic patient, mucormycosis may cause this clinical appearance.*
Laboratory findings due to preceding infections of paranasal sinuses, mastoid, etc., are noted.
Laboratory findings due to complications (e.g., meningitis, brain abscess) are noted.

INTRACRANIAL EXTRADURAL ABSCESS

CSF shows a slight increase in neutrophils and lymphocytes (20–100/cu mm) and a slight increase in protein.
Laboratory findings due to underlying osteomyelitis of middle ear or paranasal sinus are noted.

ACUTE SUBDURAL EMPYEMA

CSF
> Cell count is increased to a few hundred with predominance of either mononuclear or polynuclear leukocytes.
> Protein is increased.
> Glucose is normal or slightly decreased.
> Bacterial cultures are negative.

WBC is usually increased (up to 25,000/cu mm).

Laboratory findings due to preceding diseases
> ENT infections, especially acute sinusitis
> Trauma
> Intracranial surgery

(*Streptococci are the most common organisms when preceding condition is sinusitis.* Staph. aureus *or gram-negative organisms are the most common organisms following trauma or surgery.*)

BRAIN ABSCESS

CSF shows increased neutrophils, lymphocytes, and RBCs (25–300 WBC/cu mm). There may be increased protein level (75–300 mg/100 ml). The sugar level is normal. Bacterial cultures are negative.

Associated primary disease

      Ear, nose, and throat diseases (e.g., frontal sinusitis, middle ear infections, mastoiditis)

      Primary septic lung disease (e.g., lung abscess, bronchiectasis, empyema)

      Congenital heart disease with septal defects and pulmonary arteriovenous shunts

TUBERCULOMA OF BRAIN

CSF shows increased protein with small number of cells. The tuberculoma may be transformed into tuberculous meningitis with increased protein and cells (50–300/cu mm), decreased sugar and chloride.

Laboratory findings due to tuberculosis elsewhere are noted.

SPINAL CORD TUMOR

CSF protein is increased. It may be very high and associated with xanthochromia when there is a block of the subarachnoid space.

See Table 23, p. 203.

EPIDURAL ABSCESS OF SPINAL CORD

Spinal fluid protein is increased (usually 100–400 mg/100 ml), and WBCs (lymphocytes and neutrophils) are relatively few in number.

MYELITIS

Spinal fluid may be normal or may show increased protein and cells (20–1000/cu mm—lymphocytes and mononuclear cells).

See primary disease

      Poliomyelitis

      Herpes zoster

      Tuberculosis, syphilis, parasites, abscess

      Postvaccinal myelitis

      Multiple sclerosis

      Etc.

INFARCTION OF SPINAL CORD

Laboratory findings due to causative condition

      Polyarteritis nodosa

      Dissecting aneurysm of aorta

      Arteriosclerosis of aorta with thrombus formation

Iatrogenic (e.g., aortic arteriography, clamping of aorta during cardiac surgery)

CSF

Changes same as in cerebral hemorrhage or infarction

CHRONIC ADHESIVE ARACHNOIDITIS
(due to spinal anesthesia, syphilis, etc.)

CSF protein may be normal or increased.

CERVICAL SPONDYLOSIS

CSF shows increased protein in some cases.

POLYNEURITIS OR POLYNEUROPATHY

Due To

Infectious mononucleosis—CSF shows increased protein and up to several hundred mononuclear cells

Diphtheria—CSF protein = 50–200 mg/100 ml

Leprosy

Metabolic condition (e.g., pellagra, beriberi, combined system disease, pregnancy, porphyria)—CSF usually normal

Uremia—CSF protein = 50–200 mg/100 ml; occurs in a few chronic cases of uremia

Neoplasm (leukemia, multiple myeloma, carcinoma)—CSF protein often increased; may be associated with an occult primary neoplastic lesion outside of CNS

Amyloidosis—CSF protein often increased

Sarcoidosis

Polyarteritis nodosa—CSF usually normal; nerve involvement in 10% of cases

Toxic condition caused by drugs and chemicals (especially lead, arsenic, etc.)

Alcoholism—CSF usually normal

DISEASES CAUSING NEURITIS OF ONE NERVE OR PLEXUS

Due To

Diphtheria

Herpes zoster

Sarcoidosis

Leprosy

Tumor (leukemias, lymphomas, carcinomas—may find tumor cells in spinal fluid

Serum sickness

Bell's palsy

Idiopathic cause

MULTIPLE CRANIAL NERVE PALSIES

Laboratory findings due to causative disease

Trauma

Aneurysms

Tumors (e.g., meningioma, neurofibroma, carcinoma, chole-steatoma, chordoma)

Herpes zoster

Benign polyneuritis associated with cervical lymph node tuberculosis or sarcoidosis

FACIAL PALSY

Laboratory findings due to causative disease
Bell's palsy—occasional slight increase in cells in CSF
Herpes zoster
Pontine lesions (tumor or vascular)
Tumors invading the temporal bone
Acoustic neuromas
Sarcoidosis (uveoparotid fever or Heerfordt's syndrome)
Leprosy
Acute infectious polyneuritis

TRIGEMINAL NEURALGIA (TIC DOULOUREUX)

Laboratory findings due to causative disease
Usually idiopathic
May also stem from multiple sclerosis, herpes zoster

OPHTHALMOPLEGIA

Laboratory findings due to causative disease
Diabetes mellitus
Myasthenia gravis
Hyperthyroid exophthalmos

VON RECKLINGHAUSEN'S DISEASE (MULTIPLE NEUROFIBROMAS)

CSF findings of brain tumor if acoustic neurinoma occurs

BITEMPORAL HEMIANOPSIA

Laboratory findings due to causative disease
Usually pituitary adenoma
Also metastatic tumor, sarcoidosis, Hand-Schüller-Christian disease, meningioma of sella, aneurysm of circle of Willis

RETROBULBAR NEUROPATHY

CSF is normal or may show increased protein and up to 200 lymphocytes.

Three-quarters of these patients ultimately develop multiple sclerosis.

GLOMUS JUGULARE TUMOR

CSF protein may be increased.

29

Musculoskeletal Diseases

MYASTHENIA GRAVIS

Serum enzymes are normal.
Complete blood count and ESR are normal (occasional cases of associated macrocytic anemia).
Serum electrolytes are normal.
Thyroid function tests are normal (may be associated with, but independent of, hyperthyroidism or hypothyroidism).

High frequency of associated diabetes mellitus is seen especially in older patients; therefore GTT should be performed with or without cortisone.
Always rule out cancer of lung.
Thymic tumor is present in up to 10% of patients.

POLYMYOSITIS

Total eosinophil count is frequently increased. WBC may be increased in fulminant disease.
Mild anemia may occur.
ESR is moderately to markedly increased; may be normal.
Thyroid function tests are normal.
Serum enzymes are increased. The degree of increase reflects the activity of the disease; the level frequently becomes normal with steroid therapy or in chronic myositis.
> Serum CPK is increased in two-thirds of the patients. Levels may vary greatly. In childhood very high levels may occur.
> Serum aldolase is increased in three-quarters of the patients.
> Serum LDH is increased in about one-quarter of the patients.
> Serum SGOT is increased in about one-quarter of the patients.
> Serum hydroxybutyric dehydrogenase (HBD) may be increased, paralleling the increased LDH.
> Serum MDH may be increased but offers no additional diagnostic value.

Continued on page 221.

Table 25. Laboratory Findings in the Differential Diagnosis of Some Muscle Diseases

Disease	Complete Blood Count	ESR	Thyroid Function Tests	Percent of Patients with Increase in Various Serum Enzyme Levels	Muscle Biopsy	Comment
Myasthenia gravis	N	N	N	N	Lymphorrhages	**Cancer of lung should always be ruled out; high frequency of associated diabetes mellitus, especially in older patients. Serum electrolytes N**
Polymyositis	Total eosinophil count frequently I	Moderate to marked I; occasionally N	N	CPK in 65%; levels may vary greatly and become N with steroid therapy; marked I may occur in childhood ALD in 75%, LDH in 25%, SGOT in 25%; HBD parallels LDH; MDH offers no additional diagnostic value	Necrosis of muscle with phagocytosis of muscle fibers, infiltration of inflammatory cells	Associated cancer in up to 17% of cases (especially lung; also breast) LE preparation and latex fixations occasionally positive; serum alpha 2 and gamma globulin may be increased.
Muscular dystrophy	N	N	N	In active phase: CPK in 50%, ALD in 20%, LDH in 10%, SGOT in 15%	Various degenerative changes in muscle; late muscle atrophy; no cellular infiltration	

N = normal; I = increased.

Polymyositis (*continued*)

Urine shows a moderate increase in creatine and a decrease in creatinine. Myoglobinuria occurs occasionally in severe cases.

LE tests are usually negative. Latex fixation rheumatoid factor— (RA) tests may be positive in half of the cases.

Serum gamma globulins may be increased.

Muscle biopsy shows necrosis of muscle with phagocytosis of muscle fibers and infiltration of inflammatory cells.

Associated carcinoma is present in up to 20% of the cases and up to 50% of patients over 40 (especially cancer of lung and cancer of breast). The polymyositis may antedate the neoplasm by up to 2 years.

MUSCULAR DYSTROPHY

ESR is usually normal.

Thyroid function tests are normal.

Serum enzymes are increased, especially in

> Young patients. Highest levels (up to 50 times normal) are found at onset in infancy and childhood with gradual return to normal.
>
> The more rapidly progressive dystrophies such as the Duchenne type (and may be slightly or inconsistently increased in the limb-girdle and facioscapulohumeral types)
>
> The active early phase. Increased levels are not constant and are affected by patient's age and duration of disease. Enzymes may be increased before disease is clinically evident.

> Serum CPK is increased in about 50% of the patients.
>
> Serum aldolase is increased in about 20% of the patients.
>
> Serum LDH is increased in about 10% of the patients.
>
> Serum SGOT is increased in about 15% of the patients.
>
> Serum CPK is increased in about 75% of female *carriers*. It is thus possible to identify carrier state and detect clinically unaffected male infants with Duchenne type.
>
> Elevated serum enzyme levels are not affected by steroid therapy.

Muscle biopsy shows muscle atrophy but no cellular infiltration.

Urine creatine is increased; urine creatinine is decreased. These changes are less marked in limb-girdle and facioscapulohumeral types than in the Duchenne type.

MYOTONIC DYSTROPHY

Increased creatine in urine may occur irregularly.

Findings due to atrophy of testicle and androgenic deficiency are noted.

Urine 17-KS (ketosteroids) are decreased.

Thyroid function may be decreased.

Serum enzyme increases are slight and inconsistent. Female carriers may have higher levels of ALD and CPK than control females.

SERUM ENZYMES IN SOME DISEASES OF THE MUSCULOSKELETAL SYSTEM

CPK is the measurement of choice. It is more specific and sensitive than SGOT and LDH and more discriminating than ALD.

Continued on page 223.

Table 26. Increased Serum Enzyme Levels in Muscle Diseases

| Enzyme | Muscular Dystrophy | | | | | | Myotonic Dystrophy | Polymyositis |
| | Duchenne | | Limb-Girdle | | Facioscapulohumeral | | | |
	Frequency	Amplitude	Frequency	Amplitude	Frequency	Amplitude	Frequency	Frequency
CPK	>95%	65	75%	25	80%	5	50%	70%
ALD	90%	9	25%	3	30%	2	20%	75%
SGOT	90%	4	25%	2	25%	1½	15%	25%
LDH	90%	4	15%	1½	10%	1	10%	25%

Frequency = average % frequency of cases with increased serum enzyme level when blood is taken at optimal time.
Amplitude = average number of times normal that serum level is increased.

SERUM ENZYMES IN SOME DISEASES *(continued)*

Increased In
Dermatomyositis
Progressive muscular dystrophy. See Muscular Dystrophy, p. 221.
Myotonic dystrophy, see p. 221.

Normal In
Rheumatoid arthritis
Scleroderma
Acrosclerosis
Discoid lupus erythematosus
Muscle atrophy of neurologic origin (e.g., old poliomyelitis, polyneuritis)
Hyperthyroid myopathy

CREATINE AND CREATININE

Decreased creatinine excretion
Increased creatine excretion
Increased blood creatinine

Occurs In
Progressive muscular dystrophy
Decreased muscle mass in
 Neurogenic atrophy
 Polymyositis
 Addison's disease
 Hyperthyroidism
 Male eunuchoidism

MYALGIAS—DIFFERENTIAL DIAGNOSIS

Rheumatoid arthritis
Rheumatic fever
Hyperparathyroidism
Hyperthyroidism and hypothyroidism
Hypoglycemia
Renal tubular acidosis
Myoglobinuria
McArdle syndrome
Brucellosis
Other infections (bacterial, viral, rickettsial, etc.)

METABOLIC DISEASES OF MUSCLE

Hyperthyroidism
 Increased urine creatine
 Decreased creatine tolerance
 Normal serum enzyme levels
 Normal muscle biopsy

 Causes some cases of hypokalemic periodic paralysis.

Hypothyroidism (rarely associated with myotonia)
 Decreased urine creatine
 Increased creatine tolerance
 Increased serum CPK, especially when PBI $< 2.5 \ \mu g/100$ ml

Other serum enzyme levels normal
Associated with administration of adrenal corticosteroids and with
    Cushing's syndrome
        Increased urine creatine
        Increased serum enzymes (SGOT, aldolase)—uncommon, and
            may be due to the primary disease
        Muscle biopsy—degenerative and regenerative changes in scat-
            tered muscle fibers; no inflammatory cell infiltration

CONGENITAL MYOTONIA (THOMSEN'S DISEASE)

Mild creatine intolerance is found.
Urine creatine may be increased in some patients.
Muscle biopsy shows few changes that are not specific.
Serum enzymes are normal.

STIFF-MAN SYNDROME

BMR is often increased (up to +75).
Other laboratory examinations are normal.
CSF is normal.
Biopsy of muscle is normal or shows minimal nonspecific changes
    (e.g., slight atrophy).
Occasionally other alterations are present (e.g., persistent leukopenia
    with eosinophilia).

MYOTUBULAR MYOPATHY

Routine laboratory studies including measurement of serum en-
    zymes are normal; occasionally serum CPK is slightly increased.
Biopsy of muscle establishes the diagnosis.

MITOCHONDRIAL MYOPATHY

Routine laboratory studies including measurement of serum en-
    zymes are normal.
Biopsy of muscle with histochemical staining reaction demonstrates
    hyperactivity of certain mitochondrial enzymes (e.g., DPNH
    diaphorase, succinate dehydrogenase, cytochrome oxidase).

NEMALINE (ROD) MYOPATHY

Routine laboratory tests are normal.
Serum enzymes are normal; occasionally serum CPK is slightly
    increased.
Endocrine studies (including measurements of urine 17-KS and 11-
    oxysteroids) are normal.
Biopsy of muscle with appropriate special stains establishes the
    diagnosis.

MYOPATHY ASSOCIATED WITH ALCOHOLISM

Acute
        Increased serum CPK, SGOT, and other enzymes. Serum CPK
            increases in 1–2 days; reaches peak in 4–5 days. CPK in CSF
            is normal even when serum level is elevated.
        Gross myoglobinuria
        Acute renal failure (sometimes)

Chronic—may show some or all of the following changes
    Increased urine creatine
    Increased serum CPK and SGOT
    Diminished ability to increase blood lactic acid with ischemic exercise
    Abnormalities on muscle biopsy (support the diagnosis)
    Myoglobinuria

FAMILIAL PERIODIC PARALYSIS

Serum potassium is decreased during the attack.
Urine potassium excretion decreases at the same time.
Serum enzymes are normal.

Table 27. Types of Periodic Paralysis

	Hypokalemic (familial, sporadic, associated with hyperthyroidism)	Hyperkalemic (adynamia episodica hereditaria)	Normokalemic
Induced by	Glucose and insulin, ACTH, DOCA, epinephrine	KCl	KCl
Serum potassium during attack	Decreased	Increased	Normal or slightly decreased
Urine potassium excretion	Decreased	Normal	Decreased

ADYNAMIA EPISODICA HEREDITARIA (GAMSTORP'S DISEASE)

Transient increase in serum potassium occurs during the attack; attack is induced by administration of potassium.
Urine potassium excretion is unchanged during or before the attack.

NORMAL LABORATORY FINDINGS IN DISEASES OF BONE

Polyostotic fibrous dysplasia (Albright's syndrome) (occasionally increased serum alkaline phosphatase)
Giant-cell tumor of bone
Achondroplasia
Dyschondroplasias
Tietze's syndrome
Osteitis pubis

OSTEOMYELITIS

WBC may be increased, especially in acute case.
ESR is increased in less than 50% of patients but may be important clue in occult cases, e.g., intervertebral disk space infection.
Bacteriology
    Staph. aureus causes almost all infections of hip and two-thirds of infections of skull, vertebrae, and long bones. Other

bacteria may simultaneously be present and contribute to infection.

Gram-negative bacteria cause most infections of mandible, pelvis, and small bones.

Salmonella is more commonly found in patients with sickle hemoglobinopathy.

Laboratory findings due to underlying conditions

Postoperative status

Radiation therapy

Foreign body, tissue gangrene, contiguous infection, etc.

SKELETAL INVOLVEMENT ASSOCIATED WITH SOME METABOLIC ABNORMALITIES

Primary hypophosphatemia

Hypophosphatasia

Rickets

Gaucher's disease

Gargoylism (mucopolysac-charides in urine; sometimes Riley bodies in white cells)

Gout

Alkaptonuria

Phenylketonuria

Familial hyperparathyroidism

Idiopathic hypercalcemia

Osteogenesis imperfecta

Marfan's syndrome

Etc.

SKELETAL INVOLVEMENT ASSOCIATED WITH SOME HEMATOLOGIC DISEASES

Anemia

Hereditary hemolytic (e.g., sickle cell disease, thalassemia, hereditary spherocytosis)

Iron-deficiency anemia of childhood

Congenital aplastic anemia (Fanconi syndrome)

Coagulation defects (e.g., deficiency of AHG, PTC, or PTA)

Malignant lymphoma (e.g., leukemia, lymphosarcoma, Hodgkin's disease, multiple myeloma)

Primary reticulum cell sarcoma of bone

Reticuloendothelioses (e.g., Niemann-Pick disease, Gaucher's disease, Hand-Schüller-Christian disease; Letterer-Siwe disease, eosinophilic granuloma)

Myelosclerosis

Osteopetrosis (marble bone disease)

Etc.

OSTEOPOROSIS

Urine calcium may be increased, normal, or decreased but is not influenced by intake; calcium restriction does not produce the normal fall.

Laboratory tests (including serum calcium, phosphorus, and alkaline phosphatase) are normal.

In secondary osteoporosis, see primary disease for laboratory findings.

Administration of steroids

Cushing's syndrome

Acromegaly

Hyperthyroidism

Gonadal insufficiency

Hyperparathyroidism

Neoplasms

Immobilization

Hypophosphatasia

Uremia

Sprue

Etc.

RICKETS

Serum alkaline phosphatase is increased. This is the earliest and most reliable biochemical abnormality; parallels severity of the rickets. It may remain elevated until bone healing is complete.

Serum calcium is usually normal or slightly decreased.

Serum phosphorus is usually decreased. In some individuals, serum calcium and phosphorus may be normal.

Serum calcium and phosphorus rapidly become normal after institution of vitamin D therapy.

OSTEOMALACIA

Serum calcium and phosphorus may be decreased.

Serum alkaline phosphatase may be increased. This is the earliest biochemical alteration.

Blood chemistries may be normal.

IV infusion of a standard dose of calcium results in 24-hour retention of more than 60%.

Biopsy of bone. Undercalcified sections show an increased number of osteoid seams which are wider than normal. Biopsy can show a decreased rate of mineralization by oral tetracycline labeling prior to biopsy and examination of bone under fluorescent light.

Due To
Primary vitamin D deficiency
Gastrointestinal malabsorption
  Partial gastrectomy
  Diseases of the small intestine (e.g., regional enteritis)
  Pancreatic disease (e.g., chronic pancreatitis)
  Hepatobiliary disease (e.g., chronic biliary obstruction)
Primary hypophosphatemia
Renal disease
  Renal tubular diseases (e.g., renal tubular acidosis)
  Chronic renal insufficiency
Hypophosphatasia
Axial osteomalacia (see next section)
Others (e.g., hypoparathyroidism, hyperthyroidism, Paget's disease, osteoporosis, osteopetrosis, fluoride ingestion, ureterosigmoidostomy)

AXIAL OSTEOMALACIA

Axial skeleton shows x-ray changes resembling those in Paget's disease and metastatic tumor.

Bone biopsy is characteristic of osteomalacia.

Blood chemistries are normal.

There is no recognizable cause for osteomalacia.

VITAMIN D–RESISTANT RICKETS

Serum calcium is normal or only slightly decreased.

Serum phosphorus is decreased.

Serum alkaline phosphatase is increased.

Urine calcium is decreased.

Due To
See Osteomalacia, above.

VITAMIN D INTOXICATION

Serum calcium may be increased.
Serum phosphorus is usually also increased but sometimes is decreased, with increased urinary phosphorus.

FAMILIAL OSTEOECTASIA
(uncommon inherited disorder of membranous bone showing painful swelling of the periosteal soft tissue and spontaneous fractures)

Serum alkaline phosphatase is increased.
Serum acid phosphatase and aminopeptidase are also increased.

INFANTILE CORTICAL HYPEROSTOSIS (CAFFEY'S DISEASE)

WBC is increased.
ESR is increased.

A similar picture may occur in children over 1 year old because of hypervitaminosis A.

OSTEOSCLEROSIS

Due To
Osteopetrosis (see next section)
Heavy-metal poisoning (e.g., lead, bismuth)
Hypoparathyroidism
Hypothyroidism

OSTEOPETROSIS (ALBERS-SCHÖNBERG DISEASE, MARBLE BONE DISEASE)

Normal serum calcium, phosphorus, alkaline phosphatase
Serum acid phosphatase increased (sometimes)
Myelophthisic anemia (sometimes)
Laboratory findings due to complications
    Osteomyelitis
    Other infections

PAGET'S DISEASE OF BONE (OSTEITIS DEFORMANS)

Marked increase in serum alkaline phosphatase directly related to severity and extent of disease; sudden additional increase with development of osteogenic sarcoma
Normal serum calcium increased during immobilization (e.g., due to intercurrent illness or fracture)
Normal or slightly increased serum phosphorus
Frequently increased urine calcium; renal calculi common
Increased hydroxyproline in urine may be marked.

OSTEOGENIC SARCOMA

Marked increase in serum alkaline phosphatase (up to 40 times normal); reflects new bone formation and parallels clinical course (development of metastases, response to therapy, etc.)

OSTEOLYTIC TUMORS OF BONE
(e.g., Ewing's sarcoma)

Usually normal serum calcium, phosphorus, alkaline phosphatase

METASTATIC CARCINOMA OF BONE

Osteolytic metastases (especially from primary tumor of bronchus, breast, kidney, thyroid)
  Urine calcium is often increased; marked increase may reflect increased rate of tumor growth.
  Serum calcium and phosphorus may be normal or increased.
  Serum alkaline phosphatase is usually normal or slightly to moderately increased.
  Serum acid phosphatase is often slightly increased, especially in prostatic metastases.
Osteoblastic metastases (especially from primary tumor in prostate)
  Serum calcium is normal; rarely increased.
  Urine calcium is low.
  Serum alkaline phosphatase is usually increased.
  Serum acid phosphatase is increased in prostatic carcinoma.
  Serum phosphorus is variable.

FAT EMBOLISM

This occurs after trauma, e.g., fractures, insertion of femoral head prosthesis.
Unexplained fall in hemoglobin
Decreased platelet count
Free fat in urine in 50% of cases
Fat globules in sputum (sometimes)
Decreased arterial pO_2 with normal or decreased pCO_2
Increased serum lipase in 30–50% of cases. Increased free fatty acids. Not of diagnostic value.
Increased serum triglycerides
Fat globulinemia in 42–67% of patients and in 17–33% of controls
Normal cerebrospinal fluid

Laboratory findings alone are inadequate for diagnosis.

CONDITIONS ASSOCIATED WITH THE DEVELOPMENT OF AVASCULAR (ASEPTIC) NECROSIS OF THE HEAD OF THE FEMUR

Traumatic interruption of blood supply
  $> 25\%$ of patients with fracture of neck of femur
  Dislocation of hip
  Slipped femoral capital epiphysis
Nontraumatic interference with blood supply
  Caisson disease
  Sickle cell disease and trait and sickle cell-C hemoglobin disease
  Infection
  Gout
  Rheumatoid arthritis
  Systemic lupus erythematosus (SLE)
  Fabry's disease

Scleroderma
Gaucher's disease
Cushing's syndrome
Corticosteroid treatment
Alcoholism
Pancreatitis
X-irradiation
Idiopathic (Chandler's disease)

CLASSIFICATION OF ARTHRITIS*

Polyarthritis of unknown etiology
    Rheumatoid arthritis
    Juvenile rheumatoid arthritis (Still's disease)
    Ankylosing spondylitis (Marie-Strümpell disease)
    Psoriatic arthritis
    Reiter's syndrome
    Other
Collagen diseases (acquired connective tissue disorders)
    Systemic lupus erythematosus
    Scleroderma (progressive systemic sclerosis)
    Polymyositis and dermatomyositis
    Necrotizing arteritis and other forms of vasculitis (e.g., polyarteritis nodosa, hypersensitivity angiitis, Wegener's granulomatosis, Takayasu's disease, Cogan's syndrome, giant cell arteritis)
    Amyloidosis
    Other
Rheumatic fever
Degenerative joint disease (osteoarthritis)
    Primary
    Secondary
Diseases with frequently associated arthritis
    Sarcoidosis
    Relapsing polychondritis
    Schönlein-Henoch purpura
    Ulcerative colitis
    Regional ileitis
    Whipple's disease
    Sjögren's syndrome
    Familial Mediterranean fever
    Psoriatic arthritis
    Other
Associated with infectious agents
    Bacterial (e.g., *Brucella*, gonococcus, tubercle bacillus, *Salmonella*, pneumococcus, *Staphylococcus*, *Streptococcus moniliformis*, syphilis, yaws)
    Rickettsial
    Viral (especially rubella; mumps, viral hepatitis)
    Fungal (especially coccidioidomycosis; also histoplasmosis, blastomycosis, cryptococcosis, sporotrichosis)
    Parasitic

---

* Adapted from American Rheumatism Association, "Primer on the Rheumatic Diseases," J.A.M.A. 224 (April 30, 1973): 662–812.

Traumatic and/or neurogenic causes
 Direct trauma
 Tertiary syphilis (tabes dorsalis)
 Diabetes mellitus with neurologic complications
 Syringomyelia
 Shoulder-hand syndrome
 Mechanical derangement of joints
Endocrine diseases
 Hyperparathyroidism
 Acromegaly
 Hypothyroidism
Biochemical and metabolic diseases
 Gout
 Pseudogout (chondrocalcinosis articularis)
 Ochronosis
 Hemophilias
 Hemoglobinopathies
 Agammaglobulinemia
 Scurvy
 Gaucher's disease
 Hemochromatosis
 Hyperlipoproteinemia type II (xanthoma tuberosum and tendinosum)
 Other
Inherited and congenital diseases
 Mucopolysaccharidoses (e.g., Hurler's syndrome, Morquio's disease)
 Homocystinuria
 Ehlers-Danlos syndrome
 Marfan's syndrome
 Osteogenesis imperfecta
 Congenital hip dysplasia
Tumors
 Multiple myeloma
 Leukemia
 Metastatic tumors
 Primary juxta-articular bone
 Synovioma
 Other
Allergy and drug reactions (e.g., serum sickness)
Miscellaneous
 Aseptic necrosis of bone
 Stevens-Johnson syndrome
 Erythema nodosum
 Hypertrophic osteoarthropathy
 Juvenile osteochondritis
 Osteochondritis dissecans
 Pigmented villonodular synovitis
 Tietze's syndrome
 Other
Nonarticular rheumatism
 Intervertebral disk and low back syndromes
 Fibrositis, myositis, tendinitis, bursitis, tenosynovitis, fasciitis
 Carpal tunnel syndrome
 Neuritis
 Panniculitis

Table 28. Synovial Fluid Findings in Various Diseases of Joints

Property		Normal	Noninflammatory[1]	Hemorrhagic[2]	Acute Inflammatory[3]			Septic		
					Acute Gouty Arthritis	Rheumatic Fever	Rheumatoid Arthritis	Tuberculous Arthritis	Gonorrheal Arthritis	Septic Arthritis[4]
Volume		3.5 ml								
Appearance		Clear, colorless	I Clear, straw	I Bloody or xanthochromic	I Turbid yellow			I Turbid yellow		
Viscosity		High	High	V	D			D		
Fibrin clot		0	Usually 0	Usually 0	+			+		
Mucin clot		Good	Good	V	Fair to poor			Poor		
WBC (no/cu mm)[5]	Range	<200	<5000	<10,000	750–45,000	300–98,000	300–75,000	2500–105,000	1500–108,000	15,600–213,000
	average				13,500	17,800	15,500	23,500	14,000	65,400
Neutrophils (%)	Range	<25	<25	<50	48–94	8–98	5–96	29–96	2–96	75–100
	average				83	46	65	67	64	95
Blood-synovia glucose difference (mg/100 ml)[6]	Range	<10	<10	<25	0–41	6	0–88	0–108	0–97	40–122
	average				12		31	57	26	71
Culture[7]		0	0	0	0	0	0	See pp. 239–240.		

I = increased; D = decreased; 0 = absent; + = positive; V = variable.

1 E.g., degenerative joint disease, traumatic arthritis, some cases of pigmented villonodular synovitis.
2 E.g., tumor, hemophilia, neuroarthropathy, trauma, some cases of pigmented villonodular synovitis.
3 E.g., rheumatoid arthritis, Reiter's syndrome, acute gouty arthritis, acute pseudogout, systemic lupus erythematosus, etc.
4 E.g., pneumococcal.
5 Use saline instead of acetic acid to avoid interference with mucin clot.
6 Joint tap should be performed preferably after patient has been fasting for more than 4 hours, and a blood glucose determination should be performed simultaneously.
7 Material should be cultured aerobically and anaerobically. Culture for tubercle bacilli and guinea pig inoculation should be performed.

NEEDLE BIOPSY OF JOINT (HISTOLOGIC EXAMINATION OF SYNOVIA)

May Be Useful In
Gout
Pseudogout
Ochronosis
Tuberculosis
Coccidioidomycosis
Pyogenic arthritis
Rheumatoid arthritis
Osteoarthritis
Reiter's syndrome
Systemic lupus erythematosus

Provides major diagnostic assistance in about one-third of patients with early or difficult diagnosis.

OSTEOARTHRITIS

ESR may be slightly increased (possibly because of soft-tissue changes secondary to mechanical alterations in joints).
Complete blood count, ESR, serum protein electrophoresis, rheumatoid factor, serum uric acid, calcium, phosphorus, alkaline phosphatase, VDRL tests, etc., are normal.

RHEUMATOID ARTHRITIS

Serologic tests for rheumatoid factor (e.g., using latex, bentonite, or sheep or human RBCs). Tests become positive after disease active for more than 6 months. Positive in 75% of "typical" cases; positive in 95% of patients with subcutaneous nodules; high titers in patients with splenomegaly, vasculitis, or neuropathy; positive in 10–20% of juvenile cases. Persistent positive result may indicate an unfavorable course. Positive in up to 5% of normal population. False positive in other diseases (e.g., SLE, sarcoidosis, liver diseases, bacterial endocarditis, syphilis, leprosy, tuberculosis). Negative in osteoarthritis, gout, ankylosing spondylitis, rheumatic fever, suppurative arthritis, arthritis associated with ulcerative colitis.
Anemia is moderate in degree, of the normocytic hypochromic type, and not responsive to administration of iron, folic acid, or vitamin B_{12}, or to splenectomy.
Serum iron is decreased.
WBC is usually normal; there may be a slight increase early in the active disease.
Increased ESR and positive C-reactive protein (CRP) test are rough guides to activity and to therapy.
Serum protein electrophoresis shows increase in globulins, especially in gamma and alpha$_2$ globulins, and decreased albumin.
Positive LE test in up to 20% of patients is usually weakly reactive. Antinuclear factors are present in up to 65% of patients, depending on sensitivity of the test.
Serum calcium, phosphorus, alkaline phosphatase, uric acid, and ASOT are normal.
Synovial biopsy is especially useful in monarticular form to rule out tuberculosis, gout, etc.
For synovial fluid examination see Table 28, p. 232.
See Amyloidosis, p. 433.

Table 29. Synovial Fluid Findings in Acute Inflammatory Arthritis of Various Etiologies

Disease	WBC	Complement Activity	Rheumatoid Factor (RF)	Crystals*	Other Findings
Acute gouty arthritis	I	I	0	Monosodium urate; within PMN during acute stage	
Acute chondrocalcinosis (pseudogout)	I	I	0	Calcium pyrophosphate	
Reiter's syndrome	Marked I	Marked I	0		Macrophages with ingested leukocytes
Rheumatoid arthritis	I	Low	Usually +		
Juvenile rheumatoid arthritis	I	Low	0		Abundant lymphocytes (sometimes more than 50%); immature lymphocytes and monocytes present
Systemic lupus erythematosus	Usually very low	Low or 0	V	0	LE cells may be present
Arthritis associated with psoriasis, ulcerative colitis, ankylosing spondylitis	I	I			

I = increased; 0 = absent; V = variable; PMN = polynuclear leukocyte; + = positive.

*Crystals should be identified using polarized light microscopy. Finding of characteristic crystals is diagnostic of gout and of chondrocalcinosis.

Table 30. Comparison of Rheumatoid Arthritis and Osteoarthritis

Rheumatoid Arthritis	Osteoarthritis
Synovial fluid has high WBC and low viscosity	Effusions infrequent Synovial fluid has low WBC and high viscosity
ESR more markedly increased	ESR may be mildly to moderately increased
Rheumatoid factor (RF) usually present	RF usually absent
Positive biopsy of subcutaneous rheumatoid nodule and of synovia	Rheumatoid changes in tissue absent

JUVENILE RHEUMATOID ARTHRITIS (STILL'S DISEASE)

Serologic tests for rheumatoid factor are positive in only 10–20% of patients.
WBC may be normal or increased up to 50,000/cu mm.
Hypochromic anemia is frequent; varies from mild to severe.
Other findings are similar to those in adult rheumatoid arthritis.
  Increased ESR and CRP parallels degree of inflammation.
  Serum protein electrophoresis shows increased globulin, especially gamma.
  Secondary amyloidosis appears in long-standing active disease (see Amyloidosis, p. 433)

Table 31. ESR in Differential Diagnosis of Juvenile Rheumatoid Arthritis

Disease	ESR Falls to Normal
Untreated acute rheumatic fever	9–12 weeks
Salicylate-treated acute rheumatic fever	5 weeks
Steroid-treated acute rheumatic fever	2 weeks
Chronic rheumatic fever	Occasionally shows persistent elevation
Juvenile rheumatoid arthritis	May remain elevated for months or years despite therapy

FELTY'S SYNDROME

The syndrome occurs in 5–10% of cases of rheumatoid arthritis associated with splenomegaly and leukopenia.
Rheumatoid arthritis is far advanced.
Serologic tests for rheumatoid factor are positive; RF may be present in high titers.
Positive LE test is more frequent than in rheumatoid arthritis.
Leukopenia is present. Anemia and thrombocytopenia may occur; they respond to splenectomy.

SJÖGREN'S SYNDROME

This immunologic abnormality is associated with decreased secretion of exocrine glands.

One-half of patients have rheumatoid arthritis.

Mild anemia and leukopenia occur in one-third of patients.

ESR is usually increased.

Serologic tests for rheumatoid factor are positive even in patients without arthritis.

LE test is positive in 10% of patients all of whom have arthritis.

Serum protein electrophoresis shows increased globulin, largely due to 7S gamma globulin.

Occasionally nonthrombocytopenic purpura occurs.

The syndrome may be associated with Waldenstrom's macroglobulinemia, collagen diseases (lupus erythematosus, polyarteritis, etc.), and Felty's syndrome.

Rule out other causes of Mikulicz's syndrome (e.g., sarcoid, tuberculosis, cirrhosis, leukemia).

ANKYLOSING RHEUMATOID SPONDYLITIS (MARIE-STRÜMPELL DISEASE)

ESR is increased in up to 80% of cases.

Mild to moderate hypochromic anemia appears in up to 30% of cases.

Serologic tests for rheumatoid factor are positive in less than 15% of patients with arthritis of only the vertebral region.

CSF protein is moderately increased in up to 50% of cases.

Secondary amyloidosis appears in 6% of patients.

Laboratory findings of carditis and aortitis with aortic insufficiency, which occur in 1–4% of patients, are noted.

Laboratory findings of frequently associated diseases
    Chronic ulcerative colitis
    Regional ileitis
    Psoriasis

ARTHRITIS ASSOCIATED WITH PSORIASIS

Arthritis occurs in 2% of patients with psoriasis. There is no correlation between activity of skin and of joint manifestations; either one may precede the other.

Increased serum uric acid is due to increased turnover of skin cells in psoriasis.

Serologic tests for rheumatoid factor are negative.

ARTHRITIS ASSOCIATED WITH ULCERATIVE COLITIS OR REGIONAL ENTERITIS

There may be rheumatoid arthritis, ankylosing spondylitis, or acute synovitis (monarticular or polyarticular—absent rheumatoid factor).

Joint fluid is sterile bacteriologically and microscopically. It is similar to fluid of rheumatoid arthritis and Whipple's disease (cell count, differential count, specific gravity, viscosity, protein, sugar, poor mucin clot formation). Joint fluid examination is principally useful in monarticular involvement to rule out suppurative arthritis.

Synovial biopsy is similar to rheumatoid arthritis biopsy.

ARTHRITIS ASSOCIATED WITH WHIPPLE'S DISEASE

This is a nonspecific synovitis.

HEMOCHROMATOSIS-ASSOCIATED ARTHRITIS

Laboratory findings of hemochromatosis
Negative RA factor
No subcutaneous nodules
Biopsy of synovia—iron deposits in synovia lining but not in cartilage, little iron in deep macrophages

> *Hemarthrosis:* iron diffusely distributed in macrophages (e.g., in hemophilia, trauma, and pigmented villonodular synovitis)
> *Osteoarthritis:* small amount of iron that is limited to deep macrophages
> *Rheumatoid arthritis:* iron in both deep macrophages and lining cells

Chondrocalcinosis frequently associated

REITER'S SYNDROME

This triad of arthritis, urethritis, and conjunctivitis has additional features: dermatitis, buccal ulcerations, circinate balanitis, and keratosis blennorrhagica.
Increased ESR parallels the clinical course.
WBC is increased (10,000–20,000/cu mm), as are granulocytes.
Serum globulins are increased in long-standing disease.
Nonbacterial cystitis, prostatitis, or seminal vesiculitis is found (significance of culturing pleuropneumonia-like organisms is not determined).

GOUT

Serum uric acid is increased. Several determinations may be required to establish elevated values; beware of serum levels reduced to normal range by recent aspirin ingestion.
Serum uric acid levels are increased in about 25% of asymptomatic relatives.
Moderate leukocytosis and increased ESR occur during acute attacks; normal at other times.
Crystals of monosodium urate from tophi and joint fluid (viewed under polarized light) will be seen.
See Tables 28 and 29, pp. 232, 235.
Uric acid crystals and amorphous urates are normal findings in urinary sediment.
Uric acid stones are found in the urinary system in 15% of the cases.
Low-grade proteinuria occurs in 20–80% of gouty individuals for many years before further evidence of renal disease appears.
Histologic examination of gouty nodule should be made.
Diabetes mellitus develops with increased frequency.
See also sections on renal diseases.

DISEASES ASSOCIATED WITH GOUT

Hypertension in one-third of patients with gout
Diabetes mellitus

Familial hypercholesterolemia
Acute intermittent porphyria
von Gierke's disease
Sarcoidosis
Etc.

SECONDARY GOUT

Occurs In
Lead intoxication
Hematologic diseases (e.g., leukemia, polycythemia vera, secondary
  polycythemia, malignant lymphomas). *Blood dyscrasias are found
  in about 10% of patients with clinical gout.*
Psoriasis

CHONDROCALCINOSIS ("PSEUDOGOUT")

Joint fluid contains crystals of calcium pyrophosphate dihydrate
  inside and outside of WBCs; differentiated from urate crystals
  under polarized light.
Blood and urine findings are normal.
See Tables 28, p. 232, and 29, p. 235.

CONDITIONS WHICH MAY PRESENT AS ACUTE ARTHRITIS

Beware of conditions which may present as acute arthritis.
> Acute leukemia in children
> Hypertrophic pulmonary osteoarthropathy (clubbing) in lung
>   tumors—may have acute onset and be painful
> Drug reaction causing lupus erythematosus–like syndrome (e.g.,
>   procaine amide)
> Aortic insufficiency starting with back pain and symptoms of
>   spondylitis

SEPTIC ARTHRITIS (SUPPURATIVE OR PURULENT ARTHRITIS)

Laboratory findings due to preexisting infections (e.g., subacute
  bacterial endocarditis, meningococcic meningitis, pneumococcal
  pneumonia, typhoid, gonorrhea, tuberculosis) are noted.
See Table 28, p. 232.

Joint fluid
> In purulent arthritis
>> Gram stain is particularly useful for establishing diagnosis
>>   promptly and in cases in which cultures are negative.
>> Culture may be negative because of prior administration of
>>   antibiotics.
> In tuberculous arthritis
>> Gram stain and bacterial cultures are negative, but acid-
>>   fast stain, culture for tubercle bacilli, guinea pig inocula-
>>   tion, and biopsy of synovia confirm the diagnosis.

PIGMENTED VILLONODULAR SYNOVITIS

Complete blood count, ESR, blood cholesterol, and urinalysis are
    normal.
See Table 28, p. 232.

POLYMYALGIA RHEUMATICA

ESR is usually markedly increased.
Mild hypochromic or normochromic anemia is commonly found.
WBC count is usually normal.
Abnormalities of serum proteins are frequent although there is no
    consistent or diagnostic pattern. Most frequently the albumin is
    decreased with an increase in alpha$_1$ and alpha$_2$ globulins and
    fibrinogen. Cryoglobulins are sometimes present.
Rheumatoid factor is present in serum in 7.5% of cases.
LE test is negative.
Serum enzymes (e.g., SGOT, CPK, aldolase) are normal.
Muscle biopsy is usually normal or may show mild nonspecific
    changes.
Temporal artery biopsy is often positive because of the high
    incidence of associated cranial arteritis.

HYPERTROPHIC OSTEOARTHROPATHY (CLUBBING; HYPERTROPHIC "PULMONARY" OSTEOARTHROPATHY)

Due To
Pulmonary diseases (especially bronchogenic carcinoma, bronchiec-
    tasis, lung abscess)
Pleural disease (especially tumors, empyema)
Mediastinal lesions (e.g., malignant lymphoma, aortic aneurysm)
Cardiac diseases (especially subacute bacterial endocarditis, cya-
    notic congenital heart disease)
Hepatic disease (especially cholangiolitic cirrhosis)
Intestinal diseases (especially tuberculosis, amebic infection, re-
    gional enteritis, ulcerative colitis, neoplasms)
Rare hereditary and idiopathic causes

CARPAL TUNNEL SYNDROME

Rule out underlying conditions.
    Amyloidosis
    Pregnancy
    Acromegaly
    Rheumatoid inflammation
    Many others (e.g., fibrosis, trauma)

NORMAL LABORATORY FINDINGS IN DISEASES OF JOINTS

Slipped femoral epiphysis
Aseptic (avascular) necrosis of bone
Juvenile osteochondritis
Osteochondritis dissecans

Hypertrophic osteoarthropathy
Congenital dysplasia of hip
Joint mice
Intervertebral disk syndrome

NORMAL LABORATORY FINDINGS IN DISEASES OF MUSCULOSKELETAL SYSTEM

Fibrositis
Fasciitis
Bursitis
Capsulitis
Tenosynovitis
Tendinitis
Dupuytren's contracture

30

Hematologic Diseases

CLASSIFICATION OF ANEMIAS ACCORDING TO PATHOGENESIS

Marrow hypofunction with decreased RBC production

    Marrow replacement (myelophthisic anemias due to tumor or granulomas, e.g., tuberculosis)

> *In absence of severe anemia or leukemoid reaction nucleated RBCs in blood smear suggest miliary tuberculosis or marrow metastases.*

    Marrow injury (hypoplastic and aplastic anemias)

    Nutritional deficiency (e.g., megaloblastic anemias due to lack of vitamin B_{12} or folic acid)

    Endocrine hypofunction (e.g., pituitary, adrenal, thyroid)

Marrow hypofunction due to decreased hemoglobin production (hypochromic microcytic anemias)

    Deficient heme synthesis (iron-deficiency anemia, pyridoxine-responsive anemias)

    Deficient globin synthesis (thalassemias, hemoglobinopathies)

Excessive loss of RBCs (hemolytic anemias due to genetically defective RBC)

    Abnormal shape (hereditary spherocytosis, hereditary elliptocytosis)

    Abnormal hemoglobins (sickle cell anemia, thalassemias, hemoglobin C disease)

    Abnormal RBC enzymes (G-6-PD deficiency, congenital nonspherocytic hemolytic anemias)

Excessive loss of RBCs

    Hemolytic anemias with acquired defects of RBC and positive Coombs' test (autoantibodies as in SLE, malignant lymphoma; or exogenous allergens as in penicillin allergy)

Excessive loss of normal RBCs

    Hemorrhage

    Hypersplenism

    Chemical agents (e.g., lead)

    Infectious agents (e.g., *Clostridium welchii*, *Bartonella*, malaria)

Miscellaneous diseases (e.g., uremia, liver disease, cancers)
Physical agents (e.g., burns)
Mechanical trauma (artificial heart valves, tumor microemboli)

(Blood smear shows fragmented bizarre-shaped RBC s in patients with artificial heart valves.)

Table 32. Red Blood Cell Indices

Type of Anemia	Mean Corpuscular Volume (MCV) (cu μ)	Mean Corpuscular Hemoglobin (MCH) (μμg)	Mean Corpuscular Hemoglobin Concentration (MCHC) (gm/100 ml)
Normal	82–92	27–31	32–36
Normocytic anemias	82–92	25–30	32–36
Macrocytic anemias	95–150	30–50	32–36
Microcytic (usually hypochromic) anemias	50–80	12–25	25–30

Mean corpuscular volume (MCV) (cu μ) = $\frac{\text{hematocrit}}{\text{RBC}}$

Mean corpuscular hemoglobin (MCH) (μμg) $\frac{\text{hemoglobin}}{\text{RBC}}$; represents weight of hemoglobin in average RBC. Not as useful as MCHC.

Mean corpuscular hemoglobin concentration (MCHC) (gm/100 ml) = $\frac{\text{hemoglobin}}{\text{hematocrit}}$; represents concentration of hemoglobin in average RBC.

MCHC is increased only in hereditary spherocytosis. MCHC is not increased in pernicious anemia.

RED BLOOD CELL INDICES IN VARIOUS ANEMIAS

Macrocytic (MCV > 95; MCHC > 30)
    Megaloblastic anemia
        Pernicious anemia
        Sprue (including steatorrhea, celiac disease, intestinal resection or fistula, etc.)
        Macrocytic anemia of pregnancy
        Megaloblastic anemia of infancy
        Fish tapeworm infestation
        Carcinoma of stomach, following total gastrectomy
        Antimetabolite therapy
        Orotic aciduria
        Di Guglielmo's disease
        Etc.
    Miscellaneous macrocytic nonmegaloblastic anemias that are usually normocytic
        Anemia of hypothyroidism
        Chronic liver disease
        Etc.
Normocytic (MCV = 80–94; MCHC > 30)
    Following acute hemorrhage
    Hemolytic anemias

Anemias due to inadequate blood formation
  Myelophthisic
  Hypoplastic
  Aplastic
  Associated with various chronic infections, neoplasms, uremia, etc.
  Etc.
Microcytic (usually hypochromic) (MCV < 80; MCHC < 30)
  Iron deficiency
    Inadequate intake
    Poor absorption
    Excessive iron requirements
    Chronic blood loss
    Etc.
  Pyridoxine-responsive anemia
  Thalassemia (major or combined with hemoglobinopathy)

MYELOPHTHISIC ANEMIA

Anemia is present.

Increased nucleated RBCs and normoblasts in peripheral smear are out of proportion to the degree of anemia and may be found even in the absence of anemia. Polychromatophilia, basophilic stippling, and increased reticulocyte count may also occur.

WBC may be normal or decreased; occasionally it is increased up to a leukemoid picture; immature WBC may be found in peripheral smear.

Platelets may be normal or decreased, and abnormal forms may occur. Abnormalities may occur even when WBC is normal.

Bone marrow demonstrates primary disease.
  Metastatic carcinoma of bone marrow (especially breast, lung, prostate, thyroid)
  Hodgkin's disease
  Multiple myeloma (5% of patients)
  Gaucher's, Niemann-Pick, and Hand-Schüller-Christian diseases
  Osteopetrosis
  Myelofibrosis

MYELOFIBROSIS
(including agnogenic myeloid metaplasia)

Normocytic anemia is usual.

Peripheral smear shows anisocytosis; poikilocytosis may be marked; polychromatophilia and occasional nucleated RBCs are found.

Reticulocyte count is increased (up to 10%).

WBC may be normal (one-half of patients), increased, or decreased. Immature cells (up to 15%) are usual. Basophils and eosinophils may be increased.

Platelets may be normal or decreased, and abnormal forms may occur.

Repeated bone marrow aspiration produces no marrow elements. Surgical biopsy of bone for histologic examination shows fibrous replacement of marrow with few residual islands of marrow elements.

Needle puncture of spleen and a lymph node shows extramedullary hematopoiesis.

Leukocyte alkaline phosphatase is increased; may be marked.
Serum uric acid is often increased.
Cephalin flocculation and thymol turbidity may be abnormal.
Laboratory findings due to complications
> Hemorrhage
> Hemolytic anemia
> Infection

Rule out underlying poisoning (e.g., phosphorus, fluorine, estrogens).

PURE RED CELL ANEMIA (AREGENERATIVE ANEMIA; IDIOPATHIC HYPOPLASTIC ANEMIA; PRIMARY RED CELL APLASIA; ETC.)

Normochromic normocytic anemia is present which is refractory to all treatment except transfusion and sometimes ACTH or corticosteroids.
Reticulocytes are decreased or absent.
WBC and differential blood count are normal.
Platelet count is normal.
There is no evidence of hemolysis.
Bone marrow usually shows marked decrease in erythroid series but sometimes is normal.
Plasma iron (^{59}Fe) clearance is markedly reduced.
RBC uptake of ^{59}Fe is markedly decreased.
The disease may be related to thymus tumors (see p. 247); leukemia, which develops in 10% of patients; chemicals; bronchogenic carcinoma (rarely); kwashiorkor; etc.

PANCYTOPENIA

Anemia
Leukopenia—absolute myeloid decrease may be associated with relative lymphocytosis or with lymphocytopenia
Thrombocytopenia
Laboratory findings due to causative disease

Due To
Hypersplenism
> Congestive splenomegaly
> Malignant lymphomas
> Histiocytoses
> Infectious diseases (tuberculosis, kala-azar, sarcoidosis)
> Primary splenic pancytopenia

Diseases of marrow
> Metastatic carcinoma
> Multiple myeloma
> Aleukemic leukemia
> Osteopetrosis
> Myelosclerosis, myelofibrosis, etc.

Aplastic anemias
> Physical and chemical causes (e.g., ionizing radiation, benzol compounds)
> Idiopathic causes (familial; isolated. *"Isolated" accounts for half of all cases of pancytopenia.*)

Megaloblastic macrocytic anemias (e.g., pernicious anemia)
Paroxysmal nocturnal hemoglobinuria (rare)

APLASTIC ANEMIA

Laboratory findings represent the whole spectrum from the most severe condition of the classic type, with marked leukopenia, thrombocytopenia, anemia, and acellular bone marrow, to cases with involvement only of erythroid elements; in some cases the marrow may be cellular or hyperplastic.

Due To
Ionizing radiation (x-ray, radioisotopes)
Benzene family chemicals
Cytotoxic drugs (e.g., nitrogen mustards, busulfan)
Antimetabolite drugs (e.g., 6-mercaptopurine, antifolates)
Others (e.g., arsenic)
Various agents which are less frequently responsible (especially chloramphenicol, phenylbutazone, Atabrine, gold compounds, anticonvulsant drugs, antibiotics, etc.)

HEMATOLOGIC EFFECTS OF CHEMICALS THAT INJURE BONE MARROW
(especially benzene; also trinitrotoluene and others)

In order of decreasing frequency
> Anemia
> Macrocytosis
> Thrombocytopenia
> Leukopenia
> Others (e.g., decreased lymphocytes, increased reticulocytes, increased eosinophils)

Varying degrees of severity up to aplastic anemia
Hemolytic anemia is sometimes produced.

HEMATOLOGIC EFFECTS OF RADIATION
(depends on amount of radiation received)

Severe
> Severe leukopenia with infection
> Thrombocytopenia and increased vascular fragility, causing hemorrhage; begins in 4–7 days, peak severity in 16–22 days
> Aplastic anemia if patient survives 3–6 weeks; laboratory findings due to complications such as hemorrhage, infection, dehydration

Mild (less than 300 R)
> Increased neutrophils within a few hours with onset of radiation sickness
> Decreased lymphocytes after 24 hours, causing decrease in total WBC
> No anemia unless dose of radiation is greater; may appear in 4–8 weeks (*Early appearance of anemia with greater radiation is due to hemorrhage and changes in fluid homeostasis rather than marrow injury.*)
> Platelets slightly decreased (some cases)

Chronic (occupational)
    Decreased granulocytes
    Increased lymphocytes, relative or absolute
    Varying degrees of leukocytosis and leukemoid reactions
    Varying degrees of anemia, normocytic or macrocytic; erythro-
        cytosis
    Thrombocytopenia
Late
    Increased incidence of leukemia (e.g., in survivors of atomic
        bomb explosions)
    Increased incidence of visceral malignancy (e.g., liver cancer
        due to Thorotrast, bone cancer due to radium)

TUMORS OF THYMUS

Associated With

Cushing's syndrome associated with malignant thymoma

Congenital hypogammaglobulinemia

Combinations of lymphopenia with dysgammaglobulinemia or nor-
mogammaglobulinemia or agammaglobulinemia and histologic
abnormality of thymus associated with marked increase in susceptibility to infection (e.g., widespread moniliasis, death following
BCG vaccination)

Acquired hypogammaglobulinemia. Ten percent of adults with this
condition have an associated thymoma. The condition does not
respond to thymectomy.

Myasthenia gravis. In 10–20% of patients there is associated thymoma, malignant in a quarter of the cases. Three-quarters of
myasthenia patients show thymic hyperplasia. Response to thymectomy is usually unpredictable and varies from marked improvement to worsening.

Aregenerative anemia of unknown etiology (not autoimmune),
usually of the normocytic normochromic type, occasionally macrocytic. Tumor may be present for many years before onset of
anemia. Anemia may not be prevented or corrected by thymectomy (thymectomy causes remission in 30% of cases) or steroid
therapy.

Laboratory Findings

WBC is usually normal. Lymphocytes may be increased. In 15% of
cases there is also associated leukopenia or thrombocytopenia or
both. Occasionally pancytopenia occurs.

Bone marrow shows selective erythroid hypoplasia with normal
myeloid and megakaryocytic elements.

PERNICIOUS ANEMIA

Anemia sometimes shows RBC as low as 500,000/cu mm.

MCV is increased (95–110 cu μ).

Poikilocytosis is moderate to marked; always present in relapse.

Anisocytosis is moderate to marked; always present in relapse.

Reticulocyte count is decreased or normal.

Blood smear may show polychromatophilia, stippled RBC, Howell-
Jolly bodies, Cabot's rings, etc. Large hypersegmented leukocytes
("shift to the right") are usually present and may precede RBC
abnormalities. Occasionally there is moderate eosinophilia.

Thrombocytopenia is present; abnormal and giant forms may be seen.

Leukopenia is usual (4000–5000/cu mm).

RBC survival is decreased.

Marrow shows megaloblastic and erythroid hyperplasia and abnormalities of myeloid and megakaryocytic elements.

Achlorhydria occurs even after administration of histamine—this is virtually essential for diagnosis. Decreased volume of gastric juice, high pH, and decreased or absent pepsin and rennin are also shown.

Schilling test is diagnostic.

Serum vitamin B_{12} is decreased.

Serum iron is almost always increased during relapse unless there is complicating iron deficiency. Total iron-binding capacity (TIBC) is normal or slightly decreased.

Serum indirect bilirubin is increased (less than 4 mg/100 ml).

Urine urobilinogen and coproporphyrin I are increased.

Stool urobilinogen is increased.

Serum LDH is markedly increased.

Serum alkaline phosphatase is decreased; increases after treatment.

Serum cholesterol is moderately decreased.

Cholinesterase activity in RBC, plasma, and whole blood is decreased.

There is a characteristic therapeutic response to vitamin B_{12} administration.

RESPONSE OF LABORATORY TESTS TO SPECIFIC TREATMENT OF PERNICIOUS ANEMIA

Increased urinary urobilinogen and coproporphyrin I immediately revert to normal, preceding reticulocyte response.

Serum folate decreases at the same time reticulocytosis takes place.

Serum iron decreases to normal or less than normal at the same time reticulocytosis takes place.

Serum uric acid increases; peak precedes maximum reticulocyte count by about 24 hours; remains increased as long as rapid RBC regeneration goes on.

Serum LDH falls but is not yet normal by eighth day.

Serum cholesterol rises to greater than normal levels; most marked at peak of reticulocyte response.

RBC count reaches normal between eighth and 12th week regardless of severity of anemia; hemoglobin concentration may rise at a slower rate, producing hypochromia with microcytosis.

Reticulocyte response is proportional to severity of anemia. This response is characteristic: reticulocyte count begins to rise by fourth day after treatment and reaches maximum on eighth to ninth day; returns to normal by 14th day.

Megaloblasts disappear from marrow in 24–48 hours.

Achlorhydria persists.

RBC cholinesterase activity increases.

Serum alkaline phosphatase increases to normal.

MACROCYTIC ANEMIA OF SPRUE, CELIAC DISEASE, STEATORRHEA

See p. 171.

Table 33. Laboratory Tests in Differential Diagnosis of Causes of Vitamin B_{12} Deficiencies.

| | Gastric Juice | | Schilling Test | |
| | | | | |
Condition	HCl	Intrinsic Factor Assay	Without Intrinsic Factor	With Intrinsic Factor
Lack of intrinsic factor (usually pernicious anemia)	O	O	D	N
Intestinal lesion	P or O	P	D	D
Nutritional	P or O	P	N	N

O = absent; P = present; N = normal; D = decreased.
Presence of free HCl in gastric juice always rules out pernicious anemia (except for very rare cases); absence of HCl is not helpful.

MEGALOBLASTIC ANEMIA OF PREGNANCY AND PUERPERIUM

Anemia may have been present during previous pregnancy with spontaneous remission after delivery.
Hematologic abnormalities are less marked than in pernicious anemia (see pp. 247-248).
If achlorhydria is present, it often disappears after delivery.
Therapeutic response to folic acid but usually not to vitamin B_{12}
Urinary excretion of formiminoglutamic acid (FIGLU) is increased.

MEGALOBLASTIC ANEMIA OF INFANCY (AGE, 6–12 MONTHS)

Morphologic findings in peripheral blood smear are similar to, but less severe than, those of pernicious anemia.
Bone marrow shows megaloblastic dysplasia that varies from mild to marked.
Urine FIGLU is increased; disappears after folic acid treatment.

HEREDITARY OROTIC ACIDURIA

This disorder of pyrimidine metabolism is due to a defect in the conversion of orotic acid to uridylic acid.
The severe megaloblastic anemia is refractory to vitamin B_{12} and folic acid but responsive to oral prednisone and yeast extract containing uridylic and cytidylic acids.
Anemia is hypochromic or normocytic; there is marked anisocytosis.
Leukopenia is present with increased susceptibility to infection.
Orotic acid in urine is increased.
RBC orotidylic decarboxylase activity is decreased (< 5.5 units).

ANEMIA IN HYPOTHYROIDISM

Occurs in one-third to two-thirds of patients with hypothyroidism; usually mild (hematocrit reading > 35)

Continued on p. 252.

Table 34. Laboratory Tests in Differential Diagnosis of Vitamin B_{12} and Folic Acid Deficiencies

Deficiency	Macrocytosis	Leukopenia and Thrombocytopenia	Serum B_{12}	Serum Folate	Urinary Excretion of FIGLU*	MMA†
Vitamin B_{12}	More marked	More constant	Marked D	N	I or N	I
Folic acid	Less marked	Inconstant	N or slight D	D	I	N

D = decreased; I = increased; N = normal.
* FIGLU = formiminoglutamic acid after histidine load; not a reliable test (since B_{12} is needed for normal folic acid metabolism).
† MMA = methylmalonic acid.

Table 35. Laboratory Tests in Differential Diagnosis of Microcytic (MCV <80) and Hypochromic (MCHC <30) Anemias

First: Determine serum iron and TIBC (and also perhaps do iron stain on bone marrow smear – the most reliable index of iron deficiency).
Second: If serum iron and TIBC are both normal, hemoglobin electrophoresis will establish the diagnosis of thalassemia. If serum iron is abnormal, the cause may be iron deficiency (e.g., blood loss, dietary deficiency) or normochromic microcytic anemia of chronic disease.

Type of Anemia	Serum Iron	TIBC	Transferrin Saturation	Marrow Hemosiderin	Sideroblasts	Type of Hemoglobin	Anemia
Normal values	65–180 µg/100 ml	250–410 µg/100 ml	20–55%		30–50%	AA	—
Iron deficiency	D	I	D	O	D	AA	Hypochromic, normocytic, or microcytic
Normochromic normocytic or microcytic of chronic disease	D	D or N	D or N	N or I	D	AA	Normochromic, normocytic, or microcytic
Thalassemia							
Major	I	D	I	I	I	20–90% F	Hypochromic
Minor	N or I	N	N or I	N or I	I	2–8% F A$_2$ is I	Microcytic
Sideroblastic	N	D or N	I	I	I	AA	Hypochromic microcytic, or normochromic normocytic

O = absent; D = decreased; I - increased; N = normal.

Iron depletion: Early – serum iron is normal; TIBC may be increased. Later – serum iron decreases; anemia is often normocytic when mild or of rapid onset; anemia first becomes microcytic, then hypochromic.
Iron deficiency may occur without anemia (transferrin saturation < 15%; decreased marrow iron and sideroblasts).

Anemia in hypothyroidism   (*continued*)

Macrocytic or normocytic (*If hypochromic, rule out associated iron deficiency.*)
No anisocytosis or poikilocytosis
Decreased total blood volume and plasma volume
Normal RBC survival
Responds to treatment of hypothyroidism

IRON-DEFICIENCY ANEMIA

Due To   (usually a combination of these factors)

Chronic blood loss (e.g., menometrorrhagia; bleeding from gastrointestinal tract, especially from carcinoma of colon, hiatus hernia, peptic ulcer, parasites in intestine)
Decreased food intake (e.g., poverty, emotional factors)
Decreased absorption (e.g., steatorrhea, gastrectomy, achlorhydria)
Increased requirements (e.g., pregnancy, lactation)

Laboratory Findings
Hemoglobin is decreased (usually 6–10 gm/100 ml) out of proportion to decrease in RBC (3.5–5.0 million/cu mm); thus MCV is decreased (less than 80 cu μ), MCHC is decreased (25–30 gm/100 ml) and MCH is decreased (less than 25 $\mu\mu$g). Hypochromia and microcytosis parallel severity of anemia. Polychromatophilia and nucleated RBCs are less common than in pernicious anemia. Diagnosis from peripheral blood smear is difficult and unreliable.
Serum iron is decreased (usually less than 40 μg/100 ml), total iron-binding capacity increased (usually 350–460 μg/100 ml), and transferrin saturation decreased (less than 15%).
Bone marrow shows normoblastic hyperplasia with decreased, and later absent, hemosiderin and decreased percentage of sideroblasts.
Reticulocytes are normal or decreased unless there is recent hemorrhage.
WBC is normal or may be slightly decreased; may be increased with fresh hemorrhage.
Serum bilirubin is not increased.
Platelet count is normal or may be slightly increased.
Coagulation studies are normal.
RBC fragility is normal or (often) increased to 0.21%.
RBC life span is normal.
Laboratory findings may disclose causative factors (e.g., GI bleeding).

ATRANSFERRINEMIA
(isolated absence of transferrin)

Iron-deficiency anemia is unresponsive to therapy.
Hemosiderosis follows transfusions with involvement of adrenals, heart, etc.
Serum protein electrophoresis shows marked decrease in beta globulins.
Absence of transferrin is demonstrated with immunoelectrophoresis.

ANEMIAS OF CHRONIC DISEASES
Due To
Subacute or chronic infections (especially tuberculosis, bronchiectasis, lung abscess, empyema, bacterial endocarditis, brucellosis)

Neoplasms
Chronic liver diseases
Rheumatoid arthritis (*anemia parallels activity of arthritis*)
Rheumatic fever, SLE
Uremia (BUN $>$ 70 mg/100 ml)

Laboratory Findings
Anemia is usually mild (hemoglobin $>$ 9 gm/100 ml).
Anemia is usually normocytic, normochromic. If hypochromic or microcytic, it is always less marked than in iron-deficiency anemia.
Moderate anisocytosis and slight poikilocytosis are present.
Reticulocytosis, polychromatophilia, and nucleated RBCs are absent (*may be present with severe anemia or uremia*).
Serum iron is decreased. TIBC and transferrin saturation are decreased or normal.
Marrow hemosiderin is increased or normal; sideroblasts are decreased.
RBC survival is slightly decreased in patient but not in normal recipient.
See Table 35, p. 251.

SIDEROBLASTIC (SIDEROACHRESTIC) ANEMIAS

This miscellaneous group of diseases is characterized by increased sideroblasts in marrow.

Due To
Hereditary factors
Certain drugs (e.g., isoniazid and PAS in treatment of tuberculosis)
Preleukemia
Unknown cause

See Table 35, p. 251.

PYRIDOXINE-RESPONSIVE ANEMIA

Severe hypochromic microcytic anemia is present.
Blood smear shows anisocytosis, poikilocytosis with many bizarre forms, target cells, hypochromia. Polychromatophilia and reticulocytosis are not increased.
Serum iron is increased; TIBC is somewhat decreased; transferrin saturation is markedly increased. Marrow sideroblasts and blood siderocytes are increased. Marrow and liver biopsy show increased hemosiderin.
Bone marrow usually shows normoblastic hyperplasia; occasionally it is megaloblastic.
Response to pyridoxine is always incomplete. Even when hemoglobin becomes normal, morphologic changes in RBCs persist.

LABORATORY SCREENING FOR HEMOGLOBINOPATHIES

Normocytic normochromic RBC except
    Thalassemia syndromes—microcytic hypochromic
    Hemoglobin C, D, E diseases—microcytic normochromic
Osmotic fragility—normal or decreased (especially in thalassemia)
    Symmetric shift in Hb C, D, E diseases
    Asymmetric shift in other Hb diseases

Target cells—in many of hemolytic diseases due to Hb diseases; up
  to 50% of RBCs in Hb C, D, E diseases
Sickle cell test—proves presence of Hb S
Inclusion bodies—in Hb H and C disorders
Hb electrophoresis
Alkali denaturation for Hb F

SICKLE CELL DISEASE

Sickle cell trait (heterozygous sickle cell or hemoglobin AS disease—
  occurs in about 10% of American Negroes)
  Hemoglobin electrophoresis: Hemoglobin S is 20–40% and
    hemoglobin A is 60–80%, small amount of hemoglobin F (up
    to 2%) may be present.
  Sickle cell preparation is positive.
  Blood smear shows only a few target cells.
  No anemia or hemolysis or jaundice is present.
  Anoxia may cause systemic sickling (see below, Sickle cell
    anemia). *Beware anesthesia, airplane flights, etc.*
Sickle cell anemia (homozygous hemoglobin SS disease)
  Hemoglobin electrophoresis: Hemoglobin S is 80–100% and
    hemoglobin F is the rest (see Fetal Hemoglobin, p. 00);
    hemoglobin A is absent.
  The anemia is normocytic normochromic (hemoglobin 5–10
    gm/100 ml).
  Sickle cell preparation is positive.
  Blood smear shows a variable number of RBCs with abnormal
    shapes, nucleated RBCs, Howell-Jolly bodies, target cells,
    spherical cells.
  Reticulocyte count is increased.
  WBC is increased (10,000–30,000/cu mm), with normal differ-
    ential or shift to the left.
  Platelet count is increased (300,000–500,000/cu mm), with
    abnormal forms.
  Bone marrow shows hyperplasia of all elements.
  Decreased ESR becomes normal after blood is aerated.
  Osmotic fragility is decreased (more resistant RBC).
  Mechanical fragility of RBC is increased.
  RBC survival time is decreased.
  Indirect serum bilirubin is increased (up to 6 mg/100 ml).
  Urine contains increased urobilinogen but is negative for bile.
  Urobilinogen in stool is increased.
  Hemosiderin appears in urine sediment.
  Hematuria is frequent.
  Renal concentrating ability is decreased.
  Serum uric acid may be increased.

  Laboratory findings due to complications
    Infarction of lungs, spleen, brain, bowel, etc.
    Stasis and necrosis of liver—increased bile in urine, in
      creased direct serum bilirubin up to 40 mg/100 ml, othe
      findings of obstructive type of jaundice. Chronic chol
      cystitis and cholelithiasis in one-third of adults.
    Salmonella osteomyelitis (see pp. 225, 382)

Continued on page 256.

Table 31. Some Laboratory Findings in Hemoglobinopathies and Thalassemia

Condition	Hb Type	Hb F (Fetal Hemoglobin) % of Total	(Stained Blood Smear) Sickling	% Target Cells	Microcytosis	Hypochromia	Severity of Anemia	Splenomegaly
Normal adult	AA	0–2	0	0	0	0	0	0
Normal newborn	AF	60–90	0	0	0	0	0	0
Sickle cell trait	AS	0–2	+	4	0	0	0	0
Sickle cell anemia	SS	2–30	++	5–30	0	0–1+	4+	2+
Sickle cell–thalassemia	SF	2–20	+	20–40	3+	3+	3–4+	2+
Sickle cell–Hb C	SC	2–8	+	20–85	0	1–2+	2–3+	2+
Sickle cell–Hb D	SD	0–2	+	1+	0–1+	1–2+	3–4+	0
Sickle cell–Hb G	SG	0–2	+	0	0	0	0	0
Sickle cell–hereditary spherocytosis	SA	0–2	+	1+	1+	0	1–4+	2+
Thalassemia minor	AA$_2$	0–8	0	1+	2–3+	2–3+	1+	±
Thalassemia major	AF	10–100	0	10–35	2–4+	2–4+	3–4+	4+
Hb C–thalassemia	CA	0–2	0	3+	1+	1+	0–1+	0
Hb E–thalassemia	EF	20–40	0	10–40	2+	2+	1+	3+
Hb G–thalassemia	EG	0–2	0	1+	1+	1+	1+	0
Hb H–thalassemia	AH	0–2	0	2+	1+	2+	2+	±
Hb C trait	AC	0–2	0	1–100	0	1+	0	0
Hb C disease	CC	0–5	0	30–100	0–1+	3+	1+	2+
Hb C–elliptocytosis	AC	0–2	0	1+	1+	2+	0–1+	0
Hb D trait	AD	0–2	0	0	0	0	0	0
Hb E trait	AE	0–2	0	0	0	0	0	0
Hb E disease	EE	0–9	0	25–60	2+	0	0–1+	±
Hb G trait	AG	0–2	0	0	0	0	0	0
Hb G disease	GG	0–2	0	0	0	0	0	0
Hb I trait	AI	0–2	0	0–2	0	0	0	0

1+ to 4+ = amounts present.

Sickle cell disease (*continued*)

> *Anemia and hemolytic jaundice are present throughout life; hemolysis and anemia are* not *increased during crises.*

Hemoglobin SC disease

    Hemoglobin electrophoresis: Hemoglobin A is absent; hemoglobin S predominates (30–60%) with hemoglobin C present; hemoglobin F is 2–15%.

    Blood smear shows tetragonal crystals within RBC in 70% of patients.

    Other findings are the same as for sickle cell anemia but there is less marked destruction of RBCs, anemia, etc., and the disease is less severe clinically. *Crises may cause a more marked fall in RBC than occurs in hemoglobin SS disease.*

Sickle cell–thalassemia disease

    Hemoglobin electrophoresis: Hemoglobin S is 20–80%; hemoglobin F is 2–20%; hemoglobin A is 0–50%.

    Anemia is hypochromic microcytic; target cells are prominent; serum iron is normal.

    Other findings resemble those of sickle cell anemia.

Sickle cell-persistent high fetal hemoglobin

    Hemoglobin electrophoresis: Hemoglobin F is 20–40%; deceased hemoglobin A and A_2 and combined hemoglobin S.

    Findings are intermediate between those of sickle cell anemia and of sickle cell trait.

Sickle cell–hemoglobin D disease

    Findings are intermediate between those of sickle cell anemia and of sickle cell trait.

THALASSEMIA

Thalassemia trait

    There are decreased hemoglobin and hematocrit values, with normal or increased RBC (5–7 million/cu mm) causing slight hypochromic microcytic anemia.

    Blood smear changes are less marked than in thalassemia major but disproportionately more marked than in anemia.

    Reticulocyte count is increased (2–10%).

    Cellular marrow contains stainable iron.

    Serum iron is normal or increased.

    Osmotic fragility is decreased.

    Beta type of thalassemia minor has increased A_2 hemoglobin (3–6%) on starch or agar electrophoresis and a slight increase in hemoglobin F (2–10%); A_2 and F hemoglobins are absent in the alpha type of thalassemia.

Thalassemia major

    Fetal hemoglobin is 10–90%; Hb A is decreased; Hb A_2 is not increased.

    There is marked hypochromic microcytic regenerative hemolytic anemia.

    Blood smear shows marked anisocytosis, poikilocytosis, target cells, spherocytes, and hypochromic, fragmented, and bizarre RBCs; also many nucleated RBCs: basophilic stippling, Cabot's rings, siderocytes.

    Reticulocyte count is increased.

    WBC increase is slight, with normal differential, or marked, shift to the left.

Platelets are normal.
Bone marrow is cellular and shows erythroid hyperplasia and contains stainable iron.
Serum iron is normal or increased.
Indirect serum bilirubin is increased (2–6 mg/100 ml).
Urine urobilinogen is increased without bile.
Stool urobilinogen is increased.
RBC survival time is decreased.
Osmotic fragility is decreased.
Mechanical fragility is increased.

Hemoglobin E–thalassemia
Findings resemble those in thalassemia major.

HEMOGLOBIN C DISEASE

Hemoglobin C trait (occurs in 2% of American Negroes; less frequently in other Americans)
Blood smear shows variable number of target cells.
No other abnormalities are seen.

Hemoglobin C disease
Mild hypochromic anemia is present.
Blood smear shows many target cells, occasional nucleated RBCs, a few tetragonal crystals within RBCs which increase following splenectomy.
Reticulocyte count is increased (2–10%).
Osmotic fragility is decreased.
Mechanical fragility is increased.
RBC survival time is decreased.
Hb F is slightly increased.

Hemoglobin SC disease (see under Sickle Cell Disease, p. 254)

HEMOGLOBIN D DISEASE

Homozygous hemoglobin D disease
Mild microcytic anemia
Target cells
Decreased RBC survival time

Heterozygous hemoglobin D trait
No findings

Sickle cell–hemoglobin D disease
Findings intermediate between those of sickle cell anemia and of sickle cell trait

HEMOGLOBIN E DISEASE

Homozygous hemoglobin E disease
Mild hypochromic hemolytic anemia
Hb F sometimes slightly increased

Heterozygous hemoglobin E trait
No findings

Hemoglobin E–thalassemia
Findings like those in thalassemia major

METHEMOGLOBINEMIA

Due To
Drugs and chemicals, especially aniline derivatives (e.g., acetanilid, phenacetin, certain sulfonamides, various clothing dyes)

Abnormal hemoglobin M (several different Ms)
Inherited enzyme deficiency (e.g., methemoglobin reductase)

Laboratory Findings
Freshly drawn blood is chocolate-brown; does not become red after exposure to air.
Starch block electrophoresis identifies the hemoglobin M.
Spectroscopic absorption analysis. Band at 630 mμ disappears on addition of 5% KCN.
RBC is slightly increased; no other hematologic abnormalities are found; there is no jaundice.

Patient is cyanotic clinically but in apparent good health.

SULFHEMOGLOBINEMIA

Due To
Drugs, especially phenacetin (including Bromo-Seltzer) and acetanilid

Laboratory Findings
Spectroscopic absorption analysis. Band at 618 mμ does not disappear on addition of 5% KCN.
Laboratory findings due to associated bromide intoxication. Both conditions may be due to excessive intake of Bromo-Seltzer.

OVALOCYTOSIS (HEREDITARY ELLIPTOCYTOSIS)

Blood smear shows 25–90% of RBCs are oval.
No other hematologic abnormalities are seen in most patients; about 12% of patients show decreased RBC survival time, moderate anemia, increased serum bilirubin, and increased reticulocyte count.
Hemoglobin electrophoresis is normal.
Osmotic fragility and autohemolysis are normal.
Mechanical fragility is increased.

HEREDITARY SPHEROCYTOSIS

Defective RBC membrane is abnormally permeable to sodium, causing water inflow and rupture.
Anemia (hemolytic type) is moderate (RBC = 3–4 million/cu mm), microcytic (MCV = 70–80 cu μ) and hyperchromic (MCHC = 36–40 gm/100 ml).
Anisocytosis is marked; poikilocytosis slight.
Spherocytes are present.
Reticulocytes are increased.
Increased WBC is moderate.
Increased platelet count is moderate.
Bone marrow shows marked erythroid hyperplasia; moderate hemosiderin is present.
Indirect serum bilirubin is increased.
Stool urobilinogen is usually increased.
Haptoglobins are decreased or absent.
Coombs' test is negative.
RBC survival time is decreased (using ^{51}Cr).

Osmotic fragility is increased; when normal in some patients, the incubated fragility test shows increased hemolysis.

Autohemolysis (sterile defibrinated blood incubated for 48 hours) is increased (10–20% compared to normal of less than 4% of cells).

Abnormal osmotic fragility and autohemolysis are reduced by 10% glucose.

Mechanical fragility is increased.

HEREDITARY NONSPHEROCYTIC HEMOLYTIC ANEMIAS

This is a heterogeneous group. Some are due to deficiency of G-6-PD; others to unknown cause or to other rare congenital enzyme defects, e.g., glutathione.

Anemia is of the hemolytic type; may be severe; may begin in newborn; may be precipitated by certain drugs.

RBCs show Howell-Jolly bodies, Pappenheimer bodies, Heinz bodies, basophilic stippling; there may be slight macrocytosis.

Increase in reticulocyte count is marked even with mild anemia.

Bone marrow shows marked erythroid hyperplasia; normal hemosiderin is present.

WBC, platelet count, hemoglobin electrophoresis, osmotic fragility, and mechanical fragility are normal.

Autohemolysis is present in some cases but not in others; reduction by glucose is less than in normal blood.

GLUCOSE-6-PHOSPHATE DEHYDROGENASE (G-6-PD) IN RBC

Decreased In
American Negro males, 13%
American Negro females, 3% (20% are carriers)
Other racial groups (e.g., Greeks, Sardinians, Sephardic Jews)

May be associated with at least four clinical syndromes
> Some drug-induced acute hemolytic anemias (e.g., primaquine, sulfonamides, antipyretics)
> Favism
> Nonimmunologic hemolytic disease of the newborn
> Some cases of congenital nonspherocytic hemolytic anemia

Other Findings
Higher frequency of coronary heart disease and of cholelithiasis
Higher risk in presence of some other diseases (e.g., diabetes mellitus, viral hepatitis, pneumonia)

Increased In
Pernicious anemia to 3 times normal level; remains elevated for several months even after administration of vitamin B_{12}
ITP (Werlhof's disease); becomes normal soon after splenectomy
Also reported in hepatic coma, hyperthyroidism, myocardial infarction (first week after), other megaloblastic anemias, and chronic blood loss

ERYTHROCYTE PYRUVATE KINASE DEFICIENCY

Congenital inherited nonspherocytic hemolytic anemia showing
> Icterus
> Anemia

Reticulocytosis
Macrocytosis
Few or no spherocytes
Occasional "tailed poikilocytes"
Varying abnormalities of incubated RBC osmotic fragility
Deficiency of erythrocyte pyruvate kinase

PAROXYSMAL NOCTURNAL HEMOGLOBINURIA (MARCHIAFAVA-MICHELI SYNDROME)

Hemoglobinemia is present; increases during sleep.
Hemoglobinuria is evident on arising.
Serum haptoglobin is absent during an episode.
Chronic hemolytic anemia is well developed.
Urine contains hemoglobin, hemosiderin (in WBC and epithelial cells of sediment), and increased urobilinogen.
Osmotic fragility is normal.
Serum iron may be decreased.
WBC is usually decreased.
Leukocyte alkaline phosphatase activity is decreased.
Platelet count is usually decreased but shows thrombotic rather than hemorrhagic complications.
Autohemolysis is increased.
RBC fragility is increased in acid medium (Ham test) and in hydrogen peroxide; amount of change is related to clinical severity.
RBC acetylcholinesterase activity is decreased.

PAROXYSMAL COLD HEMOGLOBINURIA

Sudden hemoglobinuria follows exposure to cold environment.
Findings are of acute hemolytic anemia.
Cold autohemolysin is present in blood.
Positive direct Coombs' test is present only during the attack.
There may be a biologic false positive test for syphilis, or the attack may be due to congenital syphilis.

ACQUIRED HEMOLYTIC ANEMIA

Laboratory findings due to increased destruction of RBC
> RBC survival time differentiates intrinsic RBC defect from factor outside RBC.
> Blood smear may have a few spherocytes.
> Slight abnormality of osmotic fragility is shown.
> There is increased indirect serum bilirubin (less than 6 mg/100 ml because of compensatory excretory capacity of liver).
> Urine urobilinogen is increased (may vary with liver function; may be obscured by antibiotic therapy altering intestinal flora). Bile is absent from urine.
> Stool urobilinogen is increased.
> Hemoglobinemia and hemoglobinuria are present when hemolysis is very rapid.
> Haptoglobins are decreased or absent in chronic hemolytic diseases (removed following combination with free hemoglobin in serum).

Laboratory findings due to compensatory increased production of RBC
>   There is a degree of anemia. MCV reflects immaturity of circulating RBC. Polychromatophilia is present.
>   Reticulocyte count is increased.
>   Erythroid hyperplasia of bone marrow is evident.

Laboratory findings due to mechanism of RBC destruction
>   Coombs' tests are positive.
>   Warm antibodies are found.
>   Cold agglutinins are found.
>   There is a biologic false positive test for syphilis.

Laboratory findings due to underlying condition
>   Malignant lymphoma
>   Disseminated lupus erythematosus
>   Idiopathic cause
>   Etc.

LABORATORY FINDINGS DUE TO INTRAVASCULAR HEMOLYSIS

Plasma hemoglobin increases transiently with return to normal in 8 hours. Determinations lack accuracy and precision.

Plasma haptoglobin level decreases in 6–10 hours and lasts for 2–3 days after lysis of 20–30 ml blood. Determination is relatively reliable and very sensitive.

Urine hemosiderin occurs 3–5 days after hemolysis with positive Prussian blue staining of renal tubular epithelial cells. It may be difficult to detect a single episode. Urine hemosiderin is commonly found in paroxysmal nocturnal hemoglobinuria.

Hemoglobinuria occurs 1–2 hours after severe hemolysis and lasts up to 24 hours. It is a transient finding and is relatively insensitive. False positive is due to myoglobinuria or to lysis of RBCs in urine.

Schumm's test for methemalbuminemia becomes positive 1–6 hours after hemolysis of 100 ml blood and lasts 1–3 days. Methemalbuminemia also occurs in hemorrhagic pancreatitis.

Serum bilirubin increase depends upon liver function and amount of hemolysis. With normal liver function, it is increased 1 mg/100 ml in 1–6 hours to maximum in 3–12 hours following hemolysis of 100 ml blood.

Fecal urobilinogen may be increased but is not useful because of wide normal range and variability.

Urine urobilinogen is similarly insensitive and unreliable as an index of hemolysis.

Extravascular hemolysis may cause increases in serum bilirubin and urine and fecal urobilinogen and a decrease in serum haptoglobin.

HEMOLYTIC DISEASE OF THE NEWBORN (ERYTHROBLASTOSIS FETALIS)
(due to destruction of fetal RBCs by maternal antibodies caused by isoimmunization of pregnant mother)

Serum indirect bilirubin shows rapid rise to high levels. May rise 0.3–1.0 mg/hour to level of 30 mg/100 ml in untreated infants to maximum in 3–5 days unless they die. Increased urine and fecal urobilinogen parallels serum levels.

Direct Coombs' test is strongly positive on cord blood RBC when due to Rh, Kell, Kidd, Duffy antibodies but is usually negative or weakly positive when due to anti-A antibodies. It becomes negative within a few days of effective exchange transfusion, but may remain positive for weeks in untreated infants. Indirect Coombs' test on cord blood may be positive because of "free" immune antibody.

At birth there is little or no anemia. In severe cases anemia may develop rapidly (RBC may decrease by 1 million/cu mm/day) to maximum by third or fourth day.

MCHC is normal; MCV and MCH are increased.

Nucleated RBCs in peripheral blood are markedly increased (10,000–100,000/cu mm) during first 2 days (normal = 200 to 2000/cu mm) and are usually very large. They tend to decrease and may be absent by third or fourth day. Normoblastosis is mild or absent when due to other antigens than Rh_o.

Peripheral smear shows marked polychromatophilia, macrocytic RBCs, increased reticulocyte count. In ABO incompatibility, spherocytosis may be marked, with associated increased osmotic fragility; *spherocytosis is slight or absent in Rh incompatibility*.

Hb F is decreased, and adult hemoglobin is increased.

WBC is increased (usually 15,000–30,000/cu mm).

Platelet count is usually normal; may be decreased in severe cases but returns to normal after 1 week. With decreased platelets, one may find increased bleeding time, poor clot retraction, and purpura. Prothrombin and fibrinogen deficiencies may occur.

Disease terminates in 3–6 weeks with elimination of maternal antibodies from infant's serum.

Late anemia occurs during second to fourth week of life in 5% of those receiving exchange transfusion. Reticulocyte count is low, and marrow may not show erythroid hyperplasia.

For exchange transfusion
> Use mother's serum for crossmatch.
> Use Rh-negative donor unless mother and baby are both Rh-positive.
> Use indirect Coombs' test for crossmatch.

Indications for Exchange Transfusion
Serum bilirubin in normal newborn is 1–3 mg/100 ml on first day.
> May peak up to 6 mg/100 ml on third to fifth day (mild jaundice may be evident).
> Declines to normal 1.5 mg/100 ml over 2-week period.
>> In smaller, more premature infants, jaundice tends to last longer.
> Peak up to 10–12 mg/100 ml on fifth to seventh day.
> Decline to normal may take 4–5 weeks.

Clinical jaundice before the third day is more marked than usual; after sixth day is pathologic.

Hyperbilirubinemia is most likely to produce CNS damage (kernicterus) in infants that are
> Most premature
> Lightest weight
> Afflicted with dehydration, hypoglycemia, acidosis, hypoxia, hypoalbuminemia, sepsis

Exchange transfusion is indicated if

Birth weight is	and serum bilirubin is in first 48 hours	or thereafter
_____ grams	_____ mg/100 ml	_____ mg/100 ml
Less than 1000	10	12
1000–1499	12	14
1500–2000	14	16
2001–2500	16	18
More than 2500	18	20

Transfuse at one step earlier in presence of
Serum protein less than 5 gm/100 ml
Metabolic acidosis (pH less than 7.25)
Respiratory distress (with O_2 less than 50 mm Hg)
Certain clinical findings (hypothermia, CNS or other clinical deterioration, etc.)
Other criteria for exchange transfusion are suddenness and rate of bilirubin increase and when it occurs; e.g., an increase of 3 mg/100 ml in 12 hours, especially after bilirubin has already leveled off, must be followed with frequent serial determinations, especially if it occurs on first or on seventh day rather than on third day. Beware of rate of bilirubin increase greater than 1 mg/100 ml during first day. In ABO hemolytic disease, rate of bilirubin increase is not as great as in Rh disease; if danger level for exchange transfusion is not reached by third day, it is unlikely that it will be reached.

	Continue to Follow Patient	Consider Exchange	Perform Exchange
Rh antibody titer in mother	<1:64	>1:64	
Cord hemoglobin	>14 gm/100 ml	12–14 gm/100 ml	<12 gm/100 ml
Cord bilirubin	>4 mg/100 ml	4–5 mg/100 ml	>5 mg/100 ml
Capillary blood hemoglobin	>12 gm/100 ml	<12 gm/100 ml	<12 gm/100 ml and decreasing in first 24 hours
Serum bilirubin	<18 mg/100 ml	18–20 mg/100 ml	20 mg/100 ml in first 24 hours or after 48 hours 22 mg/100 ml on two tests 6–8 hours apart

In sick premature infants, 15 mg/100 ml is upper limit to indicate exchange transfusion.

Phototherapy of Coombs' positive infants decreases exchange transfusions (from 25% to 10% of these infants); follow effect of therapy with serum bilirubin every 4–8 hours. Phototherapy is usually not begun until serum bilirubin is 10 mg/100 ml. Skin color is disguised by phototherapy, so serum bilirubin determination is even more important. Beware of untreated anemia in these infants.

Severe jaundice during first day of life indicates hemolytic disease, most probably Rh or ABO hemolytic disease. If Coombs' test is negative, the following must be ruled out:

    Hereditary spherocytosis (blood smear is not helpful since hemolytic disease of the newborn also shows spherocytes)

    Elliptocytosis (blood smear shows elliptocytes, is diagnostic)

If jaundice appears later, other causes of hemolytic disease to be ruled out are

    Glucose-6-phosphate deficiency and, less frequently, pyruvate-kinase deficiency

    Slowly developing hemolytic disease

    Sepsis

If jaundice persists or peaks late, rule out

    Hemolytic disease   Hepatitis

    Sepsis   Biliary obstruction

Rare causes of later-appearing jaundice (second to third week) are

    Pyloric stenosis

    Galactosemia

See also pp. 189-192, Crigler-Najjar syndrome, Gilbert's disease, etc.

CRITERIA FOR SELECTION OF PATIENTS FOR IMMUNOSUPPRESSION OF Rh SENSITIZATION

Mother must be Rh_0 (D) negative and D^u negative.

Mother's serum must have no Rh antibodies.

Baby must be Rh_0 (D) positive.

Baby must have negative direct Coombs' test (cord blood).

Crossmatch of mother's RBC and Rh_0 Gam (1:1000) must be compatible.

ANEMIA DUE TO ACUTE BLOOD LOSS

RBC, hemoglobin, and hematocrit level are not reliable initially because of compensatory vasoconstriction and hemodilution. They decrease for several days after hemorrhage ceases. RBC returns to normal in 4–6 weeks. Hemoglobin returns to normal in 6–8 weeks.

Anemia is normocytic. (*If hypochromic or microcytic, rule out iron deficiency due to prior hemorrhages.*)

Reticulocyte count is increased after 1–2 days, reaches peak in 4–7 days (up to 15%). Persistent increase suggests continuing hemorrhage.

Increased WBC (usually up to 20,000/cu mm) reaches peak in 2–5 hours, becomes normal in 3–4 days. Persistent increase suggests continuing hemorrhage, bleeding into a body cavity, or infection. Differential count shows shift to the left.

Platelets are increased (up to 1 million/cu mm) within a few hours; coagulation time is decreased.

BUN is increased if hemorrhage into lumen of GI tract occurs.

Serum indirect bilirubin is increased if hemorrhage into a body cavity or cystic structure occurs.

Laboratory findings due to causative disease (e.g., peptic ulcer, esophageal varices, leukemia) are noted.

ANEMIAS IN PARASITIC INFESTATIONS

Anemia due to blood loss, malnutrition, specific organ damage

Malaria
> Hemolytic anemia

Diphyllobothrium latum (fish tapeworm)
> Macrocytic anemia

Hookworm
> Hypochromic microcytic anemia due to chronic blood loss

Schistosoma mansoni
> Hypochromic microcytic anemia due to blood loss from intestine
> Macrocytic anemia due to cirrhosis of schistosomiasis

Amebiasis
> Due to blood loss and malnutrition

"ANEMIA" IN PREGNANCY

This is a normal physiologic change due to hemodilution: Total blood volume and plasma volume increase more than red cell mass.

Onset is at eighth week; full development by 16th to 22d week; rapid return to normal in puerperium.

Hemoglobin averages 11 gm/100 ml; hematocrit value averages 33.

RBC morphology is normal.

RBC indices are normal.

If hemoglobin < 10 gm/100 ml or there are hypochromic microcytic indices, rule out iron-deficiency anemia, which may occur frequently during pregnancy.

See Megaloblastic Anemia of Pregnancy, p. 249.

ANEMIA IN CHILDREN

Due To
Iron deficiency
Blood loss
Hemorrhagic disease of the newborn (hypoprothrombinemia)
Hemolytic disease of the newborn (erythroblastosis fetalis)
Hemolytic anemias (*more acute in children and show more marked anemia, erythroblastosis, reticulocytosis, jaundice, leukocytosis*)
> Thalassemia
> Hemoglobinopathies
> Hereditary spherocytosis
> Others

Anemias of chronic diseases
Megaloblastic anemia of infancy
Other hematologic diseases
> Leukemias
> Histiocytoses (e.g., Gaucher's disease, Niemann-Pick disease, histiocytosis X)
> Osteopetrosis
> Gargoylism

POLYCYTHEMIA VERA

RBC is 7–12 million; may go up to > 15 million/cu mm.
Hemoglobin is 18–24 gm/100 ml.
Hematocrit value is increased.
MCV, MCH, and MCHC are normal or decreased.
Blood volume and red cell mass are increased; plasma volume is variable.
ESR is decreased.
Blood viscosity is increased.
Osmotic fragility is decreased (increased resistance).
Platelet count is increased (often more than 1 million).
Moderate polynuclear leukocytosis is present (usually more than 15,000/cu mm; sometimes there is a leukemoid reaction).
Peripheral blood smear may show macrocytes, microcytes, polychromatophilic RBC, normoblasts, large masses of platelets, neutrophilic "shift to the left."
Reticulocyte count is normal unless there has been some recent hemorrhage.
Bone marrow shows general hyperplasia of all elements.
Serum uric acid may be increased.
Leukocyte alkaline phosphatase may be greatly increased.
Serum vitamin B_{12} is increased.
Oxygen saturation of arterial blood is normal.
BMR is increased.
Bleeding time and coagulation time are normal but clot retraction may be poor.
Urine may contain increased urobilinogen and occasionally albumin is present.

Laboratory findings of associated diseases

Gout	Cirrhosis
Duodenal ulcer	Hypertension

Laboratory findings due to complications
    Thromboses (e.g., cerebral; portal vein)
    Intercurrent infection
    Hemorrhage
    Myelofibrosis
    Chronic myelogenous leukemia (develops in 20% of patients)

SECONDARY POLYCYTHEMIA

Results from hypoxia with decreased oxygen saturation of arterial blood due to
    Decreased atmospheric pressure (e.g., high altitudes)
    Chronic heart disease
        Congenital (e.g., pulmonary stenosis, septal defect, patent ductus arteriosus)
        Acquired (e.g., chronic rheumatic mitral disease)
    Arteriovenous aneurysm
    Impaired pulmonary ventilation
        Alveolar-capillary block (e.g., Hamman-Rich syndrome, sarcoidosis, lymphangitic cancer)
        Alveolar hypoventilation (e.g., bronchial asthma, kyphoscoliosis)
        Restriction of pulmonary vascular bed (e.g., primary pulmonary hypertension, mitral stenosis, chronic pulmonary emboli, emphysema)

Abnormal hemoglobin pigments (methemoglobinemia or sulf-
hemoglobinemia due to chemicals such as aniline and coal
tar derivatives)
Associated with tumors and miscellaneous conditions
Renal disease (hypernephroma, benign tumors, hydronephrosis,
polycystic kidneys)
Pheochromocytoma
Cushing's syndrome
Hemangioblastoma of cerebellum
Uterine fibromyoma
Etc.

The polycythemia may be relative.

See Table 37, below.

RELATIVE POLYCYTHEMIA

Relative polycythemia is not secondary to hypoxia but results from
a decrease in plasma volume due to decreased fluid intake (e.g.,
dehydration) and/or excess loss of body fluids (e.g., burns, shock).

Table 37. Laboratory Tests in Differential Diagnosis of Polycythemia Vera,
Secondary Polycythemia, and Relative Polycythemia

Test	Polycythemia Vera	Secondary Polycythemia	Relative Polycythemia
Hematocrit	I	I	I
Blood volume	I	I	D or N
Red cell mass	I	I	D or N
Plasma volume	I or N	N or I	D or N
Platelet count	I	N	N
WBC with shift to left	I	N	N
Nucleated RBC, abnormal RBC	I	N	N
Serum uric acid	I	I	N
Serum vitamin B_{12}	I	N	N
Leukocyte alkaline phosphatase	I	N	N
Oxygen saturation of arterial blood	N	D	N
Bone marrow	Hyperplasia of all elements	Erythroid hyperplasia	N

I = increased; D = decreased; N = normal.

ACUTE LEUKEMIA

Peripheral blood
WBC is rarely more than 100,000/cu mm. It may be normal and
is commonly less than normal. Peripheral smear shows many
cells which resemble lymphocytes; it may not be possible to
differentiate the very young forms as lymphoblasts or myelo-
blasts. Peroxidase-positive granules may be found in some
cells in acute myeloblastic but not in acute lymphoblastic

leukemia. Prognosis is better when initial WBC < 10,000/cu mm and worse when > 100,000/cu mm.

Anemia is almost always present at clinical onset. Usually normocytic and sometimes macrocytic, it is progressive and may become severe. Normoblasts and polychromatophilia are common.

Platelet count is usually decreased at clinical onset and becomes progressively severe. May show poor clot retraction, increased bleeding time, positive tourniquet test, etc.

Bone marrow smear

Blast cells are present even when none are found in peripheral blood. (*This finding is useful to differentiate from other causes of pancytopenia.*)

There is progressively increasing infiltration with earlier cell types (e.g., blasts, myelocytes).

The myeloid:erythroid ratio is increased.

Erythroid and megakaryocyte elements are replaced.

In acute myelogenous leukemia, serum LDH and MDH are frequently but inconstantly increased; there is normal to slight increase in SGOT, SGPT, ALD.

Laboratory findings due to complications

Meningeal leukemia occurs in one-quarter to one-half of children with acute leukemia; CSF shows pleocytosis and increased pressure and LDH.

Urate nephropathy. See Chronic Myelogenous Leukemia, p. 269.

Infection causes 90% of deaths. Most important pathogens are gram-negative rods (especially *Pseudomonas aeruginosa*) and fungi (especially *Candida albicans*).

Hemolytic anemia. See pp. 260–261.

Complete remission is possible with drug therapy (e.g., prednisone in acute lymphoblastic leukemia).

WBC falls (or rises) to normal in 1–2 weeks with replacement of lymphoblasts by normal polynuclear leukocytes and return of RBC and platelet counts to normal; bone marrow may become normal. Maximum improvement in 6–8 weeks.

Amethopterin toxicity causes a macrocytic type of anemia with megaloblasts in marrow compared to leukemic normocytic anemia with blast cells in marrow.

PRELEUKEMIA

(poorly defined hematologic syndrome that sometimes precedes acute nonlymphocytic leukemia; overt leukemia seen in one-third of these cases by 6 months, one-half by 12, and three-quarters by 24 months)

Anemia, leukopenia, and thrombocytopenia in various combination are most common findings.

Leukocytosis, monocytosis, and immature granulocytes may occur.

Antisocytosis, poikilocytosis, oval macrocytes, nucleated RBCs, and normochromia are most common changes in RBC morphology.

Atypical and bizarre platelets are seen in most cases.

Bone marrow is usually hypercellular and erythroid hyperplasia occurs in 50% of cases.

CHRONIC MYELOGENOUS LEUKEMIA

Peripheral blood

Increased WBC due to increase in myeloid series is earliest change. In earlier stages the more mature forms predominate with sequentially fewer cells of the younger forms; in the later, more advanced stages the younger cells become predominant.

Eosinophilic, basophilic leukocytes may increase. Monocytes normal or only slightly increased.

Lymphocytes are normal in absolute number but relatively decreased.

WBC is usually 100,000–500,000/cu mm when disease is discovered.

Decreased number of granulocytes show positive alkaline phosphatase staining reaction.

Anemia is usually normocytic; absent in early stage and severe in late stage. Blood smear shows few normoblasts, slight polychromatophilia, occasional stippling. Reticulocyte count is usually less than 3%. Anemia is due to myelophthisis; also due to bleeding (skin and GI tract), hemolysis (autoimmune hemolytic anemia is rare), and insufficient compensatory hematopoiesis. Degree of anemia is a good index of extent of leukemic process and therefore of prognosis. Anemia improves with appropriate therapy or becomes more marked as the disease progresses.

Platelet count is normal or, commonly, increased; decreased in terminal stages with findings of thrombocytopenic purpura. Low count may increase with therapy. Bleeding manifestations are usually due to thrombocytopenia.

Bone marrow

Hyperplasia of granulocytic elements occurs, with increase in myeloid:erythroid ratio.

Granulocytes are more immature than in the peripheral blood.

The number of eosinophils and basophils is increased.

Hemosiderin deposits are increased.

Needle aspiration of spleen

The number of immature leukocytes is increased.

Normoblastosis is present.

Megakaryopoiesis is increased.

Serum and urine uric acid is increased, especially with high WBC and antileukemic therapy. Urinary obstruction may develop on account of intrarenal and extrarenal uric acid crystallization.

Serum LDH is increased; rises several weeks prior to relapse and falls several weeks prior to remission.

Increased serum LDH, MDH, SGOT, SGPT, and ALD show less elevation than in acute leukemia. SGOT, SGPT, and ALD are normal in half the cases. LDH is useful for following course of therapy.

Serum protein electrophoresis shows decreased albumin with increased alpha and gamma globulins.

BMR is increased; thyroid ^{131}I uptake normal; PBI normal.

Coombs' test is positive in one-third of patients.

Serum vitamin B_{12} level is increased (often more than 1000 μg/ml).

Philadelphia chromosome (small satellite of chromosome 21) is found in patients and asymptomatic relatives.

Laboratory findings due to leukemic infiltration of organs, e.g.

Kidney (hematuria common; uremia rare)

Heart

Liver

CHRONIC LYMPHOCYTIC LEUKEMIA

Peripheral blood
>WBC is increased (usually 50,000–250,000/cu mm) with 90% lymphocytes. These are uniformly similar, producing a monotonous blood picture of small lymphocytes with minimal cytoplasm. Blast cells are uncommon.
>
>Anemia—see preceding section. Autoimmune hemolytic anemia occurs in one-quarter of the patients.
>
>Platelet count is normal or slightly decreased but almost never increased. Platelet count is less likely to increase with therapy than in myelogenous leukemia.

Bone marrow
>Infiltration with earlier cell types is progressively increased.
>There is replacement of erythroid, myeloid, and megakaryocyte series.

Lymph node aspirate or imprint. The number of immature leukocytes, predominantly blast cells, is increased.

Uric acid levels are not increased.

Philadelphia chromosome is not found.

Serum enzyme levels are less frequently elevated and show a lesser increase than in chronic myelogenous leukemia. Even serum LDH is frequently normal.

PLASMA CELL LEUKEMIA

WBC usually more than 15,000 with over 50% plasma cells varying from typical plasmacytes to immature and atypical forms

Other findings. See under Multiple Myeloma, pp. 274–275.

INFECTIOUS MONONUCLEOSIS

Leukopenia and granulocytopenia are evident during first week. Later, WBC is increased (usually 10,000–20,000/cu mm) because of increased lymphocytes (50% or more), many of which are characteristically atypical. Peak changes occur in 7–10 days; may persist for 1–2 months.

Heterophil agglutination (Paul-Bunnell test) is usually more than 1:112; this is not decreased by more than 1 tube dilution following absorption with guinea pig kidney antigen but usually completely absorbed by beef red blood cell antigen (the reverse is true in normal individuals and in serum sickness). Peak titer occurs in 2–3 weeks; duration is for 4–8 weeks. The agglutination is not related to lymphocytosis or to clinical severity.

Evidence of mild hepatitis (e.g., increased serum transaminase, increased urine urobilinogen) is very frequent at some stage but may be transient. Clinical jaundice occurs in less than 10% of patients.

Serologic test for syphilis is transient false positive.

Occasional RBC and albumin are seen in urine.

Hemolytic anemia and thrombocytopenia are rare.

ACUTE INFECTIOUS LYMPHOCYTOSIS

Markedly increased WBC (up to 40,000/cu mm or more) is due to lymphocytosis (normal appearance, small-sized lymphocytes).

Heterophil agglutination is negative.

AGRANULOCYTOSIS

In acute fulminant form, WBC is decreased to 2000/cu mm or less—
    sometimes as low as 50/cu mm. Granulocytes are 0–2%. Granulo-
    cytes may show pyknosis or vacuolization.
In chronic or recurrent form, WBC is down to 2000/cu mm with less
    marked granulocytopenia.
There is relative lymphocytosis and sometimes monocytosis.
Bone marrow shows absence of cells in granulocytic series but
    normal erythroid and megakaryocytic series.
ESR is increased.
Hemoglobin and RBC count and morphology, platelet count, and
    coagulation tests are normal.
Laboratory findings due to infection are noted.
Laboratory findings due to underlying causes (see Aplastic Anemia,
    p. 246) are noted.

PERIODIC (CYCLIC) NEUTROPENIA

In this rare condition there is a regular periodic occurrence of
    neutropenia.
        WBC is 2000–4000/cu mm and granulocytes are as low as 0%.
        Monocytosis may occur.
        Eosinophilia may occur during recovery.
Bone marrow appearance is variable.

CHEDIAK-HIGASHI ANOMALY

This is a rare autosomal recessive genetic disease showing hypopig-
    mentation of skin, hair, and uvea.
Leukocytes contain coarse, deeply staining inclusion bodies or
    granulations in cytoplasm. Abnormal granules are present in the
    myeloid cells; inclusions are common in lymphoid and monocy-
    toid cells.
Granulocytopenia is present.
Pancytopenia appears during the (accelerated) lymphoma-like
    phase.
Laboratory findings due to frequent severe pyogenic infections and
    hemorrhage, which cause early death, are noted.

MAY-HEGGLIN ANOMALY

This is an inherited dominant abnormality of WBCs and platelets.
Large, poorly granulated platelets are associated with anomalous
    area in cytoplasm of all granulocytes. Usually no other hemato-
    logic abnormalities are present.
The lesion is an asymptomatic familial one.

PELGER-HUËT ANOMALY

This is an autosomal-dominant, usually heterozygous anomaly of
    WBCs.
Nuclei of granulocytes lack normal segmentation but are shaped like
    eyeglasses, rods, dumbbells, or peanuts. Coarse chromatin is
    evident in nuclei of granulocytes, lymphocytes, and monocytes.
    These cells are present in peripheral blood and bone marrow.
No other hematologic or clinical abnormality is present.

Occasionally cells resembling those in this anomaly are seen following administration of myelotoxic agents, in acute and chronic myelogenous leukemia.

ALDER-REILLY ANOMALY

Heavy azurophilic granulation of granulocytes and some lymphocytes and monocytes associated with mucopolysaccharidoses (see pp. 309-310) are seen.

HEREDITARY HYPERSEGMENTATION OF NEUTROPHILS
(simple dominant abnormality)

Hypersegmentation of neutrophils resembles that seen in pernicious anemia but is a permanent abnormality. Most neutrophils have four or more lobes.

There is a similar condition that affects only the eosinophilic granulocytes (hereditary constitutional hypersegmentation of the eosinophil).

There is also an inherited giant multilobed abnormality of neutrophilic leukocytes.

HYPERSPLENISM

The disease is either secondary to enlarged spleen (see following section) or "primary" (with no detectable underlying disease).

There are various combinations of anemia, leukopenia, thrombocytopenia associated with bone marrow showing normal or increased cellularity of affected elements (includes primary splenic pancytopenia and primary splenic neutropenia).

SOME CAUSES OF SPLENOMEGALY
(see appropriate separate sections)

Congestion (Banti's disease)
    Cirrhosis of the liver
    Congestive heart failure
    Thrombosis or partial occlusion of the portal or splenic veins
Hematologic diseases
    Infectious mononucleosis
    Polycythemia vera
    Leukemias and lymphomas
    Multiple myeloma, macroglobulinemia
    Myelofibrosis with myeloid metaplasia. (*Teardrop RBCs are pathognomonic.*)
    Hemolytic anemias (e.g., thalassemias, hereditary spherocytosis, acquired hemolytic anemia, hemolytic disease of newborn)
    Thrombocytopenic purpuras
    Pernicious anemia and related macrocytic anemias
    Primary hypersplenism (see preceding section)
Infections
    Bacterial (e.g., endocarditis, septicemia, *Salmonella*; granulomas, e.g., tuberculosis, tularemia, brucellosis)
    Viral (e.g., hepatitis)
    Rickettsial (e.g., Rocky Mountain spotted fever, typhus)
    Protozoal (e.g., malaria, kala-azar)

Metazoal (e.g., schistosomiasis)
Mycotic (e.g., histoplasmosis, blastomycosis, coccidioidomycosis)
Collagen diseases (e.g., SLE, polyarteritis, Felty's syndrome)
Histiocytoses
    Gaucher's disease
    Nieman-Pick disease
    Histiocytosis X (Hand-Schüller-Christian disease, Letterer-Siwe disease)
Miscellaneous (e.g., sarcoidosis, amyloidosis, gargoylism, hemochromatosis)
Tumors of spleen
    Cysts (e.g., echinococcus, neoplastic)
    Primary tumors (e.g., hemangioma, lymphangioma, lymphangiosarcoma)
Needle aspiration of spleen
    May be useful in diseases without other manifestations, especially tuberculosis, sarcoidosis, Hodgkin's disease, carcinoma, lipid storage diseases (Niemann-Pick and Gaucher's diseases)
    Contraindicated in hemorrhagic conditions, in patients with septic or tender spleen, or in unconscious patients
    Caution in presence of leukopenia or mild thrombopenia

See Spleen Scanning, p. 135.

Spontaneous rupture of spleen may occur in (see appropriate separate section)
    Malaria
    Chronic myelogenous leukemia
    Infectious mononucleosis
    Splenitis

HODGKIN'S DISEASE AND OTHER MALIGNANT LYMPHOMAS

On biopsy of lymph node the histologic findings establish diagnosis.
Blood findings may vary from completely normal to marked abnormalities. Blood changes occur relatively early compared to other lymphomas.
Moderate normocytic anemia occurs, occasionally of the hemolytic type; may become severe.
WBC is variable and may be normal, decreased, or slightly or markedly increased (25,000/cu mm). Leukopenia, marked leukocytosis, anemia are bad prognostic signs. Eosinophilia occurs in about 20% of patients. Relative and absolute lymphopenia may occur. *If lymphocytosis is present, look for another disease.* Neutrophilia may be found. Monocytosis may be found. These changes may all be absent or may even be present simultaneously or in various combinations. Rarely, Reed-Sternberg cells are found in marrow or peripheral blood smears.
Serum protein electrophoresis. Albumin is frequently decreased. Increased alpha$_1$ and alpha$_2$ globulins suggest disease activity. Decreased gamma globulin is less frequent in Hodgkin's disease than in lymphosarcoma. Gamma globulin may be increased, with macroglobulins present and evidence of autoimmune process (e.g., hemolytic anemia, cold agglutinins, positive LE test).

ESR and CRP are increased during active stages; may be normal
during remission.
BMR is increased.
Laboratory findings due to involvement of other organ systems (e.g.,
liver, kidney) are noted.
Beware of complicating infections, especially disseminated tuberculosis and fungal infections.

MYCOSIS FUNGOIDES

Biopsy of lesion (usually skin) shows microscopic findings that
parallel clinical findings.
Laboratory findings are generally not helpful.
Bone marrow may show increase in reticuloendothelial cells, mono-
blasts, lymphocytes, plasma cells.
Peripheral blood may occasionally show increased eosinophils,
monocytes, and lymphocytes.

MULTIPLE MYELOMA

Very elevated serum total protein is due to increase in globulin (with
decreased A/G ratio) in one-half to two-thirds of the patients.
Serum protein immunoelectrophoresis reveals abnormal proteins in
80% of patients.

60% of patients	IgG myeloma protein
20% of patients	IgA myeloma protein
10–20% of patients	Bence Jones protein only
1–10% of patients	No abnormal protein
< 1% of patients	IgD myeloma*

Bence Jones proteinuria occurs in one-third to one-half of the
patients.
Urinary electrophoresis is positive in half the patients.
Electrophoresis of serum or urine or both is abnormal in almost all
patients.
Bone marrow aspiration usually shows 20–50% plasma cells or
myeloma cells.
Hematologic findings
  Anemia
  Rouleaux formation (due to serum protein changes) occasion-
    ally causing difficulty in crossmatching blood
  Increased ESR and other abnormalities due to serum protein
    changes
  Usually normal WBC count and platelet count; 40–55% lym-
    phocytosis frequently present on differential count with vari-
    able number of immature lymphocytic and plasmacytic
    forms
  Cold agglutinin
See bone diseases, calcium, and phosphorus, Table 47, p. 321.
  Serum calcium is markedly increased in one-fourth to one-half
    of patients.

---

* IgD myeloma is difficult to recognize because serum levels are relatively
low; specific antiserum is required to demonstrate IgD; on electrophoresis,
IgD is often included in beta globulin peak; and clinical features are the
same as in other types of myeloma. *Bence Jones proteinuria is almost always
present and total protein is often normal.*

Serum phosphorus is usually normal.
Serum alkaline phosphatase is normal or slightly increased.
Increase may reflect amyloidosis of liver rather than bone disease.
See Kidney in Multiple Myeloma, p. 368.
BUN is increased.
Uric acid is increased.
Renal function is decreased.
Urine abnormalities appear—albumin, casts, etc.

Renal failure is usually present when there is a marked increase of Bence Jones protein in blood.

Presymptomatic phase (may last up to many years) may show only
Unexplained persistent proteinuria
Increased ESR
Myeloma protein in serum or urine
Repeated bacterial infections, especially pneumonias

See Amyloidosis, p. 433.

MACROGLOBULINEMIA

Electrophoresis of serum shows an intense sharp peak in globulin fraction, usually in the gamma zone, and takes PAS stain. The pattern is indistinguishable from that in multiple myeloma.
Acrylic gel electrophoresis shows no penetration by abnormal globulin (therefore it is a macroglobulin).
Ultracentrifugation confirms macroglobulinemia when more than 5–10% of serum components have a sedimentation constant of more than 16 Svedberg units (normally such components are less than 2%)
Total serum protein and globulin are markedly increased. Immunoelectrophoresis identifies IgM as a component of increased globulin.
ESR is very high.
Rouleaux formation is marked.
There is severe anemia, usually orthochromic normocytic, occasionally hemolytic.
WBC is decreased, with relative lymphocytosis; monocytes or eosinophils may be increased.
Bone marrow sections are always hypercellular and show extensive infiltration with atypical "lymphocytes" and also plasma cells.
Lymph node biopsy shows invasion of capsule and loss of architecture as seen in lymphosarcoma in approximately half the cases.
Spleen and liver involvement occurs in approximately half the cases.
Persistent oronasal hemorrhage occurs in approximately three quarters of the cases.
Coagulation abnormalities. There may be decreased platelets; abnormal bleeding time, coagulation time, prothrombin time, prothrombin consumption, etc.

Macroglobulinemia may be primary Waldenström's or may be associated with neoplasms, collagen diseases, cirrhosis, amyloidosis, chronic infections.

Table 38. Classification of Primary Immunologic Defects

Syndrome	Number of Circulating Lymphocytes	Number of Plasma Cells	Immunoglobulin Changes	Thymus	Lymph Node Germinal Center	Lymph Node Paracortical Zone	Other Laboratory Findings
Infantile sex-linked agammaglobulinemia (Bruton's disease)	N	O	Marked D in all	N	O	N	X
Selective inability to produce IgA	N	IgA-producing plasma cells especially in lamina propria	IgA is O; others are usually N	N	N	N	May have malabsorption syndrome, steatorrhea, bronchitis
Transient hypogammaglobulinemia of infancy	N	D	IgG is D		O or rare		X
Non-sex-linked primary immunoglobulin deficiencies (e.g., dysgammaglobulinemias — acquired, congenital)	N	V (usually D)	Present, but type and amount is V	N	Usually O Reticulum hyperplasia	Often D	X, Z; increased frequency of malignant lymphoma and autoimmune diseases
Agammaglobulinemia with thymoma (Good's syndrome)	Progressive D often to very low levels	D or O	Marked D in all	Enlarged (stromal epithelial spindle-cell type)	D or O	May be D	X, Z; thymoma (see p. 247); pure red cell aplasia may occur; eosinophils O or markedly D
Wiskott-Aldrich syndrome (immune deficiency with thrombopenia and eczema)	Usually progressive D	N	Usually present, but type and amount is V (frequently IgM is D and IgA is I)	N	May be D	Progressive D in lymphocytes	X, Z; eczema and thrombocytopenia; increased frequency of malignant lymphoma

(Ataxia telangiectasia) (Louis-Bar syndrome)	(usually slight D)	(usually present)	but type and amount is V (frequently IgA and IgE are D or O)	type (no Hassall's corpuscles or cortical medullary organization)		D		ataxia; telangiectasia in tissues; ovarian dysgenesis; increased frequency of malignant lymphoma; frequent pulmonary infections when IgA is D
Primary lymphopenic immunologic deficiency (Gitlin's syndrome)	V-D	V	Always present, but type and amount is V	Hypoplastic (Hassall's corpuscles and lymphoid cells D)		Marked D in tissue lymphocytes; foci of lymphocytes may be present in spleen and lymph nodes	Z	
Autosomal recessive alymphocytic agammaglobulinemia (Swiss type agammaglobulinemia; Glanzmann and Riniker's lymphocytophthisis)	Marked D	O	Marked D in all	Hypoplastic (Hassall's corpuscles and lymphoid cells O)		Lymphocytes O or markedly D		
Autosomal recessive lymphopenia with normal immunoglobulins (Nezelof's syndrome)	D	Present	N	Hypoplastic (Hassall's corpuscles and lymphoid cells O)	May be present	Lymphocytes markedly D	Z	
DiGeorge's syndrome (thymic aplasia)	V (usually N)	Present	N	Absent	Present	Rare paracortical lymphocytes present	Z	Absent parathyroids (tetany of the newborn); frequent cardiovascular malformations

N = normal; O = absent; D = decreased; V = variable; X = recurrent infections with pyogenic organisms; Z = frequent virus, fungus, or *Pneumocystis* infection. Source: Adapted from M. Seligmann, H. H. Fudenberg, and R. A. Good, "A Proposed Classification of Primary Immunologic Deficiencies," *Amer. J. Med.* 45 (Dec. 1968): 818–819.

HEAVY-CHAIN DISEASE
(lymphoma-like disease with excessive production of heavy-chain proteins)

Serum protein electrophoresis
>   Marked decrease in albumin
>   Gamma globulin almost absent
>   Narrow band of abnormal protein in region of beta or gamma globulin that is similar in serum and urine
>   Immunoelectrophoresis: marked decrease of IgG, IgA, IgM

Serum
>   Reversed A/G ratio
>   Positive cephalin flocculation test
>   Increased uric acid (more than 8.5 mg/100 ml)
>   Increased BUN (30–50 mg/100 ml)

Hematologic findings
>   Anemia almost always present
>   Leukopenia and thrombocytopenia common.
>   Eosinophilia sometimes marked; relative lymphocytosis
>   Vacuolated mononuclear cells sometimes seen
>   Bone marrow aspiration: many atypical plasma cells and lymphocytes (some cases)

Urine
>   Trace to 1+ protein
>   Negative for Bence Jones protein
>   Identical to abnormal serum protein on electrophoresis

WISKOTT-ALDRICH SYNDROME

This is a rare immunologic sex-linked recessive condition featuring eczema, repeated infections, and thrombocytopenia.
Platelet count is decreased, with bleeding tendency.
There is marked susceptibility to infections (e.g., bacteria, viruses, fungi, *Pneumocystis carinii*).
Serum IgM is decreased.
Serum IgA is normal or may be markedly increased.
Serum IgG is normal or increased.
Blood lymphocytes are usually decreased in number, especially the small lymphocytes.
Incidence of malignancy of the lymphoid system is increased.

HYPOANABOLIC HYPOALBUMINEMIA

This is an inherited disorder present from birth, without kidney or liver disease. Growth and development are normal. The patient is unaffected except for periodic peripheral edema.
Serum albumin is less than 0.3 gm/100 ml.
Total globulins are 4.5–5.5 gm/100 ml.
Serum cholesterol is increased.
Albumin synthesis is decreased, with decreased catabolism of IV injected albumin.

CLASSIFICATION OF HEMORRHAGIC DISORDERS

Vascular abnormalities
>   Congenital (e.g., hereditary hemorrhagic telangiectasia)

Continued on p. 282.

Table 39. Summary of Coagulation Studies in Three Main Types of Hemorrhagic Conditions

Condition	Platelet Count	Capillary Fragility (Rumpel-Leede tourniquet test)	Bleeding Time	Coagulation Time	Clot Retraction	Prothrombin Time	Partial Thrombo-plastin Time (PTT)	Prothrombin Consump-tion Time
Platelet								
Thrombocytopenic purpura	(D)	I	(I)	N	P	N	N	I
Thrombocytopathy, etc.	(N)	N or I	(I)	N	V	N	N	N or I
Coagulation disorders	N	N	N	I	N	(N or I)	(I)	I
"Vascular" disorders	N	N	N	N	N	N	N	N

○ = most useful diagnostic tests; D = decreased; I = increased; N = normal; P = poor; V = variable.
See Table 40 for further details of subcategories of hemorrhagic conditions.
PTT is the best single screening test for disorders of coagulation. When used with platelet count, prothrombin time, and bleeding time, virtually all hemorrhagic disorders will be detected.

[279]

Table 40. Summary of Coagulation Studies in Hemorrhagic Conditions

Condition	Platelet Count	Capillary Fragility (Rumpel-Leede tourniquet test)	Bleeding Time	Coagulation Time	Clot Retraction	Prothrombin Time	Partial Thromboplastin Time (PTT)	Prothrombin Consumption Time	Thromboplastin Generation Test (TGT)
Thrombocytopenic purpura	(D)	+	(I)	N	(Poor)	N	N	I	I
Nonthrombocytopenic purpura	N	V	N	N	N	N	N	N	N
Glanzmann's thrombasthenia	(N*)	+ or N	N or I	N	(Poor)	N		(I) Corrected by platelet substitute	(I)
von Willebrand's disease	N	N + in severe	(I)	V	N	N	V	I	V
AHG (Factor VIII) deficiency (hemophilia)	N	N	N I in severe	I N in mild	N	N	I	I	I Corrected by absorbed plasma
PTC (Factor IX) deficiency (hemophilia B; Christmas disease)	N	N	N I in severe	(I) N in mild	N	N	I	(I)	(I) Corrected by serum
Factor X (Stuart) deficiency	N	N	N	N or slight I	N	I	I	I	I

[280]

	1	2	3	4	5	6	7	Corrected by serum or plasma
PTA (Factor XI) deficiency	N	N	N (I in severe)	◯	N	N (I in severe)	I	I ◯ Corrected by serum or plasma
Factor XII (Hageman) deficiency	N	N	N	◯	N	N	◯ I	◯ I
Factor XIII deficiency	N	N	N	N	N	N	N	N
Fibrinogen deficiency	N	N	I in severe	I	N (I in severe)	◯ I	—	N
Hypoprothrombinemia	N	N	N or I	I	N or I	◯ I	I	N
Excess dicumarol therapy	N	+ in severe	I in severe (N)	I	N (I in severe)	◯ I	I	N
Heparin therapy	N	N	N to I	N in mild	N	N	N	N
Vascular purpura (e.g., Schönlein-Henoch, hereditary hemorrhagic telangiectasia)	N	N	N	N	N	N	N	N
Increased antithromboplastin	N		I	I	I	I	I	May be I and not corrected by absorbed plasma or aged serum
Increased antithrombin	N	N	N or I (May be I in severe)	N (May be I in severe)	I	N	N†	N†
Increased fibrinolysin	N	N	N or I	N or I	N	Lysis of clot	N†	N†

◯ = most useful diagnostic tests; D = decreased; I = increased; N = normal; V = variable.
• Platelets appear abnormal
† Not useful; may be difficult to do.

Classification of hemorrhagic disorders
(*Continued*)
       Acquired (see Nonthrombocytopenic Purpura, p. 283)
          Infection (e.g., bacterial endocarditis, rickettsial infection)
          Immunologic (e.g., allergic purpura, drug sensitivity)
          Metabolic (e.g., scurvy, uremia)
          Miscellaneous (e.g., neoplasms, amyloidosis)
Connective tissue abnormalities
   Congenital (e.g., Ehlers-Danlos syndrome)
   Acquired (e.g., Cushing's syndrome)
Platelet abnormalities (see sections on thrombocytopenic purpura, thrombocythemia, thrombocytopathies)
Plasma coagulation defects
   Causing defective thromboplastin formation
      Hemophilia (Factor VIII deficiency)
      PTC (Factor IX) deficiency (Christmas disease)
      PTA (Factor XI) deficiency
      von Willebrand's disease
   Causing defective rate or amount of thrombin formation
      Vitamin K deficiency (due to liver disease, prolonged bile duct obstruction, malabsorption syndrome, hemorrhagic disease of the newborn, anticoagulant therapy)
      Congenital deficiency of Factor II (prothrombin), Factor V (proaccelerin, labile factor), Factor VII (proconvertin, stable factor), Factor X (Stuart factor)
   Decreased fibrinogen due to intravascular clotting and/or fibrinolysis
      Obstetric abnormalities (e.g., amniotic fluid embolism, premature separation of placenta, retention of dead fetus)
      Congenital deficiency of Factor XIII (fibrin-stabilizing factor), congenital afibrinogenemia, hypofibrinogenemia, etc.
      Neoplasms (leukemia, carcinoma of prostate, etc.)
      Transfusion reactions
      Gram-negative septicemia, meningococcemia
   Circulating anticoagulants
      Heparin therapy
      Dysproteinemias, SLE, postpartum state, some cases of hemophilia, etc.

THROMBOCYTOPENIC PURPURA
Due To
Idiopathic thrombocytopenic purpura (ITP; Werlhof's disease; purpura hemorrhagica)
Hematologic disorders
   Leukemias
   Anemias (aplastic, myelophthisic, pernicious anemia, acquired hemolytic)
   Hypersplenism (e.g., Gaucher's disease, Felty's syndrome, sarcoidosis, congestive splenomegaly)
   Thrombotic thrombocytopenic purpura
   Massive blood transfusions
   May-Hegglin anomaly
   Etc.
Infections (e.g., subacute bacterial endocarditis, septicemia, typhus)
Other diseases (e.g., disseminated lupus erythematosus)
Marrow suppressive agents (e.g., ionizing radiation, benzol, nitrogen mustards and other antitumor drugs)

Drug sensitivity reactions (e.g., chloramphenicol and other antibacterial drugs, tranquilizers, antipyretic drugs, heavy metals)

Laboratory Findings
Decreased platelet count—no bleeding until $< 60,000/$cu mm
Positive tourniquet test
Increased bleeding time
Poor clot retraction
Normal coagulation time
Normal partial thromboplastin time
Normal prothrombin time
Bone marrow: normal or increased number of megakaryocytes but without marginal platelets
Blood smear: decreased number of platelets; abnormal appearance of platelets—small or giant or deeply stained
Normal WBC
Laboratory findings due to hemorrhage
 Increased WBC with shift to left
 Anemia proportional to hemorrhage, with compensatory increase in reticulocytes, polychromatophilia, etc.

NONTHROMBOCYTOPENIC PURPURA

Abnormal platelets
 Thrombocytopathies
 Thrombasthenia
 Thrombocythemia
 Etc.
Abnormal serum globulins
 Multiple myeloma
 Macroglobulinemia
 Cryoglobulinemia
 Hyperglobulinemia
 Etc.
Infections (e.g., meningococcemia, subacute bacterial endocarditis, typhoid, Rocky Mountain spotted fever)
Other diseases (e.g., amyloidosis, Cushing's syndrome, polycythemia vera, hemochromatosis, diabetes mellitus, uremia)
Drugs and chemicals (e.g., mercury, phenacetin, salicylic acid, chloral hydrate)
Allergic reaction (e.g., Schönlein-Henoch purpura, serum sickness)
Diseases of the skin (e.g., Osler-Weber-Rendu disease, Ehlers-Danlos syndrome)
von Willebrand's disease
Avitaminosis (e.g., scurvy)
Miscellaneous (e.g., mechanical, orthostatic)
Blood coagulation factors (e.g., hemophilia)

THROMBOTIC THROMBOCYTOPENIC PURPURA

Thrombocytopenic purpura (see pp. 282-283)
Hemolytic anemia with
 Increased indirect bilirubin
 Increased reticulocytes
 Microspherocytes present
 Erythroid hyperplasia of marrow
 Negative Coombs' test

Various bizarre RBC ("burr" cells) in peripheral blood smear
Increased WBC and neutrophils
Urine findings due to renal miliary infarcts (see p. 366)
Biopsy of lymph node

PRIMARY HEMORRHAGIC THROMBOCYTHEMIA

Platelets more than 800,000/cu mm
No evidence of leukemia or polycythemia in peripheral blood or
  marrow
Bone marrow: hyperplasia of all elements with predominance of
  megakaryocytes and platelet masses; eosinophilia; basophilia
Anemia
Thrombohemorrhagic disease (bleeding: skin, gastrointestinal tract,
  nose, gums)

GLANZMANN'S THROMBASTHENIA

Probably represents a heterogeneous group of conditions incom-
  pletely studied and delineated
Normal platelet count with abnormal platelet morphology (e.g.,
  variation in platelet size, increased platelet size, abnormal clump-
  ing and spreading)
May be present: poor clot retraction and increased bleeding time
Normal coagulation time
TGT and prothrombin consumption tests abnormal but corrected
  by adding platelet substitute
Capillary fragility sometimes abnormal

VASCULAR ABNORMALITIES CAUSING HEMORRHAGE

Hereditary telangiectasia (Osler-Weber-Rendu disease)
Anaphylactoid purpura (Schönlein-Henoch)
Vascular purpura (associated with uremia, diabetes mellitus, chronic
  infection, hypertension, postirradiation, etc.) (others including
  "vascular pseudohemophilia")
Pigmented purpuric eruptions (e.g., angioma serpiginosum)

ALLERGIC PURPURA

This is called Henoch's purpura when abdominal symptoms are
  predominant and Schönlein's purpura when joint symptoms are
  predominant.
Platelet count, bleeding time, coagulation time, and clot retraction
  are normal.
Tourniquet test may be negative or positive.
WBC and neutrophils may be increased; eosinophils may be in-
  creased.
Urine usually contains RBCs.
Stool may show blood.

VON WILLEBRAND'S DISEASE

This is probably the same disease as pseudohemophilia, angiohe-
  mophilia, and vascular hemophilia. It is an autosomal dominant
  hereditary deficiency of unknown plasma substance needed for
  Factor VIII synthesis and capillary hemostasis.

Bleeding time is prolonged.

Factor VIII deficiency is indicated with abnormal TGT but level of Factor VIII is extremely variable.

Platelet count is normal.

Clot retraction is normal.

Coagulation time may be normal or increased depending on level of Factor VIII.

Tourniquet test may be positive.

Platelet adhesiveness to glass beads is decreased.

Characteristic triad of prolonged bleeding time, Factor VIII deficiency, and decreased platelet adhesiveness may be present in any combination; presence or absence of these abnormalities correlates poorly with history of bleeding.

HEMOPHILIA (FACTOR VIII DEFICIENCY; AHG DEFICIENCY)

Classic hemophilia (assay of Factor VIII less than 2%) shows increased bleeding time, coagulation time, prothrombin consumption time, and partial thromboplastin time.

Moderate hemophilia (assay of Factor VIII less than 3%) shows normal coagulation time and normal prothrombin consumption time but increased partial thromboplastin time.

In mild hemophilia (assay of Factor VIII less than 16%) and "subhemophilia" (assay of Factor VIII 20–30%) these laboratory tests may be normal.

Abnormal TGT is corrected by absorbed plasma.

Laboratory findings due to hemorrhage and anemia are noted.

PTC (FACTOR IX) DEFICIENCY (CHRISTMAS DISEASE; HEMOPHILIA B)

In mild deficiency, only the TGT may be abnormal.

In more severe cases, increased coagulation time, bleeding time, prothrombin consumption time, and partial thromboplastin time are found.

Defect is corrected by frozen plasma just as well as by bank blood.

FACTOR X (STUART-PROWER) DEFICIENCY

This infrequent autosomal recessive defect resembles Factor VII deficiency; heterozygotes show mild or no clinical manifestations.

Increased prothrombin time (not corrected by use of viper venom as thromboplastin) is not corrected by administration of vitamin K. Heterozygotes may have only slight increase in prothrombin time.

Acquired form may be associated with amyloidosis.

PTA (FACTOR XI) DEFICIENCY

In mild form, coagulation may be normal, prothrombin consumption time is slightly increased, and TGT is abnormal.

In severe cases, increased coagulation time, increased prothrombin consumption time, and abnormal TGT are found.

Postoperative bleeding may not begin until several days after surgery.

FACTOR XII (HAGEMAN FACTOR) DEFICIENCY

Coagulation time and prothrombin consumption time are increased; TGT is abnormal.

No hemorrhagic symptoms occur.

CONGENITAL DEFICIENCY OF FACTOR XIII (FIBRIN-STABILIZING FACTOR)

This is an unusual disease with severe coagulation defect.
All standard clotting tests appear normal.
Patient's fibrin clot is soluble in 5M urea.
Whole blood clot is qualitatively friable.
Acquired type may occur in
> Acute myelogenous leukemia
> Liver disease
> Association with hypofibrinogenemia in obstetrical complications

FIBRINOGEN DEFICIENCY

Congenital
> Afibrinogenemia, hypofibrinogenemia, dysfibrinogenemia

Acquired (see Disseminated Intravascular Coagulation, p. 287)
> Obstetric (amniotic fluid embolism, meconium embolism, abruptio placentae, septic abortion, missed abortion with prolonged retention, eclampsia)
> Surgical procedures (e.g., prostate, T and A, open heart, lung)
> Neoplasms (e.g., carcinoma of prostate, carcinoma of lung)
> Hematologic conditions (e.g., leukemia, lymphomas, multiple myeloma, acquired hemolytic anemias, hemolytic transfusion reaction, thrombotic thrombocytopenic purpura)
> Others (cirrhosis, fat embolism, shock, burns, septicemia, drugs, snake bite, etc.)

Often associated with depletion of other coagulation factors (e.g., Factors V and VIII, platelets) and presence of circulating anticoagulants
Severe bleeding with failure of blood to clot, abnormal prothrombin time and thrombin time, lysis of clot, decreased platelets, etc.
Fibrinolysis (lysis of sterile whole blood clot in 24 hours)
> Acute hemorrhage
> Severe burns
> Postoperative, obstetric states
> Drug poisoning (e.g., phenobarbital)
> Cirrhosis of liver
> Shock

Inhibition of fibrin formation
> Dysproteinemia and paraproteinemia (e.g., multiple myeloma, macroglobulinemia, cryoglobulinemia)

CONGENITAL AFIBRINOGENEMIA

This is a rare inherited autosomal recessive congenital condition.
Plasma fibrinogen is absent.
Bleeding time is often increased (one-third of patients).
Prothrombin and thrombin times are abnormal.
Platelet-to-glass adhesiveness is abnormal unless fibrinogen is added.

CONGENITAL (CONSTITUTIONAL) HYPOFIBRINOGENEMIA

Plasma fibrinogen is decreased.
Bleeding and coagulation times are normal.
Blood clots are soft and small.

CONGENITAL DYSFIBRINOGENEMIA

A rare congenital familial condition; it may have no bleeding diathesis.
Blood clot formation is abnormally slow.

DISSEMINATED INTRAVASCULAR COAGULATION

See tabular material on p. 288.

Clotting factor assays are often variably altered; may not be easily available for immediate diagnosis.
Clotting time determinations are used to monitor heparin therapy.
Underlying conditions:
    Tissue injury: pregnancy, extensive surgery, neoplasms (especially prostate), leukemias, chemotherapy of neoplasia
    Endothelial injury: infections, prolonged hypotension
    Injury of platelets or RBCs: immunologic hemolytic anemias
    Reticuloendothelial system injury: liver disease (cirrhosis, hepatitis), postsplenectomy

Suspect clinically in patients with underlying conditions who show bleeding (frequently acute and dramatic), purpura or petechiae, acrocyanosis, arterial or venous thrombosis.

HEMORRHAGIC DISEASE OF THE NEWBORN (due to lack of vitamin K)

Prothrombin time is markedly increased.
Bleeding time and coagulation time are normal; may be slightly increased.
Capillary fragility, clotting time, prothrombin consumption, and platelet count are normal.
Laboratory findings due to blood loss are noted.

CONGENITAL HYPOPROTHROMBINEMIA

This is a very rare condition possibly representing autosomal recessive defect.
Increased prothrombin time (prothrombin level about 10% of normal) is not corrected by administration of vitamin K.
Clotting time may be normal or increased.

CONGENITAL FACTOR V DEFICIENCY (PARAHEMOPHILIA)

This is an infrequent autosomal recessive defect in which bleeding occurs only in the homozygote.
Variable increase in prothrombin time, prothrombin consumption, and coagulation time is not corrected by administration of vitamin K.

Table 40a. Disseminated Intravascular Coagulation (DIC; Consumption Coagulopathy)

Determination	% of Cases Abnormal	Abnormal Level for DIC	Mean Values for DIC	Response to Heparin Therapy	Tests
Decreased platelet count (per cu mm)	93	<150,000	52,000	None or may take weeks*	Platelet count, prothrombin time, fibrinogen level are performed first as screening tests; if all three are positive, diagnosis is considered established. If only two of these are positive, diagnosis should be confirmed by at least one of the tests for fibrinolysis.
Increased prothrombin time (seconds)	90	>15	18.0	Becomes normal or falls >5 sec in few hours to 1 day	
Decreased fibrinogen level (mg/100 ml)	71	<160	137	Rises significantly (>40 mg) in 1–3 days	
Latex test for fibrinogen degradation products (titer)	92	>1:16	1:52	Begins to fall in 1 day; if very high, may take >1 week to become normal	Tests for fibrinolysis
Prolonged thrombin time (seconds)	59	>25	27	}	
Euglobulin clot lysis time (minutes)	42	<120		Returns to normal	

*Platelet count is not a satisfactory indicator of response to heparin therapy.
Adapted from R. W. Colman, S. J. Robboy, and J. D. Minna, "Disseminated Intravascular Coagulation (DIC): An Approach," *Amer. J. Med.* 52 (May 1972): 679.

CONGENITAL FACTOR VII DEFICIENCY

With this infrequent autosomal trait bleeding occurs when the gene is homozygous; heterozygotes have little or no manifestations.

Increased prothrombin time (*normal when viper venom is used as thromboplastin; this does not correct prothrombin time in Factor X deficiency*) is not corrected by administration of vitamin K.

Bleeding time, coagulation time, clot retraction, prothrombin consumption, and TGT are normal.

CIRCULATING ANTICOAGULANTS

Various types of anticoagulants may interfere with coagulation at different stages, especially Factor VIII, heparin-like activity, antithromboplastins.

See Classification of Hemorrhagic Disorders, pp. 278, 282, and Table 40, pp. 280–281.

CRYOFIBRINOGENEMIA

Plasma precipitates when oxalated blood is refrigerated at 4°C overnight.

May cause erroneous WBC count when performed on Coulter Counter.

May be associated with increased alpha₁ antitrypsin, haptoglobin, alpha₂ macroglobulin (by immunodiffusion technique) and with increased plasma fibrinogen. Not associated with cryoglobulins.

Has been reported in association with many conditions, especially
  Neoplasms
    Thromboembolic conditions

DANGERS OF BLOOD TRANSFUSIONS

Transfusion reaction due to mismatch of donor and recipient bloods

Hyperkalemia (due to breakdown of stored RBCs); rise in serum potassium to 15–20 mEq/L 10–14 days after blood is drawn from donor

Citrate toxicity due to anticoagulant—from rapid transfusion or liver disease; sometimes decreased serum ionized calcium or acidosis followed by metabolic alkalosis

Bleeding due to decreased platelets and alteration of other coagulation factors

Infections: serum hepatitis, syphilis, malaria, brucellosis, etc.

Gram-negative toxemia due to administration of contaminated blood

Hemosiderosis due to excessive number of blood transfusions

Others: allergic, circulatory, etc.

31
Metabolic and Hereditary Diseases

METABOLIC ACIDOSIS

Due To
Increased formation of acids
> Ketosis (e.g., diabetes mellitus, starvation, hyperthyroidism, high-fat and low-carbohydrate diet, after trauma)
> Cellular hypoxia including lactic acidosis (e.g., due to pulmonary disease in which respiratory acidosis often obscures the metabolic acidosis, decreased cardiac output, cardiopulmonary bypass, shock)

Decreased excretion of H^+
> Renal failure (e.g., prerenal, renal, postrenal)
> Renal tubular acidosis, Fanconi syndrome
>> Acquired (drugs, hypercalcemia)
>> Inherited (cystinosis, Wilson's disease)
> Addison's disease

Increased acid intake (e.g., ion exchange resins, salicylates, ammonium chloride, ACD in stored blood)

Increased loss of alkaline body fluids
> Intestine (e.g., diarrhea, fistulas, aspiration of contents)
> Biliary (biliary and pancreatic fistulas)
> Renal (carbonic anhydrase inhibitors)

Secondary to other metabolic disorders (excess potassium, alkalosis)

Laboratory Findings
Serum pH is decreased (less than 7.3–7.4).

Total plasma CO_2 content is decreased. Less than 15 mEq/L almost certainly rules out respiratory alkalosis.

Serum potassium is frequently increased.

There is increased serum chloride or undetermined anion concentration. More than 14 mEq/L indicates metabolic acidosis from renal failure, diabetic ketosis, lactic acidosis, or exogenous organic acids. Undetermined anion is not increased in hyperchloremic or bicarbonate-loss acidosis.

Azotemia is frequently present (increased BUN, serum creatinine, phosphate, and potassium; decreased serum calcium) and suggests metabolic acidosis due to renal failure.

There is decreased pCO_2 when acidosis becomes well established.
Urine is strongly acid (pH = 4.5–5.2) if renal function is normal.

METABOLIC ALKALOSIS

Due To
Loss of acid
  Vomiting, gastric suction, gastrocolic fistula
  Diarrhea in mucoviscidosis (rare)
  Aciduria secondary to potassium depletion
Excess of base due to administration of
  Absorbable antacids (e.g., sodium bicarbonate)
  Salts of weak acids (e.g., sodium lactate, sodium or potassium citrate)
Some vegetable diets
Potassium depletion (causing sodium and H^+ to enter the cells)
  Gastrointestinal loss (e.g., chronic diarrhea)
  Lack of potassium intake (e.g., anorexia nervosa, IV fluids without potassium supplements for treatment of vomiting or postoperatively)
  Diuresis (e.g., mercurials, thiazides, osmotic diuresis)
  Adrenal steroids (e.g., primary aldosteronism, Cushing's disease, administration of steroids, large amounts of licorice)
  Glycogen deposition
  Chronic alkalosis
  Potassium-losing nephropathy

Laboratory Findings
Serum pH is increased.
Total plasma CO_2 is increased (bicarbonate more than 30 mEq/L).
pCO_2 is normal or slightly increased.
Serum potassium is usually decreased, which condition is the chief danger in metabolic alkalosis.
Serum chloride is relatively lower than sodium.
BUN may be increased.
Urine pH is more than 7.0 (up to 7.9) if potassium depletion is not severe and concomitant sodium deficiency (e.g., vomiting) is not present.

SALT-DEPLETION SYNDROME

Decreased serum sodium and chloride
Hemoconcentration
Increased BUN

SALT-DILUTION SYNDROME

Decreased serum sodium and chloride
No hemoconcentration
Normal BUN

HYPERTENSION ASSOCIATED WITH HYPOKALEMIA

Aldosteronism, primary and secondary
Pseudo–primary aldosteronism due to chronic licorice ingestion
Cushing's syndrome
Diuresis therapy in patients with hypertension
Potassium-losing renal disease

Table 41. Illustrative Serum Electrolyte Values in Various Conditions

Electrolyte	Normal	Metabolic Acidosis							Metabolic Alkalosis			Respiratory Acidosis*	Respiratory Alkalosis†
		Diabetic Acidosis	Fasting	Severe Diarrhea	Hyperchloremic Acidosis	Addison's Disease	Nephritis	Nephrosis	Vomiting	Pyloric Obstruction	Duodenal Obstruction		
pH	7.35–7.45	7.2	7.2	7.2	7.2	7.2	7.2	7.2	7.6	7.6	7.6	7.2	7.6
Bicarbonate	21–30	10	16	12	12	22	8	20	38	58	42	46	14
Potassium	3.5–5.5	5.6	5.2	5.2	5.2	6.5	4	5.5	5.8	5.5	5.5	5.5	5.5
Sodium	130–149	122	142	128	142	111	129	138	150	132	138	142	136
Chloride	98–106	80	100	96	116	72	90	113	94	42	49	80	112

*Respiratory acidosis may be acute (due to cardiac arrest, obstruction of airway, lung collapse, infection) or chronic (due to progressive lung disease).

†Respiratory alkalosis is due to hyperventilation (caused by emotional state, exercise, infection, drugs, liver disease).

CLASSIFICATION OF SOME INHERITED METABOLIC CONDITIONS

Disorders of carbohydrate metabolism
    Diabetes mellitus
    Pentosuria
    Fructosuria
    Familial lactose intolerance
    Galactosemia
    Glycogen-storage diseases
    Mucopolysaccharidoses
    Etc.
Disorders of amino acid metabolism
    Phenylketonuria
    Tyrosinosis
    Maple syrup disease
    Alkaptonuria
    Etc.
Disorders of purine and pyrimidine metabolism
    Gout
    Orotic aciduria
    Beta-amino-isobutyric aciduria
    Etc.
Disorders of lipid metabolism
    Essential familial hypercholesterolemia
    Inherited deficiency of lipoprotein lipase
Disorders of porphyrin metabolism
Disorders of metabolism involving metals
    Wilson's disease
    Hemochromatosis
    Periodic paralysis
    Adynamia episodica hereditaria
    Etc.
Disorders of renal tubular function
    Fanconi syndrome of cystinosis
    Vitamin D–resistant rickets of primary hypophosphatemia
    Cystinuria
    Renal glycosuria
    Etc.
Disorders of serum enzymes
    Hypophosphatasia
    Etc.
Disorders of plasma proteins
    Analbuminemia
    Agammaglobulinemia
    Atransferrinemia
    Etc.
Disorders of blood
    Coagulation diseases (e.g., hemophilias)
    RBC G-6-PD deficiency
    Hemoglobinopathies and thalassemias
    Hereditary spherocytosis
    Hereditary nonspherocytic hemolytic anemia
    Etc.

DETECTING HETEROZYGOUS CARRIERS OF SOME DISORDERS*

Disorder	Abnormality
Duchenne type of muscular dystrophy	Increased serum CPK
Gout	Increased serum uric acid
Wilson's disease	Abnormality detected by ^{48}Cu studies
G-6-PD deficiency	Decreased G-6-PD in RBCs
Orotic aciduria	Decreased orotidylic decarboxylase in RBCs
Hemoglobinopathies (e.g., thalassemia)	Abnormality detected by hemoglobin electrophoresis
Tay-Sachs disease	Decreased serum fructose-l-phosphate aldolase
Glycogen-storage disease (Type III)	Decreased amylo-l, 6-glucosidase in leukocytes
Glycogen-storage disease (von Gierke's, Type I)	Decreased glucose-6-phosphate in intestinal mucosa
Phenylketonuria	Prolonged increase in serum phenylalanine after phenylalanine load
Argininosuccinic aciduria	Decreased argininosuccinase in RBCs and increased argininosuccinic acid in urine
Cystathioninuria	Increased cystathionine in urine
Cystinuria	Increased cystine and lysine in urine
Homocystinuria	Decreased cystathionine synthetase in liver
Histidinemia	Decreased histidase in skin
Hyperoxaluria	Abnormality detected by special radioisotope study
Galactosemia	Decreased galactose-l-p-uridyl transferase in RBCs

PHENYLKETONURIA

Inherited absence of phenylalanine hydroxylase activity in liver causes increased blood and urine phenylalanine along with metabolites, associated with mental retardation.

For screening of newborn infants, urine amounts of phenylpyruvic acid may be insufficient for detection by colorimetric methods when blood level is less than 15 mg/100 ml. May not appear in urine until 2–3 weeks of age.

Preliminary blood screening tests (inhibition assay, fluorometry, paper chromatography) detect levels over 4 mg/100 ml.

To confirm diagnosis of phenylketonuria, administer 100 mg of ascorbic acid and collect blood and urine 24 hours later:
    Phenylketonuria
        Serum phenylalanine is more than 15 mg/100 ml.

---

* D. Y. Y. Hsia, "The Diagnosis of Carriers of Disease-Producing Genes," *Ann. N.Y. Acad. Sci.* 134 (1966): 946–964.

Continued on page 301.

Table 42. Comparison of Types of Hyperlipoproteinemia

Point of Comparison	Type I Rarest	Type II Relatively Common	Type III Relatively Uncommon	Type IV Most Common	Type V Uncommon
Origin	Exogenous hyperlipidemia	Essential familial hypercholesterolemia		Endogenous hyperlipidemia	Mixed endogenous and exogenous hyperlipidemia
Definition	Familial fat-induced hyperglycidemia	Essential familial hypercholesterolemia	Carbohydrate-induced hyperglycidemia with hypercholesterolemia	Carbohydrate-induced hyperglycidemia without hypercholesterolemia	Combined fat and carbohydrate-induced hyperglycidemia
Gross appearance of plasma	On standing: supernatant creamy, infranatant clear	Clear or only slightly opalescent	Clear, cloudy, or milky	Slightly turbid to cloudy Unchanged on standing	Markedly turbid On standing: supernatant creamy, infranatant milky
Serum cholesterol	Normal or slightly increased	Markedly increased; causes most, or all, of hyperlipidemia	Moderately marked	Normal or slightly increased	Increased
Serum triglycerides	Markedly increased	Mild or no increase	Markedly increased	Markedly increased	Markedly increased
Lipoprotein electrophoresis	Increased chylomicrons	Increased beta lipoproteins	Increased beta and pre-beta lipoproteins	Increased pre-beta lipoproteins	Increased chylomicrons and pre-beta lipoproteins
Other laboratory abnormalities			Hyperglycemia, abnormal glucose tolerance; increased serum uric acid. Rule out liver disease.	Abnormal glucose tolerance in many. Rule out nephrotic syndrome, hypothyroidism, pregnancy, glycogen storage disease.	

Continued on pages 296 and 297

Table 42 *(continued)*

Point of Comparison	Type I Rarest	Type II Relatively Common	Type III Relatively Uncommon	Type IV Most Common	Type V Uncommon
Lipid changes resembling primary hyperlipidemias					
Diet	—	Very-high-cholesterol diet	—	Caffeine or alcohol before testing	—
Drugs	—	Triglyceride-lowering drugs in Types III and IV	Triglyceride-lowering drugs in Type IV	Cholesterol-lowering drugs Chlorthiazide Oral contraceptives	—
Primary diseases	Diabetes Dysgamma-globulinemia	Myxedema Nephrosis Obstructive liver disease Stress Porphyria Anorexia nervosa Idiopathic hyper-calcemia	Myxedema Dysgammaglobulinemia	Diabetes	Myeloma Macroglobulinemia Nephrosis Diabetes Pancreatitis

Appearance of Lipoprotein Components Visualized by Electrophoresis	Type I Rarest	Type II Relatively Common	Type III Relatively Uncommon	Type IV Most Common	Type V Uncommon
Chylomicron					
Beta-lipoprotein					
Pre-beta-lipoprotein					
Alpha-lipoprotein					

Obtain blood only after at least 12 – 14 hours' fasting and when patient has been on usual diet for at least 2 weeks.
Rule out diabetes and pancreatitis in all groups.
Increased susceptibility to coronary artery disease occurs in Types II, III, IV.
Xanthomas appear in Types I, II, III
Abdominal pain occurs in Types I, V.
If dietary or drug treatment has begun, it may not be possible to classify the lipoproteinemia or the classification may be erroneous.

(Type IIb is overindulgence hyperlipemia: shows increased cholesterol and triglycerides, with increased beta and pre-beta; can only distinguish from Type III by detecting abnormal beta-migrating lipoprotein in serum fraction with density < 1.006.)

[297]

Table 43. Summary of Primary Overflow Aminoacidurias (increased blood concentration with overflow into urine)

Disease	Increased Blood Amino Acids	Urine Abnormalities*	Other Laboratory Findings
Phenylketonuria	Phenylalanine	O-hydroxyphenylacetic acid; phenylpyruvic, acetic, and lactic acids	Blood tyrosine does not rise after phenylalanine load
Maple syrup urine disease Severe infantile form	Valine, leucine, isoleucine, alloisoleucine	Branched chain keto acids in great excess; urine has odor of maple syrup	
Intermittent form	Same	Ketoaciduria and urine odor present only during attacks	
Hypervalinemia	Valine		
Homocystinuria	Methionine; homocystine slightly increased	Homocystine in great excess in urine	Blood cystine low; vascular accidents, Marfan-like syndrome, osteoporosis
Tryptophanemia	Tryptophan	Decreased excretion of kynurenin after tryptophan load	
Hyperlysinemia	Lysine	Ornithine, gamma-aminobutyric acid, and ethanolamine in excess	
Congenital lysine intolerance	Lysine, arginine		Ammonia intoxication
Tyrosinosis	Tyrosine; methionine may be markedly increased	p-hydroxyphenylpyruvic, acetic, and lactic acids; methionine may be prominent	Generalized aminoaciduria, renal glycosuria, renal rickets, cirrhosis; Fanconi syndrome

Cystathioninuria	Cystathionine slightly increased	Cystathionine (may be over 1 gm/day)	Congenital acidosis, thrombocytopenia, pituitary gland abnormalities
Hyperglycinemia			
Severe infantile	Glycine (other amino acids may be elevated)	Acetone	May have ammonia intoxication, ketosis, neutropenia, and osteoporosis
With hypo-oxaluria	Glycine	Decreased oxalate excretion	
Argininosuccinic aciduria	Argininosuccinic acid (about 4 mg/100 ml)	Argininosuccinic acid (2.5–9.0 gm/day)	Ammonia intoxication
Citrullinemia	Citrulline		Liver disease, ammonia intoxication; may have low BUN
Ornithinemia	Ornithine	Ornithine may be normal	Ammonia intoxication
Histidinemia	Histidine (alanine may also be increased)	Alanine may be increased; imidazolepyruvic, acetic, and lactic acids	Urocanic acid absent in sweat and urine after oral histidine load
Carnosinuria		Carnosine (20–100 mg/ day)	
Hyperbeta-alaninemia	Beta-alanine, gamma-aminobutyric acid (GABA)	Beta-aminoisobutyric acid, GABA, and taurine in excess	Beta-alanine and GABA increased in CSF
Hyperprolinemia			
Type I	Proline	Hydroxyproline, glycine elevated	May have hereditary nephritis
Type II	Proline	Δ1-pyrroline-5-carboxylate, hydroxyproline, glycine elevated	No nephritis

See footnotes on next page.

Continued on next page

Table 43 *(continued)*

Disease	Increased Blood Amino Acids	Urine Abnormalities*	Other Laboratory Findings
Hydroxyprolinemia	Hydroxyproline	No excretion of △1-pyrroline-3-hydroxy-5-carboxylate or gamma-hydroxyglutamic acid after hydroxyproline load	
Hypophosphatasia	Phosphoethanolamine slightly elevated (about 0.4 mg/100 ml)	Phosphoethanolamine (up to 150 mg/day)	Bone disease

*In addition to overflow aminoaciduria

Mental retardation is often present in these patients.

For proper interpretation of aminoaciduria: Avoid all drugs and medications for 3–4 days (unless immediate diagnosis is required) since they may cause renal tubular damage with aminoaciduria or may produce confusing spots on chromatograms. Use fresh urine specimens without urinary tract infection or else amino acid pattern may be abnormal. Since aminoaciduria may occur with various acute illnesses, repeat amino acid chromatogram after recovery from acute illness to avoid misdiagnosis.

Some aminoacidurias may not be clinically significant (e.g., newborn aminoaciduria, glycinuria, beta-aminoisobutyric aciduria).

Source: M. D. Efron and M. G. Ampola, "The Aminoacidurias," *Pediat. Clin. N. Amer.* 14 (Nov. 1967): 881–903.

Table 44. Summary of Renal Transport Aminoacidurias
(blood amino acids normal or low)

Disease	Amino Acids Increased in Urine
Oasthouse urine disease (methionine malabsorption syndrome)	Methionine (may not be much increased on normal diet but is on high-methionine diet); smaller amounts of valine, leucine, isoleucine, tyrosine, and phenylalanine
Hartnup disease	Neutral (monoamine, monocarboxylic) amino acids; basic amino acids, methionine, proline, hydroxyproline, and glycine normal or only slightly increased
Glycinuria (may be harmless; may be heterozygotes for benign prolinuria; may be associated with many conditions)	Glycine
Severe prolinuria (Joseph's syndrome)	Proline, hydroxyproline, and glycine in great excess (up to 3 gm/day proline)
Benign prolinuria	Proline, hydroxyproline, and glycine (up to 600 mg/day proline)
Cystine-lysinuria Type I (renal calculi) Type II Type III	Cystine and dibasic amino acids
Isolated cystinuria (familial hypoparathyroidism-incidental?)	Cystine

Source: M. D. Efron and M. G. Ampola, "The Aminoacidurias," *Pediat. Clin. N. Amer.* 14 (Nov. 1967): 881–903.

Phenylketonuria *(continued)*

Serum tyrosine is less than 5 mg/100 ml *(is never increased in phenylketonuria)*.

Urine phenylalanine is more than 100 μg/ml.

Orthohydroxyphenylacetic acid is present in urine.

Phenylpyruvic acid in urine is significant (gives positive ferric chloride test) but may not be present in some cases.

Abnormalities of tyrosine metabolism (e.g., incomplete development of tyrosine oxidizing system, especially in premature or low-birth-weight infants)

Serum phenylalanine is more than 4 mg/100 ml (5–20 mg/100 ml).

Serum tyrosine is between 10 and 75 mg/100 ml.

Tyrosine metabolites in urine are up to 1 mg/ml (parahydroxyphenyl-lactic and parahydroxyphenylacetic acids can be distinguished from orthohydroxyphenylacetic acid by paper chromatography).

Orthohydroxyphenylacetic acid is absent from urine.

Without administration of ascorbic acid, one-fourth of premature infants may have increased serum phenylalanine and tyrosine for several weeks (but reversed in 24 hours after ascorbic acid administration) and increased urine tyrosine and tyrosine derivatives.

Similar blood and urine findings not reversed by administration of ascorbic acid may occur in untreated galactosemia, tyrosinemia, congenital cirrhosis, and giant-cell hepatitis; jaundice occurs frequently.

Serum serotonin (5-hydroxytryptophan) is decreased.

Urine 5-HIAA excretion is decreased.

MAPLE SYRUP DISEASE (KETOACIDURIA)
(metabolic block in degradation of ketoacids of branched chain amino acids)

Urine has maple syrup odor.

Chromatography of urine shows greatly increased urinary excretion of ketoacids of leucine, isoleucine, and valine.

The disease may be severe or intermittent.

HOMOCYSTINURIA

This is an inborn error of methionine metabolism with deficient cystathionine synthetase in liver and brain with inability to change homocystine to cystathionine.

Urine excretion of homocystine is increased (positive nitroprusside screening test).

Level of homocystine and methionine is increased in serum and also increased in CSF.

Laboratory findings due to associated clinical conditions (e.g., mental retardation, Marfan's syndrome, osteoporosis, thromboembolic accidents, mild variable hepatocellular dysfunction) are noted.

TYROSINOSIS

There is increased urinary excretion of P-hydroxyphenylpyruvic acid (due to deficiency of P-hydroxyphenylpyruvic oxidase) (chromatography of urine). *Also increased in myasthenia gravis, liver disease, ascorbic acid deficiency, malignancies.*

Acetic and lactic acids and methionine may be increased in urine.

Increased blood tyrosine; methionine may be markedly increased.

Laboratory findings due to Fanconi syndrome and hepatic cirrhosis are noted.

CYSTATHIONINURIA
(rare disorder of intermediate metabolism of methionine)

Increased cystathionine in urine

HYPERGLYCINEMIA

Long-chain ketosis (without hypoglycemia) and ketonuria accentuated by leucine ingestion

Neutropenia
Thrombocytopenia
Hypogammaglobulinemia
Increased glycine in blood and urine
Osteoporosis

ARGININOSUCCINIC ACIDURIA

Argininosuccinic acid is increased in urine; may also be increased in
blood and CSF.
Serum alkaline phosphatase may be increased.
Fasting blood ammonia is normal but may be markedly increased
after eating.
Heterozygous carriers show increased argininosuccinic acid in urine
and decreased argininosuccinase in RBCs.

CITRULLINEMIA
(rare condition of metabolic block in citrulline utilization and associated mental retardation)

Increased citrulline in blood and also CSF and urine
Laboratory findings due to liver disease

HISTIDINEMIA
(rare inherited disorder)

Blood histidine is increased.
Histidine, imidazole acetic, imidazole lactic, and imidazole pyruvic
acids are increased in urine; alanine may be increased.
Urine may show positive Phenistix test because of imidazole pyruvic
acid.
With oral histidine load, no FIGLU appears in urine.

HYPERPROLINEMIA

Increased proline in blood
Increased glycine and hydroxyproline in urine

HYDROXYPROLINEMIA

Increased hydroxyproline in blood

OASTHOUSE URINE DISEASE
(distinctive odor of urine)

Increase of various amino acids in blood and also in urine (e.g.,
phenylalanine, tyrosine, methionine, valine, leucine, isoleucine)

HARTNUP DISEASE
(hereditary abnormality of tryptophan metabolism)

Urine chromatography shows greatly increased amounts of indol-
acetic acid, alpha-N (indole-3-acetyl) glutamine, and tryptophan.

JOSEPH'S SYNDROME (SEVERE PROLINURIA)

Urine shows marked increase in proline, hydroxyproline, and glycine.
Heterozygotes may show mild prolinuria.

BENIGN PROLINURIA

Increased proline, hydroxyproline, and glycine appear in urine.
Heterozygotes may show glycinuria but not prolinuria.
Prolinuria may occur in association with various diseases; may be harmless.

CYSTINURIA
(failure of renal tubular reabsorption and of intestinal uptake of cystine and of dibasic amino acids)

Increased cystine in urine (20–30 times normal)
Increased urinary arginine, lysine, and ornithine
Cystine renal stones

BETA-AMINOISOBUTYRIC ACIDURIA
(familial recessive disorder of thymine metabolism)

Increased beta-aminoisobutyric acid in urine (50–200 mg/24 hours)

FAMILIAL IMINOGLYCINURIA
(inherited autosomal defect of renal transport; may be associated with mental retardation)

Increased urine glycine
Increased urine imino acids (proline, hydroxyproline)

METHYLMALONIC ACIDURIA
(very rare inborn error of metabolism with neonatal metabolic acidosis and mental and somatic retardation)

Metabolic acidosis
Increased methylmalonic acid in urine
Long-chain ketonuria
Intermittent hyperglycinemia
All findings accentuated by high-protein diet or supplemental ingestion of valine or isoleucine

Methylmalonic aciduria also occurs in vitamin B_{12} deficiency.

PRIMARY OXALOSIS
(rare familial disease)

Increased serum and urinary oxalic acid
Increased urinary glycolic and glyoxylic acid
Calcium oxalate renal calculi and nephrocalcinosis with extrarenal deposition of calcium oxalate
Uremia causes death.

Manifestations of hyperoxaluria are the same but extrarenal calcium oxalate deposits are absent.[*]

---

[*] Boquist, L., Lindqvist, B., Ostberg, Y., and Steen, L. "Primary Oxalosis," *Amer. J. Med.* 54 (May 1973): 673–680.

L-GLYCERIC ACIDURIA
(genetic variant of primary hyperoxaluria; autosomal trait that causes disease only when homozygous)

Renal calculi composed of calcium oxalate
Increased urinary oxalic acid (3–5 times normal)
L-glyceric acid in urine (not found in normal urine)

CYSTINOSIS

Children
> Renal Fanconi syndrome
>> Phosphaturia
>> Decreased serum phosphorus
>> Decreased serum calcium (usually normal)
>> Decreased serum potassium due to high urine potassium
>> Hyperchloremic acidosis (*Renal calcinosis develops in renal tubular acidosis but not in cystinosis.*)
>> Generalized aminoaciduria (similar to that seen in lead and other heavy-metal poisoning, Wilson's disease, and vitamin D deficiency)
>> Glycosuria with normal blood sugar; frequently ketonemia and ketonuria
>> Vitamin D–resistant type of rickets (*In vitamin D–resistant rickets of primary hypophosphatemia, there is no aminoaciduria; severe rickets develops before azotemia appears.*)
>> (*Renal hypophosphatemia, aminoaciduria, and glycosuria begin at 6 months of age.*)
> Polyuria with low specific gravity; proteinuria sometimes present.
> Progressive loss of glomerular function with increasing azotemia and death from uremia, usually before age 10
> Cystine crystals in bone marrow and in tissues (especially RE system)
> Serum uric acid sometimes decreased
Adults (benign disease)
> Urinary tract calculi
> Cystinuria

SECONDARY AMINOACIDURIA

Severe liver disease
Renal tubular damage due to
> Lysol
> Heavy metals
> Maleic acid
> Burns
> Galactosemia
> Wilson's disease
> Scurvy
> Rickets
> Fanconi syndrome (outdated tetracycline, multiple myeloma, inherited)
Neoplasm
> Cystathionine excretion in neuroblastoma of adrenal; ethanolamine excretion in primary hepatoma

GALACTOSEMIA
(inherited defect of galactose-1-phosphate uridyl transferase in liver and in RBC that converts galactose to glucose; therefore accumulation of galactose-1-phosphate)

Jaundice (onset at age 4–10 days)

Liver biopsy—dilated calculus filled with bile pigment with surrounding rosette of liver cells

Galactosuria—detected by nonspecific reducing tests; identified by chromatography

General ammo-aciduria—identified by chromatography

Proteinuria

Galactosemia (equal to total reducing sugar minus glucose-oxidase sugar)

Serum glucose—*apparently* elevated in fasting state but falls as galactose increases; development of hypoglycemia possible

Galactose tolerance test—positive

Lack of RBC enzyme to utilize uridine diphosphoglucose

CONGENITAL FRUCTOSE INTOLERANCE

This is a severe familial genetic disease of infancy due to defect involving fructose-1-phosphoaldolase and fructose-1, 6-diphosphoaldolase; it resembles galactosemia.

Fructose in urine of 100–300 mg/100 ml gives a positive test for reducing substances (Benedict's reagent, Clinitest) but not with glucose-oxidase methods (Clinistix, Tes-Tape). Identify fructose by paper chromatography.

Aminoaciduria and proteinuria may be present.

Fructose tolerance test shows prolonged elevation of blood fructose and marked decrease in serum glucose. Serum phosphorus shows rapid prolonged decrease.

Hypoglycemia with convulsions and coma follows ingestion of fructose.

Increased serum bilirubin and cirrhosis may occur.

BENIGN FRUCTOSURIA

This is a benign asymptomatic disorder due to fructokinase deficiency.

Large amount of fructose in urine gives a positive test for reducing substances (Benedict's reagent, Clinitest) but not with glucose-oxidase methods (Clinistix, Tes-Tape).

Identify fructose by paper chromatography.

Fructose tolerance test shows that blood fructose increases to 4 times more than in normal persons, blood glucose increases only slightly, and serum phosphorus does not change.

ALKAPTONURIA

Recessive inherited absence of liver homogentisic acid oxidase causes excretion of homogentisic acid in urine.

Urine becomes brown-black on standing and reduces Benedict's solution and Fehling's solution in the absence of glucose.

An oral dose of homogentisic acid is largely recovered in the urine of affected patients but not in normal individuals.

SUCROSURIA

Urine specific gravity is very high (up to 1.070).
Urine tests for reducing substances are negative.
   Sucrosuria may follow IV administration of sucrose or the
   purposeful addition of cane sugar to urine.

PENTOSURIA

Pentosuria is due to a block in oxidation of glucuronic acid; the
   patient can metabolize only the sixth carbon, excreting the 5-
   carbon fraction as pentose
Urinary excretion of L-xylulose is increased (1–4 gm/day), and the
   increase is accentuated by administration of glucuronic acid and
   glucuronogenic drugs (aminopyrine, antipyrine, menthol, etc.).

Differential Diagnosis
Alimentary pentosuria—arabinose or xylose excreted after ingestion
   of large amount of certain fruits (e.g., plums, cherries, grapes)
Healthy individuals—small amounts of D-ribose in urine
Healthy individuals—trace amounts of ribulose in urine
Muscular dystrophy—small amounts of D-ribose in urine (some
   patients)

MANNOHEPTULOSURIA

Mannoheptulose in urine after a person eats avocados occurs in
   some individuals; not clinically important.

LACTOSURIA

This is a transient disorder of infancy with chronic diarrhea and
   failure to thrive due to interference with or inhibition of or late
   development of intestinal lactase.
Lactose in urine produces positive test for reducing sugars (Benedict's reagent, Clinitest) but negative test with glucose-oxidase
   methods (Tes-Tape, Clinistix).
In the oral lactose tolerance test serum glucose curves are nearly
   normal.
Stools are acid.

PHYSIOLOGIC LACTOSURIA

Occurs near the end of pregnancy and during lactation

INTESTINAL DEFICIENCY OF SUGAR-SPLITTING ENZYMES (MILK ALLERGY, MILK INTOLERANCE, CONGENITAL FAMILIAL LACTOSE INTOLERANCE, LACTASE DEFICIENCY, DISACCHARIDASE DEFICIENCY)

In this familial disease in infancy with diarrhea, vomiting, failure to
   thrive, malabsorption, etc., patient becomes asymptomatic when
   lactose is removed from diet.
Oral lactose tolerance test shows a rise in blood sugar of less than
   20 mg/100 ml (dose of 100 gm of lactose).

A dose of 50 gm each of glucose and galactose produces a rise in blood sugar of more than 25 mg/100 ml.

In diabetics, lactose ingestion may cause a greater increase in blood sugar.

After ingestion of milk or 50–100 gm of lactose, stools have a pH of 4.5–6.0 (normal pH is more than 7.0) and are sour and frothy.

Lactose in urine amounts to 100–2000 mg/100 ml. It produces a positive test for reducing sugars (Benedict's reagent, Clinitest) but a negative test with glucose-oxidase methods (Tes-Tape, Clinistix).

CLASSIFICATION OF PORPHYRIAS

I. Congenital erythropoietic porphyria (due to excess production of free uroporphyrin I by marrow RBC; very rare; onset usually before 2 years of age; extreme photosensitivity)

Urine is burgundy red and fluoresces; composed chiefly of uroporphyrin I.

Stool contains large amounts of coproporphyrin I.

Excretion of porphobilinogen and delta-aminolevulinic acid is normal.

Hypersplenism is present.

There is severe normochromic normocytic anicteric hemolytic anemia, which is improved by splenectomy.

Teeth fluoresce.

Skin shows abundant melanin in deeper epidermis.

II. Hepatic porphyria

A. Acute intermittent type is the most frequent and most severe form in the United States. The disease is mendelian dominant, has its onset in adults, and is characterized by abdominal pain and nervous system manifestations; no photosensitivity. Symptoms are due to demyelinization of nervous system. Variation is from latent to very severe.

Urine

Marked increase in porphobilinogen is seen (also increased in latent form).

Usually there is an increase in delta-aminolevulinic acid (also increased in latent).

Coproporphyrin and uroporphyrin may be increased.

May be normal color when fresh and become brown, red, or black on standing.

BSP retention is abnormal.

Serum sodium and chloride are decreased during acute attack.

Laboratory findings and symptoms may be precipitated by drugs (especially barbiturates, alcohol, sulfonamides, etc.).

B. Hereditary mixed types may be cutaneous with few or no acute manifestations, acute intermittent without cutaneous symptoms, various combinations, or latent. Cutaneous manifestations are due to excess production of porphyrins in liver. Postmortem tissues show pink fluorescence under ultraviolet light.

Variable laboratory findings

Urine uroporphyrin and coproporphyrin are usually increased (may be normal during remission).

Stool shows increased porphyrin.

In mixed type, there may also be increased delta aminolevulinic acid and porphobilinogen.

C. Constitutional type has its onset usually after age 50; family history is negative. Most patients are chronic alcoholics and may have liver disease. Disease sometimes accompanies malignant lymphoma, carcinoma, nonalcoholic cirrhosis, etc.

Urine and stool contain much increased porphyrins (mostly uroporphyrin).

D. Acquired

Due to hepatoma (in rare cases). Serum shows ultraviolet fluorescence.

Stool contains increased coproporphyrin and uroporphyrin.

Due to chemicals. An epidemic in Turkey was caused by hexachlorobenzene and mercury on wheat.

III. Protoporphyria erythropoietica (infrequent condition with photosensitivity)

RBC protoporphyrin and coproporphyrin are increased.

Fecal protoporphyrin and coproporphyrin are increased.

Urine uroporphyrin and coproporphyrin are not increased.

No anemia is seen.

No fluorescence of teeth is found.

RBC protoporphyrins are also increased in iron-deficiency anemia.

GENETIC MUCOPOLYSACCHARIDOSES

Mucopolysaccharide Type	Mucopolysaccharide Excreted in Urine
I (Hurler's syndrome)	Chondroitin sulfate B and heparitin sulfate
II (Hunter's syndrome)	Chondroitin sulfate B and heparitin sulfate
III (Sanfilippo's syndrome)	Heparitin sulfate
IV (Morquio-Ulrich syndrome)	Keratosulfate
V (Schei's syndrome)	Chondroitin sulfate B

All MPS diseases show metachromatically staining inclusions of MPS in circulating polynuclear leukocytes (Reilly granulations) or lymphocytes, cells of inflammatory exudate, and bone marrow cells (most consistently in clasmatocytes). MPS is also deposited in various parenchymal cells.

GENETIC DISEASES OF MUCOPOLYSACCHARIDE METABOLISM

Morquio-Ulrich syndrome

Excess excretion of keratosulfate in urine associated with aortic valvular disease, osteochondrodystrophy, and cloudy cornea

Schei's syndrome

Excess excretion of chondroitin sulfate B in urine associated with aortic valve disease (usually regurgitation)

Hurler's syndrome (gargoylism)
  Excess excretion of chondroitin sulfate B and mucopolysaccharide in urine
  Alder-Reilly anomaly—azurophil granules in cytoplasm of myeloid cells (occasionally lymphocytes and monocytes)
  Fibrosis of heart valves with functional changes

CLASSIFICATION OF GLYCOGENOSES (GLYCOGEN-STORAGE DISEASES – GSD)

Frequency Among GSD (%)	*Type*	*Clinical Name*	*Enzyme Defect*
20	I	Classic von Gierke's disease	Deficiency of liver glucose-6-phosphatase
20	II	Pompe's disease	Defect in lysozomal acid maltase (alpha-1, 4-glucosidase)
30	III	Forbes' disease (debrancher deficiency, limit dextrinosis)	Deficiency of amylo-1, 6-glucosidase (debranching enzyme)
Less than 1	IV	Andersen's disease (brancher deficiency, amylopectinosis)	Absence of amylo-(1,4 → 1.6)-transglucosidase (branching enzyme)
5	V	McArdle's disease of muscle	Absence of muscle phosphorylase
25	VI		Deficiency of liver phosphorylase
	VII		Deficiency of glycogen synthetase

VON GIERKE'S DISEASE (TYPE I GLYCOGEN-STORAGE DISEASE; GLUCOSE-6-PHOSPHATASE DEFICIENCY)

Blood glucose is markedly decreased.
Blood triglycerides, cholesterol, and serum-free fatty acids are markedly increased.
Blood lactic acid and pyruvate are increased.
Blood and urine acetone secondary to acidosis is increased.
Mild anemia is present.
There is increased serum uric acid (due to depressed renal tubular function by increased blood lactic acid) causing clinical gout.
Serum phosphorus and alkaline phosphatase are decreased.
Urine glucose is increased.
Urinary nonspecific amino acids are increased without increase in blood amino acids.
Other renal function tests are relatively normal.
Liver function tests (other than related to carbohydrate metabolism) are relatively normal.
Functional tests
  Administer 1 mg of glucagon intravenously after 8-hour fast. A 50–60% increase in blood glucose appears in 10–20 minutes in the normal person. No increase occurs in one with von Gierke's disease.
  Administer galactose or fructose intravenously. No rise in

blood glucose occurs in von Gierke's but normal rise occurs in limit dextrinosis (Type III GSD).

Biopsy of liver

Histology is not diagnostic; shows vacuolization of hepatic cells and abundant glycogen granules. Confirm with Best's stain.

Biochemical studies

Glycogen content is more than 4% by weight.

Glucose-6-phosphatase is absent or markedly decreased.

Glycogen is biochemically normal.

Other enzymes (other GSD) are present in normal amounts.

Biopsy of jejunum

Intestinal glucose-6-phosphatase is decreased or absent.

POMPE'S DISEASE (TYPE II GLYCOGEN-STORAGE DISEASE; GENERALIZED GLYCOGENOSIS; ALPHA-GLUCOSIDASE DEFICIENCY GLYCOGENOSIS)

Features of the disease are imbecility, varying neurologic defects, muscle hypotonia, cardiac enlargement, and frequent liver enlargement.

Fasting blood sugar, GTT, glucagon responses, and rises in blood glucose after fructose infusion are normal. No acetonuria is present.

General hematologic findings are normal.

Staining of circulating leukocytes for glycogen shows massive deposition.

Confirm diagnosis by muscle biopsy, specific enzymatic assays, glycogen structure analysis (these are special studies).

TYPE III GLYCOGEN-DEPOSITION DISEASE (FORBES'S DISEASE; DEBRANCHER DEFICIENCY; LIMIT DEXTRINOSIS)

This is a familial disease with enlarged liver, retarded growth, chemical changes, and benign course.

Serum cholesterol is increased.

Acetone appears in urine.

Fasting hypoglycemia occurs.

There is a diabetic type of glucose tolerance curve with associated glucosuria.

Infusions of galactose and fructose cause a normal hyperglycemic response.

Fasting blood sugar does not show expected rise after administration of subcutaneous glucagon.

Confirm diagnosis by biochemical findings of increased liver glycogen, abnormal glycogen structure, absence of detectable amylol, 6-glucosidase activity with normal phosphorylase and glucose-6-phosphatase.

TYPE IV GLYCOGEN-DEPOSITION DISEASE (ANDERSEN'S DISEASE; BRANCHER DEFICIENCY; AMYLOPECTINOSIS)

This extremely rare fatal condition is due to absence of amylo-(1,4 → 1,6)-transglucosidase.

Liver function tests may be altered (e.g., slight increase in bilirubin, reversed A/G ratio, increased SGOT, decreased serum cholesterol).

There may be a flat blood glucose response to epinephrine and glucagon.

There may be increased WBC and decreased hemoglobin.

Biopsy of liver may show a cirrhotic reaction to the presence of polysaccharide of abnormal structure which stains with Best's carmine and periodic acid–Schiff stain but has a very low glycogen content.

TYPE V GLYCOGEN-DEPOSITION DISEASE (McARDLE'S SYNDROME; McARDLE-SCHMID-PEARSON DISEASE; MYOPHOSPHORYLASE DEFICIENCY)

This is a familial autosomal recessive disease showing very limited ischemic muscle exercise tolerance in the presence of normal appearance of muscle.

Epinephrine or glucagon causes a normal hyperglycemic response.

Biopsy of muscle is microscopically normal in youth; vacuolation and necrosis are seen in later years. Increased glycogen is present. Absence of phosphorylase is demonstrated by various techniques.

Following exercise that quickly causes muscle cramping and weakness, the regional blood lactate and pyruvate does not increase (in a normal person it increases 2–5 times).

Myoglobinuria may occur after strenuous exercise.

TYPE VI GLYCOGEN-STORAGE DISEASE (HEPATIC PHOSPHORYLASE DEFICIENCY)

Enlarged liver present from birth is associated with hypoglycemia.

Hypoglycemia is mild to moderate.

Serum cholesterol and lactic acid are mildly increased.

Liver function tests are normal except for mobilization of glycogen.

Fructose tolerance is normal.

Response to glucagon and epinephrine is variable but tends to be poor.

Leukocyte phosphorylase activity is decreased.

TYPE VII GLYCOGEN-STORAGE DISEASE (GLYCOGEN SYNTHETASE DEFICIENCY)

Fasting hypoglycemia is marked.

Other members of family may have reduced tolerance to glucose.

Biopsy of liver shows decreased glycogen content, no detectable glycogen synthetase activity.

RBCs show decreased glycogen synthetase activity.

FAMILIAL PAROXYSMAL PERITONITIS (FAMILIAL MEDITERRANEAN FEVER; "PERIODIC DISEASE")

WBC is increased (10,000–20,000/cu mm), and there may be increased eosinophils during an attack but a return to normal between attacks.

ESR is increased during an attack but normal between attacks.

Mild normocytic normochromic anemia is occasionally seen.

Serum glycoprotein is increased in patients and their relatives.
Increased alpha$_2$ globulin and fibrinogen are common.
Amyloidosis develops in 10–40% of patients; it is not related to frequency or severity of clinical attacks.
Etiocholanolone is increased in urine and blood during attacks in a few patients.

LESCH-NYHAM SYNDROME

The syndrome appears in children, with choreoathetosis, mental retardation, tendency to self-mutilating biting and scratching.
Serum uric acid levels are very high (because of complete absence of hypoxanthine-guanine phosphoribosyltransferase).

FAMILIAL DYSAUTONOMIA (RILEY-DAY SYNDROME)

This condition is due to an autosomal recessive trait occurring in Ashkenazi Jews, who show difficulty in swallowing, corneal ulcerations, insensitivity to pain, motor incoordination, excessive sweating, diminished gag reflex, lack of tongue papillae, progressive kyphoscoliosis, pulmonary infections, etc.
Urine vanilmandelic acid (VMA) (3-methoxy-4-hydroxymandelic acid) may be low and homovanillic acid (HVA) increased.
In asymptomatic carriers, urine VMA may be lower than in healthy adults.

BATTEN'S DISEASE (BATTEN-SPIELMEYER-VOGT DISEASE)
(autosomal recessive type of juvenile amaurotic idiocy)

Azurophilic hypergranulation of leukocytes occurs in patients and in heterozygous and homozygous members of families. In Giemsa- and Wright-stained smears, it resembles toxic granulation but differs by the absence of supravital staining in Batten's disease and by normal leukocyte alkaline phosphatase activity (markedly increased in toxic granulation). The disease occurs in 15% or more of neutrophils.

TAY-SACHS DISEASE (G$_{M2}$ GANGLIOSIDOSIS; INFANTILE AMAUROTIC IDIOCY)

This condition is due to an autosomal recessive trait found predominantly (but not exclusively) in Ashkenazi Jews and is characterized by the appearance during infancy of psychomotor deterioration, blindness, "cherry-red spot" in the macula, and an exaggerated extension response to sound.
There is early marked increase of serum LDH and SGOT and decrease of serum fructose-1-phosphate aldolase. (*Serum fructose-1-phosphate aldolase is also decreased in heterozygotes.*)
SGOT and cerebrospinal fluid GOT are increased throughout course of disease and may even be increased before clinical symptoms are present; return to normal if patient lives 3–4 years. Similar changes in LDH and MDH in serum and cerebrospinal fluid with peak at second year are followed by gradual return to normal.
Serum aldolase is normal during first few months, then progressively rises to peak (of twice normal) at age 12–24 months correlating with skeletal muscle atrophy, then returns to normal in next 3–12 months.

Cerebrospinal fluid aldolase rises early and then declines slowly as disease progresses; does not parallel serum level since it originates from a different source.

Serum acid phosphatase is normal.

Occasional vacuolated lymphocytes are seen.

Liver function tests are normal.

LANDING'S DISEASE (G_{MI} GANGLIOSIDOSIS; SYSTEMIC LATE INFANTILE LIPIDOSIS)

This is a rare familial disorder due to an autosomal recessive gene with no racial predilection, characterized by psychomotor deterioration, enlargement of liver and/or spleen, and roentgenographic findings resembling those in Hunter and Hurler syndromes.

Vacuolated lymphocytes may be found.

Abnormal leukocytic granulations (Alder-Reilly bodies) may be present.

Serum LDH, SGOT, and fructose-1-phosphate aldolase are normal.

Foam cell histiocytes (resembling Niemann-Pick cells) may be seen in biopsy from bone marrow, liver, or rectum.

13(D_1)-TRISOMY SYNDROME

See Nuclear Sex Cromatin and Karyotyping, pp. 137–138.

In peripheral blood smears, most of the neutrophilic leukocytes show an increased number of anomalous nuclear projections compared to those of normal persons. The nuclear lobulation may appear abnormal (nucleus may look twisted without clear separation of individual lobes, coarse lumpy chromatin, etc.).

Fetal hemoglobin may persist longer than normal (i.e., be increased).

32

Endocrine Diseases

HYPERTHYROIDISM

Serum T-3 uptake is increased.
Serum PBI is increased.
Serum BEI is increased.
Serum PB^{131}I and conversion ratio are increased.
Serum T-4 (total thyroxine) is increased.
Serum free thyroxine is increased.
Thyroid uptake of ^{131}I is increased. It is relatively more affected at 1, 2, or 6 hours than at 24 hours. It may be normal in presence of recent iodine ingestion.
Salivary excretion of ^{131}I is increased.
Urinary excretion of ^{131}I is increased.
Iodine tolerance test shows increased utilization of iodine.
BMR is increased.
Serum thyroxine-binding globulin (TBG) is normal.
Serum cholesterol is decreased.
Serum total lipids are usually decreased.
Hyperglycemia is present.
Glycosuria is present.
Glucose tolerance is decreased with early high peak and early fall.
Creatine excretion in urine and creatine tolerance are increased (normal serum creatine almost excludes hyperthyroidism).
There is increased urinary and fecal excretion of calcium with normal serum phosphorus.
Thyroid suppression test. Triiodothyronine administration decreases ^{131}I uptake in normal individuals but not in hyperthyroid individuals.
There is associated impairment of liver damage (e.g., impaired excretion of BSP).

Triiodothyronine (T-3) toxicosis
    Should be suspected particularly in patients with clinical thyrotoxicosis (with increased BMR) in whom usual laboratory tests are normal

Continued on page 318.

Table 45. Thyroid Function Tests in Various Conditions

Disease	RAIU (radioactive iodine uptake)	Free Thyroxine	T-4 (total serum thyroxine)	Serum PBI	Serum T-3 Uptake	Serum TBG (thyroxine-binding globulin)	Serum Cholesterol	BMR
Hypothyroidism	D	D	D	D	D	N or I	I	D
Hyperthyroidism	I	I	I	I	I	N	D	I
Administration of								
Thyroxine (factitious hyperthyroidism) *no goiter*	D	I	I	I	I	N	D	I
Inorganic iodine	D	N	N	I	N	N	N	N
Radiopaque contrast media	D	N	N	I	N	N	N	N
Estrogen and antiovulatory drugs	I	N	I	I	D	I	V	V
ACTH and corticosteroids	D	N	D	D	I	D	V	V
Dilantin or large doses of salicylates		N	D	D	I	D		
Pregnancy	*	N	I	I	D	I	V	V
With hyperthyroidism	*	I	I	I	N	I		
With hypothyroidism	*	D	D–N	D–N	D	I		
Hereditary increase of TBG in euthyroid state	I	N	I	I	D	I	V	V
Hereditary decrease of TBG in euthyroid state	D	N	D	D	I	D	V	V

[316]

Thyroiditis	V	V	V	V	V	V	V
Adenomatous thyroid goiter	N	N	N	N	N	N	N
Thyroid neoplasm (non-functional)	N	N	N	N	N	N	N
Nephrosis	May be I	N	D	D	I	I	I

N = normal; D = decreased; I = increased; V = variable.
*Contraindicated.
Normal T-3 does not rule out hypothyroidism since about half of hypothyroid patients fall in the normal range. Very high PBI and very low RAIU probably means ingestion of iodine. Moderately high PBI and low RAIU suggests thyroiditis. PBI is highest when the thyroiditis is maximum.

Hyperthyroidism   *(continued)*

       Serum T-4 is normal.
       TBG and TBPA (thyroxine-binding albumin) are normal.
       ^{131}I uptake is autonomous (not suppressed by T-3 adminis-
         tration).
       Serum T-3 (measured by radioimmunoassay) is increased.
Increased serum T-3 is associated with increased T-4 in
       Graves' disease
       Toxic adenoma
       Toxic multinodular goiter
       Factitious hyperthyroidism
Increased serum T-3 is associated with normal or low T-4 in
       T-3 hyperthyroidism
       TBG deficiency with hyperthyroidism
       Ingestion of T-3 alone or combined with T-4
       Premonitory clinical hyperthyroidism
Decreased serum T-3 is associated with decreased T-4 in
       Hypothyroidism, primary or secondary
Decreased serum T-3 is associated with normal T-4 in
       Newborn (first week of life)
       Fetus at term

HYPOTHYROIDISM

Serum T-3 uptake is decreased. (May be normal in up to half of
   hypothyroid patients.)
Serum PBI is decreased.
Serum BEI is decreased.
Serum PB^{131}I and conversion ratio are decreased.
Serum T-4 (total thyroxine) is decreased.
Serum free thyroxine is decreased.
Thyroid uptake of ^{131}I is decreased.
Serum alkaline phosphatase is increased (originates from bone).
Serum calcium is sometimes increased.
Salivary excretion of ^{131}I is decreased.
Urinary excretion of ^{131}I is decreased.
Iodine tolerance test shows decreased utilization of iodine.
BMR is decreased.
Serum thyroxine-binding globulin (TBG) is normal.
Serum cholesterol is increased (chiefly useful to follow effect of
   therapy, especially in children).
Fasting blood sugar is decreased.
Glucose tolerance is increased (oral GTT is flat; IV GTT is normal).
TSH stimulation (20 units/day for 3 days) increases ^{131}I uptake to
   about normal (20%) in secondary (pituitary) hypothyroidism but
   not in primary hypothyroidism.
Serum thyrotropin is increased in primary hypothyroidism and
   decreased in secondary (pituitary) hypothyroidism.
Normocytic normochromic anemia is found.
Serum carotene is increased.
Laboratory findings indicative of pernicious anemia and primary
   adrenocortical insufficiency occur with increased frequency in
   primary hypothyroidism.

When hypothyroid patient becomes euthyroid after treatment
     PBI is low (usually 2 μg/100 ml) when treated with triiodothy-
     ronine (Cytomel).

PBI is often high normal or slightly increased when treated with thyroxine (Synthroid).

PBI is normal when treated with desiccated thyroid (Thyroid U.S.P.).

PBI may be below normal when treated with thyroglobulin (Proloid).

Table 46. Laboratory Tests in Differential Diagnosis of Primary and Secondary Hypothyroidism

Test	Panhypopituitarism	Primary Myxedema
Urine 17-KS	Absent	Low
Response to insulin	Prompt decrease in blood sugar; fails to return to normal	Usually delayed fall in blood sugar and sometimes delayed return to normal
Response to administration of thyrotropic hormone	Responds with increase in 131I uptake, BMR, etc.	No response
Serum thyrotropin	Decreased	Increased
BMR	More marked decrease (e.g., minus 40–50)	Less marked decrease

THYROID FUNCTION DURING PREGNANCY

Normally during pregnancy BMR increases 10–25% above nonpregnant level and serum cholesterol also increases; these are therefore not useful in differential diagnosis. Radioactive iodine uptake (RAIU) is contraindicated.

PBI reaches upper limit of normal 3–6 weeks after conception; if PBI does not rise early in pregnancy, abortion is probable. PBI may reach 10–12 µg/100 ml. *Beware of falsely increased PBI due to prior administration of x-ray contrast media (even many years before) and of drugs.*

In hyperthyroidism, both serum T-3 uptake and T-4 are increased, but in the pregnant euthyroid patient or euthyroid patient taking birth control pills or estrogens, the T-4 is increased and the T-3 uptake is decreased. Hyperthyroidism may be indicated by the failure of the T-3 uptake to decrease during pregnancy.

T-3 uptake gradually decreases (as early as 3–6 weeks after conception) until the end of the first trimester and then remains relatively constant. It returns to normal 12–13 weeks postpartum. Failure to decrease by the eighth to tenth week of pregnancy may indicate threatened abortion (one should know the patient's normal nonpregnant level).

THYROID FUNCTION DURING NEONATAL PERIOD

Neonatal Hyperthyroidism

Laboratory findings due to present or past maternal hyperthyroidism are noted.

If there was hyperthyroidism in the past, all laboratory tests may be normal except that administration of thyroid fails to produce the normal expected depression of thyroid function.

Laboratory findings due to increased susceptibility to infection are noted.

Laboratory findings of hyperthyroidism are noted (see p. 315).

Neonatal Hypothyroidism

Decreased serum alkaline phosphatase and PBI are the most important indications.

These tests should always be done whenever there is suspicion of hypothyroidism (e.g., prolonged icterus neonatorum, anemia, birth weight more than 9 lb, various clinical findings).

Increased serum cholesterol may be found and is a useful confirmation in borderline cases.

Occasionally RAIU may be indicated (shows little or no uptake) because of the need to make early diagnosis to avoid permanent brain damage.

Laboratory findings of maternal hypothyroidism are often present.

ACUTE STREPTOCOCCAL THYROIDITIS

WBC and polynuclear leukocytes are increased.

ESR is increased.

The 24-hour uptake of ^{131}I is usually decreased but sometimes is normal.

Serum PBI is usually normal but may be increased or decreased.

BEI is lower than PBI because with thyroid necrosis iodine-containing proteins enter the blood; these are included in the PBI determination but not in the BEI because they are not soluble in butanol.

HASHIMOTO'S THYROIDITIS (STRUMA LYMPHOMATOSA)

Thyroid function may be normal; 15–20% of patients develop hypothyroidism; occasionally a patient passes through a hyperthyroid stage.

Serum antithyroglobulin antibodies (tanned RBCs) are positive at a titer of 1:25,000, but lower titers may be significant. Half the patients may have a significant titer.

PBI may be decreased, normal, or increased and may vary over a period of time (because of thyroid destruction and regeneration). *Suspect Hashimoto's thyroiditis when PBI is increased or normal but BEI and T-4 are decreased (gland is making iodoprotein but decreased amounts of thyroxine).* ^{131}I may be higher than expected in hypothyroidism.

Radioiodine scan may show involvement of only a single lobe (more common in younger patients).

Response to TSH distinguishes primary and secondary hypothyroidism. If thyroid uptake for each lobe is measured separately after TSH, a difference between the lobes may demonstrate lobar thyroiditis when total uptake is apparently normal.

Laboratory findings of hypothyroidism, when present (see p. 318), are noted.

Biopsy of thyroid may be performed.

Table 47. Laboratory Findings in Various Diseases of Calcium and Phosphorus Metabolism

Disease	Serum Calcium* (>11 in 90%)	Serum Phosphorus (<3 in 90%)	Serum Alkaline Phosphatase	Urine Calcium†	Urine Phosphorus
Hyperparathyroidism	I	D	I (N if no bone disease)	I	I
Hypoparathyroidism	D	I	N	D	D‡
Pseudohypoparathyroidism	D	I	N, occ. D	D	D‡
Pseudopseudohypoparathyroidism	N	N	N	N	N
Secondary hyperparathyroidism (renal rickets)	V	I	I or N	D or I	D
Vitamin D excess	I	I or D	N or I	I	I
Rickets and osteomalacia	D or N	D or N	I	D	D
Osteoporosis	N	N	N	N or I	N
Polyostotic fibrous dysplasia	N	N or I	N or I	N	N
Paget's disease	N	N or I	I	N or I	I
Metastatic neoplasm to bone	N or I	V	N or I	V	I
Multiple myeloma	N or I	V	N or I	N or I	N or I
Sarcoidosis	N or I	N or I	N or I	I	I
Fanconi syndrome or renal loss of fixed base	D or N	D	N or I	I	I
Histiocytosis X (Letterer-Siwe, Hand-Schüller-Christian, eosinophilic granuloma)	N	N	N or I	N or I	N
Hypercalcemia and excess intake of alkali (Burnett's syndrome)	I	I or N	N	N	N
Solitary bone cyst	N	N	N	N	N

N = normal; D = decreased; I = increased; V = variable; occ. = occasionally.
* Serum calcium. Repeated determinations may be required to demonstrate abnormalities. Serum protein level should always be known. See also response to corticoids on p. 115.
† Urine calcium: patient should be on a low calcium diet (e.g., Bauer-Aub).
‡ See Ellsworth-Howard test on p. 76.

DE QUERVAIN'S THYROIDITIS (SUBACUTE THYROIDITIS) (probably of viral origin)

^{131}I uptake is decreased; may be zero in early stages. It is not increased by TSH administration during active phase. It may be over 50% for several weeks after recovery.

PBI is normal to increased; BEI may be less than 80% of PBI.

ESR is increased.

WBC is normal or decreased.

Biopsy of thyroid confirms diagnosis.

Antithyroglobulin antibodies (tanned RBCs) may be present for up to several months at levels of about 1:320 but the titer is never as high as in Hashimoto's thyroiditis. The level falls with recovery.

RIEDEL'S CHRONIC THYROIDITIS

Biopsy of thyroid confirms diagnosis.

Some patients may have laboratory findings of hypothyroidism.

SIMPLE NONTOXIC DIFFUSE GOITER

No specific laboratory findings.

SINGLE OR MULTIPLE NODULAR GOITERS

Isotope scanning of thyroid may show decreased ("cold") or increased ("hot") uptake.

Functioning solitary adenoma may produce hyperthyroidism.

MALIGNANT TUMORS OF THYROID

No specific laboratory findings

Histologic examination of tissue

PRIMARY HYPERPARATHYROIDISM

Serum calcium is increased (may be as high as 20 mg/100 ml). Repeated determinations may be required to demonstrate increased serum calcium levels. Rapid decrease after excision of adenoma may cause tetany during next few weeks, especially when serum alkaline phosphatase is increased.

Serum total protein must always be measured simultaneously as marked decrease may cause a decrease in calcium.

Normal calcium level may occur with coexistence of conditions that decrease serum calcium level (e.g., high phosphate intake, malabsorption, acute pancreatitis, nephrosis, infarction of parathyroid adenoma); also beware of laboratory error as a cause of "normal" serum calcium.

High phosphate intake can abolish increased serum and urine calcium and decreased serum phosphorus; low-phosphate diet unmasks these changes.

Serum phosphorus is decreased (less than 3 mg/100 ml). It may be normal in the presence of high phosphorus intake or renal damage with secondary phosphate retention. It may be normal in one-half of patients, even without uremia.

Serum alkaline phosphatase is normal or may be markedly increased in the presence of bone disease. There is a slow decrease to normal after excision of adenoma.

Urine calcium is increased (more than 400 mg on a normal diet; 180 mg on a low-calcium diet). Urine calcium increase is found in only 70% of patients with hyperparathyroidism.

Urine phosphorus is increased unless there is renal insufficiency or phosphate depletion (especially due to commonly used antacids containing aluminum). Phosphate loading unmasks the increased urine phosphorus of hyperparathyroidism.

Polyuria is present, with low specific gravity.

Cortisone administration (150 mg daily for 10 days)

> Usually does not affect the increased serum calcium of parathyroid adenoma.

> Within 2 weeks lowers the increased serum calcium of multiple myeloma, metastatic carcinoma, vitamin D intoxication, infantile hypercalcemia, sarcoidosis.

Serum chloride is increased (more than 100 mEq/L; less than this in other types of hypercalcemia).

Serum alpha$_2$ and beta$_1$ globulins are slightly increased but return to normal after parathyroidectomy. *Serum protein electrophoresis should always be performed in hyperparathyroidism to rule out multiple myeloma and sarcoidosis.*

Uric acid is increased in more than 15% of patients. Uric acid level is not affected by cure of hyperparathyroidism, but a postoperative gout attack may occur.

Increased hydroxyproline in serum and urine may occur with bone disease but is not as useful as serum alkaline phosphatase for detection of bone disease.

Frequently anemia, decreased WBC, and sometimes decreased platelets due to bone marrow depression are found.

Serum parathyroid hormone level (measured by radioimmunoassay) is elevated in all patients with hyperparathyroidism. Intravenous infusion of calcium sufficient to induce hypercalcemia suppresses the level of serum parathyroid hormone in primary hyperplasia of the parathyroids and in secondary hyperparathyroidism due to renal insufficiency but does not suppress the serum parathyroid hormone level due to parathyroid adenoma.

Serum parathyroid hormone level rises above baseline level after neck massage only on the side of the adenoma, thereby aiding preoperative localization of the adenoma.

Hyperparathyroidism must always be ruled out in the presence of

> Renal colic and stones or calcification (2–3% have hyperparathyroidism)

> Peptic ulcer (occurs in 15% of patients with hyperparathyroidism)

> Calcific keratitis

> Bone changes (*present in one-fifth of patients with hyperparathyroidism*)

> Jaw tumors

> Clinical syndrome of hypercalcemia (nocturia, hyposthenuria, polyuria, abdominal pain, adynamic ileus, constipation, nausea, vomiting) (*present in one-fifth of patients with hyperparathyroidism; only clue to diagnosis in 10% of patients with hyperparathyroidism*)

Multiple endocrine adenomatosis (e.g., islet cell tumor of pancreas, pituitary tumor, pheochromocytoma)

Relatives of patients with hyperparathyroidism or "asymptomatic" hypercalcemia

Mental aberrations

"Asymptomatic" hyperparathyroidism (routine serum calcium screening) is found in 0.09% of patient population.

In parathyroid hormone–secreting cancer (usually bronchus, kidney, ovary, colon)

Laboratory findings are the same as when due to adenoma except

Nephrolithiasis is rare.

Serum chloride is usually low.

X-ray changes are absent even with increased serum alkaline phosphatase.

Hypercalcemia responds to cortisone in 23% of patients.

Laboratory findings due to malignancy are noted.

See sections on decreased tubular reabsorption of phosphate, increased phosphate clearance, negative calcium tolerance test, serum calcium and phosphorus changes induced by phosphate deprivation, all on p. 77.

SECONDARY HYPERPARATHYROIDISM

This is a diffuse hyperplasia of parathyroid glands usually secondary to chronic advanced renal disease.

Laboratory findings due to underlying causative disease are noted.

Laboratory findings like those in primary hyperparathyroidism are noted, but

Serum calcium is usually not increased in osteomalacia, rickets, renal rickets, steatorrhea.

Serum calcium may be slightly increased in pituitary basophilism, multiple myeloma, metastatic carcinoma of bone, osteogenesis imperfecta, etc.

HYPOPARATHYROIDISM

Serum calcium is decreased (as low as 5 mg/100 ml). *More than a third of these patients may present as "epileptics."* Hypoparathyroidism should be ruled out in presence of mental and emotional changes, cataracts, faulty dentition in children, associated changes in skin and nails (e.g., moniliasis is frequent).

Serum phosphorus is increased (usually 5–6 mg/100 ml; as high as 12 mg/100 ml).

Serum alkaline phosphatase is normal or slightly decreased.

Urine calcium is decreased (Sulkowitch's test is negative).

Urine phosphorus is decreased. Phosphate clearance is decreased (see p. 77).

Injection of potent parathyroid extract (200 units IV) causes urine phosphorus to increase 10 times or more within 3–5 hours. In a normal person the increase in urine phosphorus is 5–6 times. In pseudohypoparathyroidism the urine phosphorus is not increased more than 2 times (see Ellsworth-Howard test, p. 76).

Alkalosis is present.

Serum uric acid is increased.

There is a flat oral GTT (due to poor absorption).

CSF is normal even with mental or emotional symptoms or with calcification of basal ganglia.

PSEUDOHYPOPARATHYROIDISM

Serum calcium, phosphorus, and alkaline phosphatase are the same as in hypoparathyroidism but cannot be corrected by (or they respond poorly to) administration of parathyroid hormone (see reference to Ellsworth-Howard test in the section on hypoparathyroidism just preceding).

PSEUDOPSEUDOHYPOPARATHYROIDISM

Serum and urine calcium, phosphorus, and alkaline phosphatase are normal.

Response to parathyroid hormone is normal.

Clinical anomalies are the same as in pseudohypoparathyroidism.

PRIMARY HYPOPHOSPHATEMIA

This is a familial but occasionally sporadic condition of intrinsic renal tubular defect in phosphate resorption.

Serum phosphorus is always decreased in the untreated patient.

Serum calcium is usually normal.

Serum alkaline phosphatase is often increased.

Bone biopsy shows a characteristic pattern of demineralization around osteocyte lacunae.

HYPOPHOSPHATASIA

This rare genetic disease of bone mineralization with x-ray changes and clinical syndromes is found in infants and children, and adults.

Serum alkaline phosphatase is decreased to about 25% of normal (may vary from 0 up to 40% of normal); is not correlated with severity of disease.

Serum and urine levels of phosphoethanolamine are increased (may be normal in asymptomatic heterozygotes).

Serum calcium is increased in severe cases.

Treatment with corticosteroids usually causes an increase in serum alkaline phosphatase (but it never attains normal level) with a marked fall in serum calcium; phosphoethanolamine excretion in urine continues high.

PSEUDOHYPOPHOSPHATASIA
(clinical syndrome resembling hypophosphatasia)

Serum alkaline phosphatase is normal.

IDIOPATHIC HYPERPHOSPHATASIA OF INFANCY (FAMILIAL OSTEOECTASIA)

This condition is characterized by excessive osteoblastic activity but almost no formation of normal cortical bone.

Serum alkaline phosphatase is increased.

IDIOPATHIC HYPERCALCEMIA OF INFANCY WITH FAILURE TO THRIVE

Characteristics are mental retardation, elfin face, and chemical changes.
Serum calcium is increased.
Serum cholesterol is increased.

NEONATAL HYPOCALCEMIA
(age 1–4 weeks; serum calcium less than 8 mg/100 ml)

Age 1–2 days—associated with
Prematurity and low birth weight (occurs in up to 50% of infants)
Maternal diabetes (occurs in up to 25% of infants)
Age 5–10 days—associated with
Feeding of cow's milk (increased serum phosphorus and decreased serum calcium)
Rarely associated with
Maternal hypercalcemia or hyperparathyroidism
Congenital absence of parathyroid glands
Hypoproteinemia (e.g., nephrosis, liver disease)
Maternal osteomalacia
Renal disease (primary renal tubular defect; decreased glomerular filtration rate causing phosphate retention)
Iatrogenic disorders (e.g., citrate administration during exchange transfusion)

When tetany syndrome is associated with a normal serum calcium or not relieved by administration of calcium, rule out decreased serum magnesium (normal = 1.51 ± 0.12 mEq/L).
Serum phosphorus is more than 8 mg/100 ml when neonatal hypocalcemia is due to high phosphate feeding. BUN is increased when neonatal hypocalcemia is due to severe renal disease.

SYNDROME OF FAMILIAL HYPOCALCEMIA, LATENT TETANY, AND CALCIFICATION OF BASAL GANGLIA

This rare clinical syndrome has features resembling those of pseudohypoparathyroidism, pseudopseudohypoparathyroidism, and basal cell nevus syndrome.
Hypocalcemia is not responsive to parathormone administration.
Parathormone administration produces a phosphate diuresis.

DECREASED TISSUE CALCIUM WITH TETANY

The tetany, associated with normal serum calcium, magnesium, potassium, and CO_2 responds to vitamin D therapy.
Special radioactive calcium studies show decreased tissue calcium pool that returns toward normal with therapy.

VITAMIN D INTOXICATION

Serum calcium may be increased.
Serum phosphorus is usually also increased but sometimes is decreased, with increased urinary phosphorus.

MAGNESIUM-DEFICIENCY TETANY SYNDROME

Serum magnesium is decreased (usually less than 1 mEq/L).
Serum calcium is normal (slightly decreased in some patients)
Blood pH is normal.
Tetany responds to administration of magnesium but not of calcium.

DIABETES MELLITUS

When glycosuria is present, diabetes mellitus must always be ruled out.
Elevated fasting blood sugar (FBS) may be normal in mild diabetes; therefore it is not adequate for case finding.
Elevated 2-hour postprandial blood sugar alone is superior to FBS alone for routine screening for diabetes.
Glucose tolerance test (GTT) is most useful for detecting latent or incipient diabetes. If GTT is normal but diabetes mellitus is clinically suspected, test should be repeated. Cortisone GTT increases the sensitivity of the test.

> With fasting hyperglycemia, prolonged increase of blood sugar follows glucose ingestion.

> ✳ With normal FBS, a 1-hour blood sugar over 170 mg/100 ml and 2-hour blood sugar over 150 mg/100 ml indicates diabetes mellitus.

> More severe diabetes produces a more abnormal curve.

> Some cases of mild diabetes show hypoglycemia at 4–5 hours.

> When only one of the blood sugar levels at 1-, 2-, or 3-hour intervals is abnormal, 50% of the patients become diabetic.

> *A diabetic type of GTT curve may result if the patient has had inadequate caloric and carbohydrate diet; therefore, during the preceding 3 days, he should have a carbohydrate intake of 300 gm/day.*

Hypoglycemic episodes may occur in the prediabetic state. Half the patients with hypoglycemic episodes have a positive family history of diabetes.

Primary diabetes mellitus
> Inherited metabolic defect with impaired production, release, or effectiveness of insulin

Secondary diabetes
> Pancreas
>> Chronic pancreatitis, hemochromatosis, carcinoma of pancreas, postpancreatectomy
> Endocrine
>> Hyperthyroidism, hyperadrenalism (Cushing's syndrome, primary aldosteronism, pheochromocytoma), acromegaly

See sections on diabetic nephrosclerosis, papillary necrosis, infection of genitourinary tract, lipoproteins, etc.

DIABETIC KETOACIDOSIS

Blood glucose is increased (usually more than 300 mg/100 ml).
Plasma acetone is present.

There is hemoconcentration due to dehydration and electrolyte changes.

Azotemia is present.

Blood pH is decreased.

WBC is increased (often more than 20,000/cu mm without infection).

Urine contains increased sugar, ketones, protein, and casts.

See Metabolic Acidosis, pp. 290–292.

Look for precipitating factors, especially infection.

SOME HETEROGENEOUS GENETIC DISEASES ASSOCIATED WITH HYPERGLYCEMIA

Alstrom's syndrome
Ataxia-telangiectasia
Diabetes mellitus
Friedreich's ataxia
Hemochromatosis
Herrmann's syndrome
Hyperlipoproteinemias (three different types)
Isolated growth hormone deficiency
Laurence-Moon-Biedl-Bardet syndrome
Lipoatrophic diabetes
Myotonic dystrophy
Optic atrophy
Prader-Willi syndrome
Refsum's syndrome
Schmidt's syndrome
Werner's syndrome

PRADER-WILLI SYNDROME

This condition is characterized by mental retardation, muscular hypotonia, obesity, short stature, and hypogonadism associated with diabetes mellitus.

Diabetes mellitus frequently develops in childhood and adolescence but is insulin-resistant, responds to oral hypoglycemic drugs, and is not accompanied by acidosis.

ISLET CELL TUMORS OF PANCREAS—CLASSIFICATION

Insulin-secreting beta cell tumor (may be benign or malignant, primary or metastatic) produces hyperinsulinism with hypoglycemia. (See next section, Hyperinsulinism, for laboratory findings and differential diagnosis.)

Non-insulin-secreting non-beta cell tumor (benign or malignant, primary or metastatic) may produce several types of syndromes.

Zollinger-Ellison syndrome (see next page)

Profuse diarrhea with hypokalemia and dehydration

Profuse diarrhea with hypokalemia (and sometimes periodic paralysis) may occur as a separate syndrome without peptic ulceration. (*Some of the patients have histamine-fast achlorhydria.*) Diabetic glucose tolerance curves may occur in some of them because of chronic potassium depletion. May be associated with multiple endocrine adenomas.

Nonspecific diarrhea
Steatorrhea (due to inactivation of pancreatic enzymes by acid
pH)

HYPERINSULINISM
(due to hyperfunctioning islet cell tumor of pancreas or islet cell hyperplasia)

Blood glucose is less than 40 mg/100 ml at time of symptoms.
Symptoms are relieved by administration of glucose. Frequent
blood glucose determinations may be required. It may be necessary to provoke symptoms by fasting for 72 hours and determining glucose levels whenever symptoms develop. (*This procedure
may have to be repeated as some tumors secrete insulin intermittently.*)
Note that 24% of patients with islet cell tumor have a positive family
history of diabetes; 25% of patients with diabetes have a positive
family history of diabetes; and 3–6% of nondiabetics have a
positive family history of diabetes.

*In functional hypoglycemia, blood glucose is often not less than 60
mg/100 ml.* See Tolbutamide Tolerance Test, p. 73.

Dumping syndrome shows normal blood glucose level.
See sections on advanced liver disease, hypopituitarism, hypoadrenalism, glycogen-storage disease, alcoholism, hypoglycemia associated with neoplasms, etc.

ZOLLINGER-ELLISON SYNDROME

There is a large volume of highly acid gastric juice in the absence of
pyloric obstruction; it is refractory to vagotomy and subtotal
gastrectomy.* (See Serum Gastrin, p. 70.)
Hypokalemia is frequently associated with chronic severe diarrhea
that may be a clue to this diagnosis.
Steatorrhea occurs rarely.
Laboratory findings due to peptic ulcer of stomach, duodenum, or
proximal jejunum (e.g., perforation, fluid loss, hemorrhage) are
noted. *Up to one-quarter of these patients have ulcers in unusual
locations or have multiple ulcerations. A tendency toward rapid or
severe recurrence of ulcer after adequate therapy is a clue to
Zollinger-Ellison syndrome.*

Tumors are solitary benign adenomas in 28% of patients.
Adenomas are multiple in 29% of patients and may be ectopic
(e.g., in duodenal wall).
Tumors are malignant in 62% of patients; 44% of patients have
metastases.
Diffuse hyperplasia occurs in 10% of patients.

*This syndrome is associated with adenomas of other endocrine glands,
especially adrenal and pituitary, in more than 20%.*

---

* 12-hour nocturnal secretion shows acid of more than 100 mEq/L and
volume of more than 1500 ml. Basal secretion is more than 60% of the
secretion caused by histamine or betazole stimulation.

ADRENAL FUNCTION TESTS

Daily infusion of 50 units of ACTH for 5 days, with before and after measurement of 24-hour urines for 17-KS, 17-OHKS (*Protect possible Addison's disease patient with 1 mg of dexamethasone.*)

    Complete primary adrenal insufficiency (Addison's disease)—no increase in urine steroids or increase of less than 2 mg/day

    Incomplete primary adrenal insufficiency—less than normal increases on all 5 days or slight increase on first 3 days which may be followed by decrease on days 4 and 5

    Secondary adrenal insufficiency due to pituitary hypofunction—"staircase" response of progressively higher values each day

    Secondary adrenal insufficiency due to chronic steroid therapy—may require prolonged ACTH testing to elicit the "staircase" response; may produce increments only in 17-OHKS but not in 17-KS

    Normal = 3–5 times increase on first day and further increase next day

Do not do metyrapone test until this test proves that adrenals are sensitive to ACTH.

Measurement of circulating eosinophil count before and after ACTH stimulation (see above)

    Normal

        Decrease of 80% if previous baseline was more than 100 cells/cu mm and no parasitic eosinophilia

    Adrenal insufficiency

        Decrease of less than 25%

LABORATORY TESTS FOR EVALUATION OF ADRENAL-PITUITARY FUNCTION IN PATIENTS WITH HYPERADRENALISM

Adrenal-Cortical Reserve (stimulation of adrenal cortex by administration of ACTH)

Functioning adrenal cortex is indicated by increased blood and urine 17-OHKS above patient's previous baseline level.

    Normal adrenal-cortical reserve. An increase of 3–5 times is shown the first day and a further increase the next day.

    Adrenal cortical hyperplasia. This is often not helpful in diagnosis of Cushing's syndrome.

    Hypopituitarism. A slight increase is shown the first day and a greater increase the next day.

Nonfunctioning adrenal cortex is indicated by no increase of blood and urine 17-OHKS.

    Adenoma of adrenal cortex. Lack of response almost always means autonomous tumor.

    Carcinoma of adrenal cortex. Lack of response almost always means autonomous tumor; there is an associated characteristic marked increase over baseline of urinary neutral 17-KS.

    Also: Addison's disease

Pituitary-Adrenal Suppression (suppression of pituitary ACTH secretion by administration of dexamethasone)

Functioning pituitary-adrenal system is indicated by decrease in blood and urine 17-OHKS.

> Normal pituitary-adrenal system. Urinary level falls to less than 50% of baseline level following lower or higher dose of dexamethasone. Plasma cortisol decreases (less than 5 $\mu g/100$ ml) after both lower and higher dose schedules of dexamethasone.

> Adrenal hyperplasia. Urinary level falls to less than 50% only after higher but not after lower dose of dexamethasone. Plasma cortisol decreases (less than 5 $\mu g/100$ ml) only after higher dose of dexamethasone; remains above 10 $\mu g/100$ ml after low dose of dexamethasone in Cushing's syndrome.

Failure of pituitary control of adrenal-cortical secretion is indicated by *no* decrease in blood and urine 17-OHKS.

> Adenoma or carcinoma of adrenal cortex. Lack of response to high and low doses of dexamethasone confirms diagnosis of Cushing's syndrome and differentiates autonomous tumor from adrenal hyperplasia due to pituitary dysfunction.

> Adrenal hyperfunction due to extra-adrenal tumor (e.g., cancer of bronchus). There is a lack of response to high or low doses of dexamethasone.

Pituitary Reserve (adrenal suppression of pituitary secretion of ACTH inhibited by administration of metyrapone)

Functioning adrenal-pituitary system is indicated by increased urine 17-OHKS (to twice the previous baseline).

> Normal adrenals

> Adrenal-cortical hyperplasia

Nonfunctioning adrenal-pituitary system (Long-standing production of excessive cortisol by adrenal tumor decreases pituitary reserve and responsiveness. Therefore ACTH is not secreted and there is no increase in urinary 17-OHKS and 17-KS.)

> Adenoma or carcinoma of adrenal cortex

> Adrenal hyperfunction due to extra-adrenal tumor (e.g., cancer of bronchus)

> Also: Addison's disease, hypopituitarism

CUSHING'S SYNDROME*

> Glucose tolerance is diminished.
> GTT is frequently diabetic in type.
> Glycosuria appears in 50% of cases.
> FBS may be elevated.
> Insulin tolerance is increased.
> Occasional polydipsia and polyuria are seen.

Usually moderate increase in serum sodium and decrease in serum potassium are found.

> Hypokalemic alkalosis occurs in about 10% of cases.

> *(Hypokalemic alkalosis may indicate extra-adrenal neoplasia*

---

*T. Nichols, C.A. Nugent, and F.H. Tyler, "Steroid Laboratory Tests in the Diagnosis of Cushing's Syndrome." *Amer. J. Med.* 45 (1968): 116–128.

such as bronchogenic carcinoma causing increased production of ACTH with increased secretion of mineralocorticoids and glucocorticoids; occurs in 30–50% of such patients.)

Urine potassium is increased; sodium decreased.
Salivary sodium: potassium ratio is decreased.
Hematologic changes are as follows.
  WBC is normal or increased.
  Relative lymphopenia is frequent (differential is usually less than 15% of cells).
  Eosinopenia is frequent (usually less than 100/cu mm).
  Hematocrit is usually normal; if increased, it indicates an androgenic component.
Osteoporosis causes changes.
  Serum and urine calcium may be increased.
BUN and NPN may be increased.
Urine creatine is increased.
Serum gammaglobulin may be decreased and alpha$_2$ globulin may be moderately increased.
Urinary 17-ketosteroids (17-KS) levels are usually increased (more than 25 mg/24 hours).
Urinary 17-hydroxysteroid (17-OH) levels are increased (more than 10 mg/24 hours).
  The night collection sample is equal to or greater than the day sample (opposite pattern in normal person).
  ACTH stimulation produces the lowest urinary 17-OH in Cushing's syndrome due to adrenal carcinoma and the highest urinary 17-OH due to adrenal hyperplasia, with intermediate urinary 17-OH due to adrenal adenoma.
Plasma 17-OH is increased and remains high late in day (in normal person, plasma 17-OH falls by more than half late in day).
Dexamethasone suppression of adrenal cortex. In normal person given small doses of dexamethasone, the urinary 17-OH falls to less than 4 mg/24 hours (often less than 2 mg/24 hours). Cushing's syndrome due to adenoma or carcinoma shows little or no fall in urinary 17-OH; with adrenal hyperplasia large doses of dexamethasone suppress urinary 17-OH to less than 50% of baseline, but there is less or no suppression with small doses of dexamethasone. (*See below: There are cases in both categories which do not follow these general rules.*) No suppression is seen in Cushing's syndrome due to nonendocrine neoplasm even when large doses of dexamethasone are given.
Serum ACTH is high when Cushing's syndrome is of pituitary or hypothalamic origin and low when it is due to adrenal tumor or hyperplasia.
Metyrapone test. See Table 48, p. 333.
Various steroid tests are abnormal in 55–100% of patients with Cushing's syndrome and up to 36% of patients without Cushing's syndrome. They are more than 40% above normal in 28–96% of patients with Cushing's syndrome and up to 5% of patients without Cushing's syndrome.
Therefore the clinician should remember that in Cushing's syndrome, as in all other complex clinical problems, the diagnosis should not be established or ruled out on the basis of only 1 or 2 laboratory tests.

Continued on page 334.

Table 48. Laboratory Tests in Differential Diagnosis of Cushing's Syndrome of Different Etiologies

Condition	Component	Basal	After ACTH Stimulation	Dexamethasone Suppression 2 mg/day	Dexamethasone Suppression 8 mg/day	Metyrapone Test
Normal	17-OH in urine	N	I	D	D	Marked I
	Plasma cortisol*	N	I	D	D	Marked I
Adrenal hyperplasia due to Pituitary dysfunction	17-OH in urine	I	I	Not D	D	
	Plasma cortisol	N or I	I	Not D	D	Marked I
Extra-adrenal tumor (e.g., cancer of bronchus)	17-OH in urine	I	Usually NC (may be I)	Not D	Not D	Marked I
	Plasma cortisol	I	Usually NC (may be I)	Not D	Not D	
Adrenal adenoma	17-OH in urine	I	†	Not D	Not D	Not I
	Plasma cortisol	I	†	Not D	Not D	Not I
Adrenal carcinoma	17-OH in urine	I	Not I	Not D	Not D	Not I
	Plasma cortisol	I	Not I	Not D	Not D	
Steroid therapy	17-OH in urine	D	NC or I	Not D	Not D	Not I
	Plasma cortisol	I	NC	Not D	Not D	

I = increased; D = decreased; N = normal; NC = no change.
*Plasma cortisol is higher in morning than afternoon in normal person; no diurnal variation in Cushing's syndrome.
†NC with autonomous tumor; I with incompletely autonomous tumor.

[333]

Cushing's Syndrome (*continued*)

Best steroid tests for identifying patients with Cushing's syndrome are the suppression of urinary 17-OH by low dose of dexamethasone and suppression of plasma 17-OH by a single dose of dexamethasone.

No single test can establish the cause of Cushing's syndrome with certainty.

Suppression of urinary 17-OH by high dose of dexamethasone is positive in 80% of patients with adrenal hyperplasia due to excessive pituitary secretion of ACTH without tumor; a positive result is very uncommon in adrenal tumors.

Increased urinary 17-OH by metyrapone administration is positive in

100% of adrenal hyperplasias without tumor
50% of adrenal adenomas
25% of adrenal carcinomas

Increased urinary 17-KS > 4 times normal in

50% of adrenal carcinomas
15% of extrapituitary tumors that secrete ACTH
3% of adrenal hyperplasias without tumors

Urinary 17-KS are normal or low in

70% of adrenal adenomas
50% of adrenal hyperplasias
10% of adrenal carcinomas

Increased urinary 17-OH > 4 times normal in

63% of patients with Cushing's syndrome
3% of patients without Cushing's syndrome
65% of Cushing's syndrome due to extrapituitary tumors that secrete ACTH
3% of Cushing's syndrome due to adrenal hyperplasia without tumor

ADRENOGENITAL SYNDROMES

Pregnanetriol is almost always elevated in all cases of adrenogenital syndrome; it is the most specific diagnostic procedure for adrenogenital syndrome.

Plasma cortisol is low in all types.

Urinary 17-ketogenic steroids (17-KGS) are elevated in all types (17-OH included).

ACTH stimulation causes marked increase in 17-KGS, 17-KS, and pregnanetriol; little or no change in Porter-Silber (P-S) chromagens.

Metyrapone test causes increase in 17-KGS but subnormal increase in P-S chromagens.

See Table 49, p. 336.

ADRENAL FEMINIZATION

This condition occurs in adult males with adrenal tumor (usually unilateral carcinoma, occasionally adenoma) that secretes estrogens.

Urinary estrogens are markedly increased.

17-KS are normal or moderately increased and cannot be suppressed by low doses of dexamethasone when due to adrenal tumor.

17-OH are normal.
Biopsy of testicle shows atrophy of tubules.

ALDOSTERONISM (PRIMARY)

Excessive mineralocorticoid hormone secretion by adrenal cortex causes renal tubules to retain sodium and excrete potassium. The classic biochemical abnormalities are urinary aldosterone, plasma renin, and serum potassium measurements.

Urinary aldosterone is increased on normal-salt diet (not detectable on all days); cannot be reduced by high sodium intake and DOCA administration.

Plasma renin is markedly decreased (normal or increased in secondary aldosteronism). It cannot be stimulated by use of salt restriction and upright posture to deplete plasma volume.

Hypokalemia (usually < 3.0 mEq/L) is allevaited by administration of spironolactone* and by sodium restriction but not by potassium replacement therapy.

Saline infusion causes significant fall in serum potassium and in corrected potassium clearance. This hypokalemia induced by sodium loading is a reliable screening test.

Urine is neutral or alkaline (pH > 7.0) and not normally responsive to ammonium chloride load. Its large volume and low specific gravity are not responsive to vasopressin or water restriction (decreased tubular function, especially reabsorption of water). Proteinuria is intermittent or persistent. There is hyperkaluria even with low potassium intake. Sodium output is reduced.

There is absence of hyponatremia or slight hypernatremia, hypochloremia, and alkalosis (CO_2 content > 25 mEq/L; blood pH tends to increase).

Glucose tolerance is decreased in up to half of patients.

Ketosteroids and 17-hydroxysteroids are normal.

Serum magnesium falls.

Total blood volume increases because of increased plasma volume.

Sodium level in sweat is low.

Salivary Na:K ratio less than 0.65 is consistent with diagnosis but a higher ratio does not exclude it.

Measurement of aldosterone in blood from periphery and both adrenal veins confirms diagnosis by elevated level from side of lesion; opposite side has level close to that in peripheral blood. This also distinguishes unilateral adenoma from bilateral adenomas and hyperplasia and indicates location of lesion for surgeon.

Caused By
Single benign cortical adenoma—70%
Multiple benign cortical adenomas—15%
Bilateral cortical hyperplasia—9%
Normal size adrenal with normal architecture or focal nodular hyperplasia—6%
Rarely, adrenal carcinoma or heterotopic adrenal tissue

---

*Administration of spironolactone for 3 days increases serum potassium more than 1.2 mEq/L. It also increases urine sodium and decreases urine potassium. Negative potassium balance recurs in 5 days. It increases urinary aldosterone (this is variable in hypertensive and normal people).

Table 49. Laboratory Tests in Differential Diagnosis of Adrenogenital Syndromes of Different Etiologies*

Syndrome	Urinary 17-KS	Urinary 17-OH	Urinary (others)	Suppression by Dexamethasone	Blood Electrolytes
Congenital syndrome with salt-losing	Moderate I	D	Pregnanetriol is I in 21-hydroxylation block; tetrahydro-11-deoxycortisol is I in 11-β-hydroxylation block (also causes increase in Porter-Silber chromagens)	Marked D in 17-KS and 17-OHKS on 8 mg/day; no suppression on 2 mg/day (in normal person, suppression on 2 or 8 mg/day)	Sodium D, potassium I
Congenital syndrome with hypertension	Moderate I	Usually I			
Tumors	Marked I; in cancer, urine dehydroepiandrosterone (DHA) is I	Normal or slight I		NC in 17-KS or 17-OHKS	N

N = normal; I = increased; D = decreased; NC = no change.

*Due to excessive adrenocortical secretion of androgenic steroids; in congenital form, there may be an associated deficiency of glucocorticoids and an excess or a deficiency of mineralocorticoids. Occur at any age when due to benign or malignant tumor; usually before 1 year of age (but may be later in life) when due to inborn metabolic error in production of cortisol.

Table 50. Laboratory Differentiation of Primary and Secondary Aldosteronism

Testing Procedure	Primary	Secondary
Etiology	Usually due to tumor (adenoma more frequent than carcinoma); may be due to bilateral hyperplasia	1. Edematous conditions (e.g., cirrhosis, nephrosis, congestive heart failure) 2. Hypertension (e.g., essential, malignant, renovascular renal artery stenosis) 3. Renal tubular dysfunction (e.g., renal tubular acidosis, Fanconi syndrome) 4. Hemorrhage
Blood electrolytes	Hypokalemia, usually with acidosis and hypernatremia	Depends on underlying condition
Plasma renin	Marked D	N or I
Urinary 17-OH and 17-KS	Usually N; may be I in adrenal carcinoma	N
Urinary aldosterone	Marked I	Marked I
Aldosterone administration	Escapes from sodium retention after initial rise in serum sodium	Causes increased edema
Salt-loading	Does not suppress aldosterone secretion (as in normal person) and increases potassium excretion	
Low-sodium diet	Usually reduces potassium excretion	
Deoxycorticosterone administration (DOCA)	In adenoma, aldosterone level is *not* suppressed; in bilateral adrenal hyperplasia, aldosterone level *is* suppressed	

D = decreased; N = normal; I = increased.

ALDOSTERONISM (SECONDARY)

Due To
Congestive heart failure
Cirrhosis with ascites (aldosterone 2000–3000 mg/day)
Nephrosis
Toxemia of pregnancy
Malignant hypertension
Low-sodium diet
Renin-producing renal tumor (see pp. 370–371)

NORMOTENSIVE SECONDARY HYPERALDOSTERONISM (BARTTER'S SYNDROME)

Blood vessels are unable to respond normally to angiotensin; therefore there is no hypertension. To maintain blood pressure, juxtaglomerular apparatus secretes increased amounts of renin.

Increased urinary aldosterone with associated findings (hypokalemic alkalosis, inability to concentrate urine, proteinuria, etc.)

Increased plasma renin concentration

PSEUDOALDOSTERONISM DUE TO INGESTION OF LICORICE (AMMONIUM GLYCYRRHIZATE)
Excessive ingestion causes hypertension due to sodium retention.

Decreased serum potassium

Decreased aldosterone excretion in urine

Decreased plasma renin activity

PHEOCHROMOCYTOMA

Blood and urine levels of norepinephrine and, to a lesser extent, epinephrine are increased, usually even when patient is asymptomatic and normotensive; rarely are increases found only following a paroxysm.

Urine VMA (vanilmandelic acid, a catecholamine metabolite) excretion is considerably increased. This determination is simpler than for catecholamines and therefore is more commonly used. Beware of false increase due to foods (e.g., vanilla, fruits, especially bananas, coffee, tea) and drugs (e.g., vasopressor agents) taken in prior 72 hours. (See p. 114.) Beware of nonspecific techniques for VMA assay that fail to detect 30% of cases of pheochromocytoma.

Hyperglycemia and glycosuria are found in half of patients during an attack.

Glucose tolerance test frequently shows a diabetic type of curve.

Elevated BMR (more than +20%) occurs in about half of these patients, but other thyroid function tests are normal.

Urine changes are secondary to sustained hypertension.

Up to 15% of pheochromocytomas are malignant; 15% are extra-adrenal; 10% are multiple. Family inheritance in 10–20% of patients. Extensive surgical exploration may be required. Rarely, this syndrome is due to hyperplasia of the adrenal medulla.

"Incidental" pheochromocytomas have been discovered.

Five percent of patients with pheochromocytoma have normal blood pressure most or all of the time.

Table 51. Laboratory Tests in Differential Diagnosis of Benign Pheochromocytoma and Neural Crest Tumors (Neuroblastoma, Ganglioneuroma)

Urinary Levels Of	Pheochromocytoma	Neural Crest Tumor (Neuroblastoma, Ganglioneuroma)
Catecholamines	I	I
VMA	I	I
Metanephrines	I	I
Dopamine	N*	I
HVA	N*	I

I = increased; N = normal.

*I in malignant pheochromocytoma

NEUROBLASTOMA, GANGLIONEUROMA, GANGLIOBLASTOMA

Urinary levels of catecholamines (norepinephrine, normetanephrine, dopamine, VMA, and HVA [homovanillic acid]) are increased. Excretion of epinephrine is not increased.

Not all methods include dopamine in measurement of total catecholamines.

Not all patients have increased urinary levels of catecholamines, VMA, and HVA.
  If only 1 of these substances is measured, only about 75% of cases are diagnosed.
  If VMA and HVA or VMA and total catecholamines are measured, 95–100% of cases are diagnosed.
These tests are also useful for differential diagnosis of Ewing's tumor versus metastatic neuroblastoma of bone and to show response to therapy (surgery, radiation, or chemotherapy), which should bring return to normal in 1–4 months. Continued elevation indicates need for further treatment.

Table 52. Laboratory Differentiation of Primary and Secondary Adrenal Insufficiency

Determination	Primary Adrenal Insufficiency	Adrenal Insufficiency Secondary to Hypopituitarism
After ACTH stimulation (see p. 330)		
Urinary 17-OH and 17-KS levels	No responsive increase	Marked "staircase" response
Eosinophil count (falls 80–90% daily in normal person)	Falls less than 20%	Fall depends on degree of insufficiency
Blood ACTH level	Increased	Decreased

ADDISON'S DISEASE
(chronic adrenal insufficiency)

Serum potassium is increased.
Serum sodium and chloride are decreased.
Sodium:potassium ratio is less than 30:1.
Blood volume is decreased; hematocrit level is increased (because of water loss).
BUN is increased.
Fasting hypoglycemia is present, with a flat oral glucose tolerance curve and insulin hypersensitivity. IV GTT shows a normal peak followed by severe prolonged hypoglycemia. Lymphocytosis, usually relative, is seen.
Eosinophilia is present (300/cu mm). (*A total eosinophil count of less than 50 is evidence against severe adrenal-cortical hypofunction.*)
Normocytic anemia is slight or moderate but difficult to estimate because of decreased blood volume.

Blood cortisol level is markedly decreased.
Urine 17-hydroxycorticoids are absent or markedly decreased.
Urine 17-ketosteroids are markedly decreased.
Urine 17-ketogenic steroids are markedly decreased.
See Table 52 for blood ACTH levels and response to ACTH stimulation of eosinophil count and of urinary steroids.
The Robinson-Power-Kepler water tolerance test used as a screening procedure for Addison's disease and the Cutler-Power-Wilder sodium chloride deprivation test have been replaced by the ACTH stimulation tests, which are more direct and more useful and avoid the risk of crisis which may be precipitated by the former tests.

WATERHOUSE-FRIDERICHSEN SYNDROME

This is an acute adrenal insufficiency with degenerative changes in adrenal cortex; patient often dies before progression to cortical hemorrhage.
Dehydration occurs.
Azotemia is due to dehydration and shock affecting renal function.
Serum sodium and chloride are decreased and potassium is increased in some cases.
Hypoglycemia occurs regularly.

LABORATORY TESTS FOR EVALUATION OF FUNCTION OF OVARY

Estrogens
Increased in
    Granulosa cell tumor of ovary
    Theca-cell tumor of ovary
    Luteoma of ovary
    Pregnancy
Decreased in
    Primary hypofunction of ovary
    Secondary hypofunction of ovary

Pregnanediol
Increased in
    Luteal cysts of ovary
    Arrhenoblastoma of ovary
Decreased in
    Amenorrhea
    Threatened abortion (sometimes)
    Fetal death
    Toxemia of pregnancy

Pituitary Gonadotropins
Increased in
    Primary hypogonadism
    Menopause
Decreased in
    Secondary hypogonadism

17-Ketosteroids
Increased in
    Virilizing ovarian tumors (e.g., adrenal rest tumor, granulosa

cell tumor, hilar cell tumor, Brenner tumor, and most frequently arrhenoblastoma); increased in about half of patients and normal in half of patients

Decreased in
Primary ovarian agenesis

OVARIAN TUMORS

Feminizing Ovarian Tumors (e.g., granulosa cell tumor, thecoma, luteoma)

Pap smear of vagina and endometrial biopsy show high estrogen effect and no progestational activity; no signs of ovulation during reproductive phase.

Urinary FSH is decreased (inhibited by increased estrogen).

Urine 17-KS and 17-OHKS are normal.

Pregnanediol is absent.

Masculinizing Ovarian Tumors (e.g., arrhenoblastoma, hilar cell tumors, adrenal rest tumors)

Pap smear of vagina shows decreased estrogen effect.

Endometrial biopsy shows moderate atrophy of endometrium.

Urine FSH (gonadotropins) are low.

Urine 17-KS are normal or may be slightly increased in arrhenoblastoma. They may be markedly increased in adrenal tumors of ovary ("masculinovoblastoma"). They may be moderately increased in Leydig cell tumors.

> *In arrhenoblastoma there may be an increase of androsterone, testosterone, etc., excreted in urine even though the 17-KS are not much increased.*
>
> *In adrenal cell tumors of ovary, laboratory findings may be the same as in hyperfunction of adrenal cortex with Cushing's syndrome, etc.*

BMR is normal.

In some cases there are no endocrine effects from these tumors.
Some cases of arrhenoblastoma with masculinization also show evidence of increased estrogen formation.

Struma Ovarii

About 5–10% of cases are hormone-producing. Classic findings of hyperthyroidism may occur. These tumors take up radioactive iodine. (*Simple follicle cysts may also take up radioactive iodine.*)

Primary Chorionepithelioma of Ovary

Urinary chorionic gonadotropins are markedly increased.

Estrogen and progesterone secretion may be much increased.

Nonfunctioning Ovarian Tumors

Only effect may be hypogonadism due to replacement of functioning ovarian parenchyma.

PRECOCIOUS PUBERTY IN GIRLS

Due To

Diseases of central nervous system (usually floor of the third ventricle) with involvement of the posterior hypothalamus (e.g.,

tuberculous meningitis, epidemic encephalitis, other inflammations, tumors, tuberous sclerosis—more frequent in boys)
Polyostotic fibrous dysplasia (Albright's syndrome)
Ovarian tumors
Teratomatous choriocarcinomas, granulosa cell tumors, theca-cell tumors, luteomas
Adrenal adenoma or carcinoma, which may secrete estrogen and be associated with feminization without virilization in rare cases.
Iatrogenic cause or accidental ingestion or inunction of estrogens.

LABORATORY FINDINGS

Pap smear of vagina indicates estrogen effect.
Pituitary gonadotropin is usually low, with ovarian and adrenal lesions.
Increased 17-KS and estrogen excretion (above normal adult level) occur, with feminizing adrenal tumors.
Chorionic gonadotropin titers are increased in choriocarcinoma. (*Not all choriocarcinomas produce gonadotropin.*)

STEIN-LEVENTHAL SYNDROME

Urinary androsterone, dehydroandrosterone, etiocholanolone, pregnanetriol, and 11-oxypregnanetriol are usually increased.
Urinary 17-KS are normal or slightly increased.
Urinary pregnanediol is normal.
Urinary gonadotropin is normal or slightly increased.
Dexamethasone administration does not decrease urinary 17-KS.
Chorionic gonadotropin administration increases urinary 17-KS.
Plasma testosterone is near upper limit of normal.

"CONSTITUTIONAL" HIRSUTISM IN WOMEN

With normal menses and fertility, urine 17-KS is normal.
With amenorrhea, hypomenorrhea, or oligomenorrhea, urine 17-KS may be slightly increased.

LABORATORY TESTS IN DIFFERENTIAL DIAGNOSIS OF PATIENTS WITH HIRSUTISM AND DIMINISHED MENSES

Urine 17-OHKS
Normal
Constitutional hirsutism
Stein-Leventhal syndrome
Mild adrenogenital syndrome
Masculinizing tumor of ovary
Increased
Cushing's syndrome

URINE 17-KS

Normal
Constitutional hirsutism
Stein-Leventhal syndrome
Masculinizing tumor of ovary
Cushing's syndrome

Slight increase
    Constitutional hirsutism
    Stein-Leventhal syndrome
    Mild adrenogenital syndrome
    Cushing's syndrome
Marked increase
    Masculinizing tumor of ovary
    Adrenogenital syndrome

Urine 17-KS Decreased by Daily Prednisone
Poor response
    Constitutional hirsutism
    Stein-Leventhal syndrome
    Masculinizing tumor of ovary
Good response
    Adrenogenital syndrome

Urine 17-KS Further Decreased by Daily Stilbestrol and Prednisone
No response
    Constitutional hirsutism
    Masculinizing tumor of ovary
    Adrenogenital syndrome
Response
    Stein-Leventhal syndrome (testosterone level also decreases)

TURNER'S SYNDROME (OVARIAN DYSGENESIS)

Barr chromatin inclusions are negative (male) in 80% of cases.
Chromosomal pattern: 45 chromosomes (monosomy X with XO; or, if XX, one X is abnormal; or XO mosaic)
Biopsy of ovary shows connective tissue stroma with rare follicular structure.
Vaginal smear and endometrial biopsy are atrophic.
17-KS and 17-OH are normal.
ACTH is normal.
FSH is increased.
BMR, PBI, T-3, etc., are usually normal.

About 50% of patients with primary amenorrhea have Turner's syndrome or sometimes testicular feminization.

TURNER'S SYNDROME IN THE MALE

Biopsy of testicle reveals dysgenetic tubules with few or no germ cells.
Chromosomal pattern: 46 chromosomes (XY pattern with very defective Y that is equivalent to XO)

MENOPAUSE (FEMALE CLIMACTERIC)

Urinary gonadotropin is increased.
Urinary estrogens are decreased.
Urinary 17-ketosteroids are decreased.
Plasma gonadotropin is increased.

Table 53. Laboratory Differentiation of Primary and Secondary (to Pituitary Defect) Hypogonadism

Determination	Primary Hypogonadism	Hypogonadism Secondary to Pituitary Defect
Level of FSH and gonadotropin in urine	High	Low
After administration of gonadotropins		
17-KS excretion	Does not increase	Increases
Clinical evidence of hypogonadism	Does not subside	Subsides with Increased sperm count
		Increased estrogenic effect in woman's Pap smear

SECONDARY OVARIAN INSUFFICIENCY

Urinary gonadotropin is decreased or absent.

CHIARI-FROMMEL SYNDROME

Patients with recent pregnancy show continuing amenorrhea and lactation with atrophy of uterus and ovaries with no recognizable cause.

Protein-bound iodine is decreased.
FSH and estrogen levels are decreased.

LABORATORY TESTS FOR EVALUATION OF FUNCTION OF TESTICLE

Chorionic Gonadotropins in Urine
Increased in
Choriocarcinoma
Seminoma

Pituitary Gonadotropins in Urine
Increased in
Primary hypogonadism
Decreased in
Secondary hypogonadism

17-Ketosteroids in Urine (indicative of adrenal rather than testicular status)
Increased in
Interstitial cell tumor
Decreased in
Primary hypogonadism
Secondary hypogonadism

Plasma Testosterone
Decreased in
Primary hypogonadism
Secondary hypogonadism

Semen Analysis
Sterile males usually show
  Volume of less than 3 ml
  Less than 20 million sperm/ml
  Less than 25% motility

Biopsy of Testicle
Evidence of atrophy in sterility study
Diagnosis of tumor

Normal spermatogenesis associated with normal endocrine findings in patient with aspermia and infertility suggests a mechanical obstruction to sperm transport that may be correctable.

Chromosome Analysis
Turner's syndrome (gonadal dysgenesis)—usually chromatin negative
Klinefelter's syndrome—chromatin positive
Pseudohermaphroditism—chromosomal sex corresponding to gonadal sex

GERMINAL APLASIA

Chromatin-negative buccal smears are normal.
Chromosomal pattern is normal.
Urinary gonadotropin is normal.
Urinary pituitary gonadotropin is increased.
17-KS are decreased.
There is azoospermia.
Biopsy of testicle shows that Sertoli's and Leydig's cells are intact and germinal cells are absent.

KLINEFELTER'S SYNDROME

Urinary gonadotropin level is elevated.
Biopsy of testicle shows atrophy, with hyalinized tubules lined only by Sertoli's cells, clumped Leydig's cells, and failure of spermatogenesis.
There is azoospermia.
About half of the patients have the chromatin-positive nuclear pattern seen in the female. (These have more marked testicular changes.)
Abnormal chromosomal pattern. XY males have an extra X; usually XXY; may have additional X, e.g., XXYY, XXXY, XXXXY.

LABORATORY STUDIES FOR AMBIGUOUS GENITALIA IN CHILDHOOD AND INFANCY

Determine sex chromatin pattern in buccal smears and urinary 17-KS excretion; biopsy of gonads may be indicated.
If buccal smear pattern positive (e.g., XX, XXY) and urinary 17-KS are normal, diagnosis may be
  Female pseudohermaphroditism, nonadrenal type
  True hermaphroditism
  Klinefelter's syndrome

If buccal smear pattern is positive and urinary 17-KS are increased, diagnosis may be

> Female pseudohermaphroditism (congenital adrenogenital or iatrogenic)
> True hermaphroditism
> Arrhenoblastoma, mother or fetus (rare)

If buccal smear pattern negative (e.g., XY, XO) and urinary 17-KS are normal, diagnosis may be

> Turner's syndrome
> Abdominal testes in male
> Feminizing testes (undescended)
> True hermaphroditism
> Absence of testes
> Male pseudohermaphroditism due to deficient testes

If buccal smear pattern is negative and urinary 17-KS are increased, diagnosis may be

> Male pseudohermaphroditism due to congenital lipoid adrenal hyperplasia (rare)

MALE CLIMACTERIC

Urinary gonadotropin level is elevated.

LABORATORY TESTS FOR EVALUATION OF FUNCTION OF PLACENTA

Chorionic Gonadotropins
Increased in
> Hydatidiform mole
> Chorionepithelioma

Decreased in
> Fetal death
> Nonpregnant state

Pregnanediol
Decreased in
> Toxemia of pregnancy
> Fetal death
> Threatened abortion (sometimes)

ACROMEGALY AND GIGANTISM
(usually due to eosinophilic adenoma of pituitary)

Serum growth hormone (measured by radioimmunoassay; still limited availability)

> Fasting level above 5 ng/ml in men is diagnostic of acromegaly; not diagnostic in women because of wide fluctuations in levels in acromegalic range.
> Most patients of both sexes show a fall of less than 50% during IV glucose tolerance test whereas normal subjects show almost complete suppression of growth hormone by induced hyperglycemia.

Glucose tolerance is impaired in most patients. Mild diabetes mellitus that is insulin-resistant is found in less than 15%.

Secretory activity of tumor is indicated by the following.

> Serum phosphorus is increased.
> Serum alkaline phosphatase may be increased.
> BMR is increased. (*PBI and RAIU are normal.*)
> Urine calcium is increased.
> Urine hydroxypyroline is increased.
> Biopsy of costochondral junction evidences active bone growth.
> Serum growth hormone level is increased (immunologic assay method is not generally available).
> IV ACTH administration may cause excessive increase in urine 17-KS but normal 17-OHKS excretion.

Adrenal virilism and increased urine 17-KS are common in women.

Urine 17-KS, ketogenic steroids, and pituitary gonadotropins are usually normal or may be slightly changed but not diagnostically useful.

Rare associated endocrinopathies are: hyperthyroidism, hyperparathyroidism, pheochromocytoma, insulinoma.

Complete blood count and ESR are normal.

In inactive cases, all secondary laboratory findings may be normal.

In late stage, panhypopituitarism may develop.

PITUITARY GROWTH HORMONE DEFICIENCY

There may be isolated deficiency with dwarfism or associated with TSH deficiency, with ACTH deficiency, or with TSH and ACTH deficiencies.

Serum growth hormone levels are decreased (measured by radioimmunoassay < 1.0 ng/ml) with no response 4 hours after oral glucose load and serum growth level < 10 ng/ml after IV insulin (0.1 unit/kg) is administered.

Decreased fasting blood sugar (less than 50 mg/100 ml) is frequent; responds to growth hormone therapy.

Unresponsiveness to insulin-induced hypoglycemia (blood sugar at 90 minutes is more than 15 mg/100 ml below the fasting level) occurs in about one-half of patients with isolated deficiency of growth hormone but almost all with combined ACTH and growth hormone deficiencies.

Serum phosphorus and alkaline phosphatase are decreased in prepubertal child but normal in adult-onset cases.

TSH deficiency (see Hypothyroidism, p. 318, and Table 46)

ACTH deficiency (see tests of adrenal function and adrenal-pituitary function, pp. 330, 331)

Gonadotropins are decreased or absent from urine in postpubertal patients (but increased levels occur in primary hypogonadism).

May Be Due To

Pituitary

> Congenital hypoplasia or absence, atrophy, fibrosis, cystic changes with calcification, etc.

Hypothalamus

> Progressive degenerative changes, which may cause multiple deficiency or isolated growth hormone deficiency types

Familial and genetic types

> Isolated growth hormone deficiency or multiple deficiency types

HYPOPITUITARISM

Due To
Pituitary necrosis secondary to postpartum hemorrhage (Sheehan's syndrome)
Craniopharyngioma, chromophobe adenoma, eosinophilic adenoma
Meningioma
Metastatic tumors (especially breast)
Granulomatous lesions (e.g., sarcoidosis, Hand-Schüller-Christian syndrome)
See sections on secondary insufficiency of gonads, thyroid, adrenals. All of these may be involved or only one (usually gonadal first).
See Diabetes Insipidus, next page.

ANOREXIA NERVOSA

BMR may be low.
PBI is usually normal.
Urine 17-KS and 17-OHKS may be low; in panhypopituitarism (Simmond's disease) these are practically absent.
Metyrapone administration shows limited pituitary ACTH reserve in about half of the patients; the rest show a normal response. Panhypopituitarism patients are unresponsive. This is a most useful procedure for distinguishing anorexia nervosa from panhypopituitarism.
Insulin tolerance test is the same as in panhypopituitarism.

DISEASES OF HYPOTHALAMUS

Due To
Neoplasms (primary or metastatic cancer; craniopharyngioma) (most frequent cause)
Inflammation (e.g., tuberculosis; encephalitis)
Trauma (e.g., basal skull fractures; gunshot wounds)
Intracranial xanthomatosis
Others

Manifestations
Sexual abnormalities are the most frequent manifestations of hypothalamic disease.
    Precocious puberty
    Hypogonadism (frequently as part of Fröhlich's syndrome)
Diabetes insipidus is a frequent but not an early manifestation of hypothalamic disease.

FRÖHLICH'S SYNDROME (ADIPOSOGENITAL DYSTROPHY)

Usually this is a transient functional disorder of the hypothalamus.
No deficiency of ACTH, TSH, or growth hormone is seen.
If there is thyroid or adrenal hypofunction, look for organic lesion, especially craniopharyngioma.

PRECOCIOUS PUBERTY IN BOYS

See Pineal Tumors (following section) and Diseases of Hypothalamus (above).

Precocious puberty occurs occasionally in boys with hepatoblastoma.

Urine contains chorionic gonadotropin-like substance.

There is secondary Leydig's cell hyperplasia.

PINEAL TUMORS

Boys: precocious puberty in 30%
Girls: delayed pubescence

Diabetes insipidus occurs occasionally.

DIABETES INSIPIDUS

Urine
> Low specific gravity (usually 1.004 or less) is found.
> Large volume (4–15 liters/24 hours) is characteristic.
> Urine does not become concentrated when fluids are withheld.
> There is no response to hypertonic NaCl IV (normal person shows decrease in urine volume during and after infusion).
> Vasopressin (Pitressin) injection decreases urine flow (does not cause decrease in nephrogenic diabetes insipidus), and specific gravity becomes normal.

Antidiuretic Response (increase in urine osmolality equal to, or more than, plasma with urine:serum ratio 1.0 or more) To Stimuli Listed Below	*Hypophyseal Diabetes Insipidus (vasopressin deficiency)*	*Nephrogenic Diabetes Insipidus (renal insensitivity to vasopressin)*	*Primary Polydipsia*
Dehydration for 8–12 hours	No response	No response	Response
Nicotine (smoke 2 cigarettes) during water diuresis	No response	No response	Response
3% NaCl given IV (10 ml/kg in 30 minutes) during water diuresis	No response	No response	Response
Administer vasopressin (25–50 mU IV or 2.5–5.0 U IM)	Response	No response	Response
Plasma vasopressin level in response to dehydration, nicotine, and 3% NaCl (see above)	Low to absent	Elevated	Elevated

INAPPROPRIATE SECRETION OF ANTIDIURETIC HORMONE

Decreased serum sodium and chloride
Normal serum potassium, CO_2, and BUN
Decreased serum osmolality
Increased urine osmolality

Increased ratio of urine:serum osmolality
Increased urine sodium
Responds to water restriction but not to administration of isotonic or even hypertonic saline
May be associated with
   Acute intermittent porphyria
   Brain tumor (primary or metastatic)
   Pneumonia
   Pulmonary tuberculosis
   Tuberculous meningitis
   Systemic neoplasms
   Others

NONENDOCRINE NEOPLASMS CAUSING ENDOCRINE SYNDROMES

Tumors secrete polypeptides that have hormonal activity.
Cushing's syndrome*
   Bronchogenic carcinoma and carcinoid
   Thymoma
   Hepatoma
   Carcinoma of ovary
   Also carcinoma of thyroid, pancreas, etc.
Hypoglycemia. Patients show variable sensitivity to tolbutamide.
   Not associated with decreased serum phosphorus as in insulin-induced hypoglycemia.
      Bronchogenic carcinoma
      Carcinoma of adrenal cortex (6%)
      Hepatoma (23%)
      Fibrosarcoma (most frequent)
Thyrotoxicosis. Signs and symptoms are rare, but PBI, RAIU, etc., are increased.
   Tumors of GI tract, hematopoietic, pulmonary, etc.
   Trophoblastic tumors in women
   Choriocarcinoma of testis
Precocious puberty in boys
   Hepatoma
Hypercalcemia simulating hyperparathyroidism†
   Renal carcinoma
   Squamous cell carcinoma of upper respiratory tract
   Carcinoma of breast (occurs in 15% of cases with bone metastases)
   Malignant lymphoma, etc.
See also Carcinoid Syndrome (next section), Precocious Puberty in Girls (p. 341), Precocious Puberty in Boys (p. 348), Secondary Polycythemia (pp. 266–267), Inappropriate Secretion of Antidiuretic Hormone (p. 350).

---

* Cushing's syndrome due to these neoplasms cannot be distinguished from Cushing's syndrome due to excessive pituitary secretion of ACTH by use of dexamethasone suppression test or metyrapone test.

† Serum calcium is up to 21 mg/100 ml; less marked increase with renal tumors. Serum phosphorus is decreased in more than half the patients. Alkaline phosphatase is frequently increased but not difficult to evaluate because of liver metastases. Serum proteins are not consistently abnormal. Urine calcium and phosphorus and renal tubular reabsorption of phosphate are not useful in differential diagnosis.

CARCINOID SYNDROME

The syndrome occurs in patients with malignant carcinoids (argentaffinomas).

Urinary level of 5-hydroxyindolacetic acid (5-HIAA) (a metabolite of serotonin) is increased, usually when tumor is far advanced (i.e., large liver metastases), but may not be increased despite massive metastases. Useful in confirming diagnosis in only 5–7% of patients with a carcinoid tumor.

Blood serotonin may be increased (more than 0.4 mg/ml).

VMA and catecholamines in urine are at normal levels.

Laboratory findings due to other aspects of carcinoid syndrome are noted (e.g., pulmonary valvular stenosis, tricuspid valvular insufficiency, heart failure, liver metastases, electrolyte disturbances).

MULTIPLE ENDOCRINE ADENOMAS (MEA SYNDROME)

	Wermer's Syndrome	*Sipple's Syndrome*
Characteristic neoplasms	Pituitary adenoma Islet cell adenoma or carcinoma Parathyroid adenoma or hyperplasia	Medullary thyroid carcinoma Pheochromocytoma Parathyroid adenoma or hyperplasia
Associated neoplasms	Adrenal cortical adenoma Renal cortical adenoma Thyroid carcinoma or hyperplasia Carcinoid Lipoma Gastric polyp Mediastinal endocrine neoplasm	Mucosal neuroma

33

Genitourinary Diseases

RENAL GLYCOSURIA
(glycosuria when serum glucose is less than 180 mg/100 ml)

Due to proximal tubular damage
    Fanconi syndrome
    Heavy-metal poisoning
    Nephrotic phase of glomerulonephritis
Due to increased glomerular filtration rate without tubular damage
    Pregnancy
Oral and IV glucose tolerance tests are normal.
Ketosis is absent.

RENAL DISEASES THAT MAY BE FOUND WITHOUT PROTEINURIA

Congenital abnormalities
Renal artery stenosis
Obstruction of GU tract
Pyelonephritis
Stone
Tumor
Polycystic kidneys
Hypokalemic nephropathy
Hypercalcemic nephropathy
Prerenal azotemia

PROTEINURIA PREDOMINANTLY GLOBULIN RATHER THAN ALBUMIN

Multiple myeloma
Macroglobulinemia
Primary amyloidosis
Adult Fanconi syndrome (some patients)

ORTHOSTATIC PROTEINURIA

First morning urine before arising shows high specific gravity but no
    protein.

Continued on page 356.

Table 54. Urinary Findings in Various Diseases

Disease	Volume	Specific Gravity	Protein*	RBC†	WBC and Epithelial Cells†	Casts‡	Comment
Normal	600–2500	1.003–1.030	0 (0.05 gm)	0–occ. (0–0.130)	0–0.65	0–occ. (2000/24 hrs)	
Acute febrile states	D	I	Trace to +			Few	
Orthostatic proteinuria	N	N	I (up 1 gm)	N (0–0.130)	0–3	V; H & G	Normal when recumbent; abnormalities after upright posture
Glomerulo-nephritis							
Acute	D	I	2–4+ (0.5–5)	1–4+ (1–1000)	1–400	2–4+; H & G; RBC, epithelial, mixed RBC & epithelial	Gross hematuria or "smoky" urine
Latent			(0.1–2)	(1–100)	1–20	RBC, H & G	
Nephrosis ("nephrotic stage")	D	I	4+ (4–40)	0–few (0.5–50)	20–1000	Epithelial, fatty, waxy; H & G	Fat-laden epithelial cells, anisotropic fat in epithelial cells and casts
Terminal	I or D	D; fixed	1–2+ (2–7)	Trace–1+ (0.5–10)	1–50	1–3+ Broad, waxy, H & G, epithelial	
Pyelonephritis							
Acute	N	N	0–2+ (0.5–2)	Few (0–1)	20–2000	WBC, H & G, bacteria	Bacteria, many WBC in clumps

Continued on next page

See footnotes on page 355.

[353]

Table 54 *(continued)*

Disease	Volume	Specific Gravity	Protein*	RBC†	WBC and Epithelial Cells†	Casts‡	Comment
Chronic	N or D	N or D	2–4+ (0–5)	Few (0–1)	0.5–50	Same as acute; often few or none	Same as acute; findings may be intermittent
Renal tuberculosis			(0.1–3)	(1–20)	1–50	WBC, H & G	Tubercle bacilli
Disseminated lupus erythematosus	V	N or D	1–4+ (0.5–20)	1–4+ (1–100)	1–100	1–4+ RBC, *fatty, waxy*; H & G	
Toxemia of pregnancy	D	I	3–4+ (0.5–10)	0–1+ (0–1)	1–5	3–4+ H & G	
Malignant hypertension	V	D; fixed	1–2+ (1–10)	Trace–1+ (1–100)	1–200	1–2+ H & G, RBC, fatty	Increasing uremia with minimal or marked proteinuria and hematuria
Benign hypertension	N or I	N or D	0–1+	0–trace (1–5)		0–1+ H & G	
Congestive heart failure	D	I	1–2+	0–1+		1+ H & G	
Intercapillary glomerulosclerosis (Kimmelstiel-Wilson syndrome)			1–4+ (2–20)	(0–1)	1–30	Epithelial, fatty, H & G	Frequently associated: pyelonephritis and nephrosclerosis

Lower nephron
nephrosis

Acute	D		1–4+	1–4+	RBC; *H & G,* epithelial
Diuretic	I	0.5–10.0	(0–1)	1–100	Broad, waxy, epithelial, **H & G**

D = decreased; I = increased; occ. = occasional; V = variable; N = normal; H & G = hyaline and granular casts.
Cast requires examination of fresh or preserved urine and acid pH.
* Protein = quantitative values in ( ) given as gm/24 hours.
† = quantitative values given as cells × 10⁶/24 hours.
‡ Italics denote most important or diagnostic finding.

Orthostatic proteinuria (*continued*)

Urine after arising may contain protein up to 3 gm/L but usually less than 1 gm/day.

Urine microscopy is normal.

Orthostatic proteinuria is usually considered benign, but some patients show pathologic changes on renal biopsy and ultimately manifest chronic renal disease.

RENAL TUBULAR ACIDOSIS IN ADULTS

Especially Proximal Tubule Due to

Multiple myeloma with Bence Jones proteinuria

Wilson's disease; other heavy-metal intoxication

Drugs—toxic effects (e.g., due to sulfonamides, degraded tetracycline, amphotericin B)

Rejection of renal transplant

Fanconi syndrome (not due to other causes)

Especially Distal Tubule Due to

Due to increased serum globulins (especially gamma) (e.g., SLE, Sjögren's syndrome, Hodgkin's disease, sarcoidosis, chronic active hepatitis, cryoglobulinemia)

Potassium depletion nephropathy

Pyelonephritis

Medullary sponge kidney

Ureterosigmoidostomy

Primary (may be hereditary)

ACUTE RENAL FAILURE

Early Stage

Urine is scant in volume (often less than 50 ml/day) for up to 2 weeks; anuria for more than 24 hours is unusual. Urine is usually bloody (because RBCs and protein are present specific gravity may be high). Sodium concentration is usually more than 50 mEq/L.

WBC is increased even without infection.

BUN rises as much as 20 mg/100 ml/day in transfusion reaction. It rises as much as 50 mg/100 ml/day in overwhelming infection or severe crushing injuries.

Disproportionately increased serum phosphorus and creatinine indicates tissue necrosis.

Serum amylase and lipase may be increased without evidence of pancreatitis.

Metabolic acidosis is present.

Second Week

Urine becomes clear several days after onset of acute renal failure, and there is a small daily increase in volume. Daily volume of 400 ml indicates onset of tubular recovery. Daily volume of 1000 ml occurs in several days or up to 2 weeks. RBCs and large hematin casts are present. Protein is slight or absent.

Azotemia increases. BUN continues to rise for several days after onset of diuresis.

Metabolic acidosis increases.

Serum potassium is increased (because of tissue injury, failure of urinary excretion, acidosis, dehydration, etc.). EKG changes are always found when serum potassium is more than 9 mEq/L but are rarely found when it is less than 7 mEq/L.

Serum sodium is often decreased, with increased extracellular fluid volume.
Anemia usually appears during second week.
Bleeding tendency is frequent, with decreased platelets, abnormal prothrombin consumption, etc.

Diuretic Stage
Large urinary potassium excretion may cause decreased serum potassium level.
Urine sodium concentration is 50–75 mEq/L.
Serum sodium and chloride may increase on account of dehydration from large diuresis if replacement of water is inadequate.
Azotemia disappears 1–3 weeks after onset of diuresis.

Later Findings
Anemia may persist for weeks or months.
Pyelonephritis may first occur during this stage.
Renal blood flow and glomerular filtration rate do not usually become completely normal.
Recovery from renal cortical necrosis complicating pregnancy may be followed by renal calcification, contracted kidneys, and death from malignant hypertension in 1–2 years.

If there is complete anuria for more than 48 hours, suspect urinary tract obstruction, bilateral renal vascular thrombi or emboli, cortical necrosis, or acute glomerulonephritis.
Suspect cortical necrosis if proteinuria is more than 3–4 gm/L, BUN does not fall, and diuresis does not occur.
Suspect urinary tract obstruction if recurrent oliguria and increasing azotemia occur during period of diuresis.

Due To
Renal parenchymal damage (usually tubular injury)
  Poisons (e.g., carbon tetrachloride, toluene, phosphorus, mercury bichloride)
  Intravascular hemolysis
  Necrotizing pyelonephritis
  Polyarteritis
  Hypersensitivity reaction (e.g., penicillin)
Decreased renal blood flow with ischemia ("lower nephron nephrosis")
  Shock due to various causes
  Renal vascular occlusion
Renal outflow obstruction
  Precipitation of sulfonamides
  Mechanical obstruction (cancer, calculi, ligation, etc.)
Often, combined mechanisms, e.g., crushing injury with myoglobinemia plus shock, shock plus intravascular hemolysis from transfusion reaction or bacteremia or infusion of distilled water during prostatectomy

Indications for Artificial Dialysis in Acute Renal Failure
Uncontrollable hyperkalemia
Increasing acidosis in which congestive heart failure contraindicates sodium administration
Simplified treatment of oliguria in presence of severe infection, tissue damage, etc.

CHRONIC RENAL INSUFFICIENCY

BUN and serum creatinine are increased and renal function tests impaired (see p. 25).

Loss of renal concentrating ability (nocturia, polyuria, polydipsia) is an early manifestation of progressive renal functional impairment. Specific gravity is usually same as that of glomerular filtrate.

Hypotonic urine unresponsive to vasopressin may occur in
> Obstructive uropathy
> Chronic pyelonephritis
> Nephrocalcinosis
> Amyloidosis
> Familial nephrogenic diabetes insipidus.

Serum sodium is decreased (because of tubular damage with loss in urine, vomiting, diarrhea, diet restriction, etc.). The decrease is indicated by increased urine sodium levels (more than 5–10 mEq sodium/L). It may occur in any renal disease, especially when polyuria is marked, but is more common with obstructive uropathy, chronic pyelonephritis, and interstitial nephritis than with chronic glomerulonephritis.

Serum potassium is increased (on account of dietary sodium restriction and increased potassium ingestion, acidosis, oliguria, tissue breakdown). Decreased serum potassium with increased loss in urine (more than 15–20 mEq/L) occurs in primary aldosteronism. It may occur in malignant hypertension, tubular acidosis, Fanconi syndrome, nephrocalcinosis, diuresis during recovery from tubular necrosis.

Acidosis (due to renal failure to secrete acid as NH_4^+ and to reabsorb filtered bicarbonate) is present.

Serum calcium is decreased (because of decreased serum albumin, increased serum phosphorus, decreased calcium absorption in intestine, etc.). Tetany is rare. Secondary parathyroid hyperplasia may occur, but hypercalcemia is not found.

Serum phosphorus increases when creatinine clearance falls to about 25 ml/minute.

Serum alkaline phosphatase may be normal or may be increased with renal osteodystrophy.

Serum magnesium increases when glomerular filtration rate falls below 30 ml/minute.

Increase in serum uric acid is usually less than 10 mg/100 ml. Secondary gout is rare. If clinical gout is present, plus family history of gout, or serum uric acid level is more than 10 mg/100 ml, rule out primary gout nephropathy.

Blood organic acids, phenols, indoles, certain amino acids, etc., are increased.

Normochromic normocytic anemia is usually proportionate to the degree of azotemia.

Bleeding tendency is evident. There may be decreased platelets, increased capillary fragility, abnormal TGT and prothrombin consumption (possible platelet defect), normal bleeding and clotting time.

Gastrointestinal hemorrhage from ulcers anywhere in GI tract may be severe.

Laboratory findings due to uremic pericarditis, pleuritis, and pancreatitis are noted. (BUN is usually more than 100 mg/100 ml.)

Serum albumin and total protein are decreased. *When there is edema without hypoproteinemia or heart failure, rule out acute glomerulo-*

nephritis, toxemia of pregnancy, excess fluid intake in oliguria during acute tubular necrosis or terminal renal failure.

Due to   (see appropriate separate sections)

Primary renal disease
  Vascular lesions
    Nephrosclerosis, benign or malignant
    Renal artery stenosis or thrombosis
    Renal vein thrombosis
    Acute ischemic tubular necrosis, renal cortical necrosis
  Glomerular lesions—glomerulonephritis
  Tubular or interstitial lesions
    Infectious—chronic pyelonephritis, tuberculosis
    Others
      Fanconi syndrome and renal tubular acidosis
      Heavy-metal poisoning
      Analgesic abuse
      Radiation nephritis
      Chronic interstitial nephritis
  Congenital
    Polycystic disease
    Congenital hypoplastic kidneys
Systemic diseases involving the kidney
  Collagen diseases
    Systemic lupus erythematosus
    Polyarteritis nodosa
    Scleroderma
    Subacute bacterial endocarditis
    Goodpasture's syndrome
    Allergic purpura, etc.
  Metabolic diseases
    Diabetes mellitus
    Gout
    Amyloidosis
    Hypercalcemic nephropathy
    Hypokalemic nephropathy
  Urinary tract obstruction
    Neoplasms (e.g., carcinoma of cervix)
    Calculi
    Retroperitoneal fibrosis
    Prostatic enlargement
    Urethral stricture
    Congenital urethral or bladder defects
  Other
    Multiple myeloma
    Sickle cell anemia
    Hemoglobinurias (e.g., paroxysmal nocturnal)

POSTSTREPTOCOCCAL ACUTE GLOMERULONEPHRITIS IN CHILDREN

Evidence of infection with Group A beta-hemolytic streptococcus by
  Culture of throat
  Serologic findings indicative of recent streptococcal infection

Antistreptolysin O (ASO) titers of more than 250 Todd
units (increased in 80% of patients)
Antihyaluronidase
Antistreptokinase
Antidesoxyribonuclease-beta
Antidiphosphopyridine-nucleotidase
Antinicotinamide-adeninedenucleotidase, etc.

Urine

Hematuria—gross or only microscopic. Microscopic hematuria
may occur during the initial febrile upper respiratory infection (URI) and then reappear with nephritis in 1–2 weeks. It
lasts 2–12 months; usual duration is 2 months.
RBC casts show glomerular origin of hematuria.
WBC casts and WBCs show inflammatory nature of lesion.
Granular and epithelial cell casts are present.
Fatty casts and lipid droplets occur several weeks later; not
related to hyperlipemia.
Proteinuria is usually less than 2 gm/day (but may be up to 6–8
gm/day). May disappear while RBC casts and RBCs still
occur.
Oliguria is frequent.

Azotemia is found in about 50% of patients.
Glomerular filtration rate usually shows greater decrease than renal
blood flow; therefore filtration factor is decreased.
PSP excretion is normal in cases of mild to moderate severity;
increases with progression of disease.
ESR is increased.
Leukocytosis is present, with increased polynuclear neutrophils.
There is mild anemia, especially when edema is present (may be due
to hemodilution, bone marrow depression, or increased destruc-
tion of RBCs).
Serum proteins are normal or there is nonspecific decrease of
albumin and increase of alpha$_2$ and sometimes of beta and gamma
globulin.
Serum cholesterol may be increased.
Serum complement falls 24 hours before onset of hematuria and
rises to normal when hematuria subsides.
Antihuman kidney antibodies are present in serum in 50% of
patients.
Decreased urinary aldosterone occurs in the presence of edema.

*Azotemia with high urine specific gravity and normal PSP excretion
usually means acute glomerulonephritis.*

Clinical Course

Patients usually recover in 2–4 weeks; 10% die within a few months.
A second attack is unusual after repeated urinalysis is normal.
Marked proteinuria for more than 4 months suggests poor prognosis.
Acute nephritis in Schönlein-Henoch anaphylactoid purpura has a
poorer initial prognosis and more often becomes chronic.
Acute glomerulonephritis in adults causes death or becomes chronic
in one-quarter to one-half of patients. There may be a long latent
period with only proteinuria and abnormal microscopical urinary
findings.

NEPHROTIC SYNDROME

Characterized By
Marked proteinuria—usually > 4.5 gm/day

Decreased serum albumin—usually < 2.5 gm/100 ml

Increased serum cholesterol (free and esters)—usually > 350 mg/100 ml (Low or normal serum cholesterol occurs with poor nutrition and suggests poor prognosis.)

Increased serum phospholipids, neutral fats, triglycerides, low-density β-lipoproteins, and total lipids

Urine containing doubly refractive fat bodies as seen by polarizing microscopy; many granular and epithelial cell casts

Hematuria—may be present but not part of syndrome

Azotemia—may be present but not part of syndrome

Changes secondary to proteinuria and hypoalbuminemia (e.g., decreased PBI, decreased serum calcium, decreased serum ceruloplasmin, increased fibrinogen)

Increased ESR due to increased fibrinogen

Changes due to primary disease (see below)

Etiology
Renal
>Glomerulonephritis ($> 50\%$ of cases)
>Lipoid nephrosis (10% of cases)

Systemic
>Systemic lupus erythematosus (20% of cases)
>Amyloidosis
>Myeloma
>Diabetic glomerulosclerosis (15% of cases)

Venous obstruction
>Renal vein thrombosis
>Obstruction of inferior vena cava (thrombosis, tumor)
>Constrictive pericarditis
>Tricuspid stenosis
>Congestive heart failure

Infections (e.g., subacute bacterial endocarditis)

Allergic (e.g., serum sickness)

Toxic (e.g., heavy metal)

CHRONIC GLOMERULONEPHRITIS

Various Clinical Courses
Early death after marked proteinuria, hematuria, oliguria, progressive increasing uremia, anemia

Intermittent or continuous or incidental proteinuria, hematuria with slight or absent azotemia, and normal renal function tests (may develop into late renal failure or may subside)

Exacerbation of chronic nephritis (with accentuation of proteinuria, hematuria, and decreased renal function) shortly following streptococcal URI

Nephrotic syndrome (see preceding section)

Compared to pyelonephritis, chronic glomerulonephritis shows lipid droplets and epithelial and RBC casts in urine, more marked

proteinuria (more than 2–3 gm/day), poorer prognosis for equivalent amount of azotemia.

NEPHROSCLEROSIS

"Benign" nephrosclerosis ("essential hypertension")
    Urine contains little or no protein or microscopical abnormalities.
    Ten percent of patients develop marked renal insufficiency.
"Accelerated" nephrosclerosis ("malignant hypertension")
    Syndrome may occur in the course of "benign" nephrosclerosis, glomerulonephritis, unilateral renal artery occlusion, or any cause of hypertension.
    Increasing uremia is associated with minimal or marked proteinuria and hematuria.

URINARY STONES
(autopsy incidence = 1.12%; cause of death = 0.38%)

Calcium is present in 90% of stones in patients in North America.
    Increased urinary calcium in 35% of stone-forming patients (30% of these have hyperparathyroidism)
        20–30% have
            Bone diseases
                Destructive (e.g., metastatic tumor)
                Osteoporosis (e.g., immobilization, Paget's disease, Cushing's syndrome)
            Milk-alkali syndrome
            Hypervitaminosis D
            Sarcoidosis
            Etc.
        50–60% have
            Idiopathic hypercalciuria—usually bilateral and occurring in males
            Usually urine pH above 6.0
Oxalate is present in 30% of renal stones (diet, urine pH, infection are not relevant in normal individuals).
    Familial oxalate stone formers (normal or increased urinary oxalate)
    Oxalosis (increased urinary oxalate; many stones)
Cystine stones form when more than 300 mg/day is present in urine in congenital familial cystinuria. Urine shows cystine crystals.
    Positive cyanide-nitroprusside test
Uric acid is present in 10% of stones.
    Gout—15% of patients with gout have stones.
    Urine is more acid than normal (e.g., patients with chronic diarrhea, ileostomy).
    More than half of patients with urate calculi have normal serum and urine uric acid levels.
Xanthine is present in children with inborn error of metabolism.
Hereditary glycinuria is a rare familial disorder associated with renal calculi.
Microscopic hematuria is found in 80% of cases.
In renal colic, hematuria and proteinuria are present, and there is an increased WBC due to associated infection.

OBSTRUCTIVE UROPATHY
(unilateral or bilateral; partial or complete)

Partial obstruction of both kidneys may cause increasing azotemia with normal or increased urinary output (due to decreased renal concentrating ability).

Partial obstruction may cause inexplicable wide variations in BUN and urine volume in patients with azotemia. PSP excretion is less in first 15-minute period than in any later period. There is considerable PSP excretion after the 2-hour test period.

In unilateral obstruction, BUN usually remains normal unless previous renal disease is present.

Laboratory findings due to superimposed infection or underlying disease are noted.

Laboratory findings due to underlying disease

> Obstruction of bladder, e.g., benign prostatic hypertrophy, carcinoma of prostate or bladder, urethral stricture, neurogenic bladder dysfunction (multiple sclerosis, diabetic neuropathy, etc.)
>
> Obstruction of both ureters, e.g., infiltrating neoplasm (especially of uterine cervix), bilateral calculi, congenital anomalies, retroperitoneal fibrosis

If ureter is obstructed more than 4 months, functional recovery is unlikely. When obstruction is relieved, most functional recovery takes place in 2–3 weeks; then there is continued improvement for several months.

PYELONEPHRITIS

Bacteriuria (see p. 106). Colony count of over 100,000/ml of urine (properly collected) indicates active infection. If the count is 10,000 to 100,000/ml it should be repeated. Bacteria seen on gram stain of uncentrifuged urine indicates bacteriuria.

A culture should be performed for identification of the specific organism and determination of antibiotic sensitivity.

Microscopical examination of urine sediment. WBC casts are very suggestive of pyelonephritis. Glitter cells are evident.

Pyuria is present in only 50% of cases of chronic urinary tract infection and asymptomatic bacteriuria. Bacteriuria and pyuria are often intermittent; in the chronic atrophic stage of pyelonephritis, they are often absent.

Urine concentrating ability is decreased relatively early in chronic infection compared to other renal diseases.

Albuminuria is usually less than 2 gm/24 hours (up to 2+ qualitative) and therefore helps to differentiate pyelonephritis from glomerular disease, in which albuminuria is usually more than 2 gm/24 hours. Albuminuria may be undetectable in a very dilute urine associated with fixed specific gravity.

There is a decrease in 24-hour creatinine clearance before rise in BUN and blood creatinine takes place.

Hyperchloremic acidosis (due to impaired renal acid excretion and bicarbonate reabsorption) occurs more often in chronic pyelonephritis than in glomerulonephritis.

Renal blood flow and glomerular filtration show parallel decrease proportional to progress of renal disease. Comparison of function in right and left kidneys shows more disparity in pyelonephritis than in diffuse renal disease (e.g., nephrosclerosis, glomerulone-phritis).

Fluctuation in renal insufficiency (e.g., due to recurrent infection, dehydration) with considerable recovery is more marked and frequent in pyelonephritis than in other renal diseases.

Laboratory findings of associated diseases, e.g., diabetes mellitus, urinary tract obstruction (stone, tumor, etc.), neurogenic bladder dysfunction, are present.

Laboratory findings due to sequelae (e.g., papillary necrosis, bacter-emia) are present.

When urine cultures are persistently negative in the presence of other evidence of pyelonephritis, specific search should be made for tubercle bacilli (e.g., culture, guinea pig inoculation).

PAPILLARY NECROSIS OF KIDNEY

Findings of associated diseases
      Diabetes mellitus
      Urinary tract infection
      Chronic overuse of phenacetin
Sudden diminution in renal function; occasionally oliguria or anuria with acute renal failure
Hematuria

RENAL ABSCESS
(due to metastatic infection not related to previous renal disease)

Urine
      Trace of albumin
      Few RBCs (may have transient gross hematuria at onset)
      No WBCs
      Very many gram-positive cocci in stained sediment
WBC high (may be more than 30,000/cu mm)

Complications
Sudden rupture into renal pelvis—urine suddenly cloudy and con-tains very many WBCs and bacteria
Renal carbuncle formation
Rupture into perirenal space
Secondary pyelonephritis

PERINEPHRIC ABSCESS

Laboratory findings due to underlying or primary diseases (see above)
      Hematogenous from distant foci (e.g., furuncles, tonsillitis) usually due to staphylococci and occasionally streptococci
      Direct extension from kidney infection (e.g., pyelonephritis, pyonephrosis) due to gram-negative rods and occasionally tubercle bacilli
      Infected perirenal hematoma (e.g., due to trauma, tumor, polyarteritis nodosa) due to various organisms
Urine changes due to underlying disease
      Urine may be normal and sterile. (*Do acid-fast smear and culture for tubercle bacilli.*)
Increased polynuclear leukocytes

Increased ESR
Positive blood culture (sometimes)

RENAL TUBERCULOSIS

Should be ruled out when there is unexplained albuminuria, pyuria, microhematuria; especially in presence of TB elsewhere
Urine culture for TB
Guinea pig inoculation

See Table 54, pp. 353–355.
See Tuberculosis, pp. 390–391, for general findings.

HORSESHOE KIDNEYS

Laboratory findings due to complications
     Calculi
     Pyelonephritis
     Hematuria

POLYCYSTIC KIDNEYS

Polyuria is common.
Hematuria may be gross and episodic or an incidental microscopical finding.
Proteinuria may be an incidental finding of routine analysis.
Renal calculi may be associated.
Superimposed pyelonephritis is frequent.
Death occurs within 5 years after BUN rises to 50 mg/100 ml.
Death usually occurs in early infancy, or in middle age when superimposed nephrosclerosis of aging or pyelonephritis has exhausted renal reserve.
Cerebral hemorrhage causes death in 10% of patients; intracranial berry aneurysms are frequently associated.

MEDULLARY CYSTIC DISEASE

Anemia
Polyuria
Salt-losing syndrome
Death from renal insufficiency (may take many years)

Urinalysis shows minimal or no proteinuria; presence of RBCs, WBCs, casts, or bacteria is rare. Specific gravity may be decreased.
Serum alkaline phosphatase may be increased when bone changes occur.

SPONGE KIDNEY

Findings due to complications
     Hematuria
     Infection
     Calculi within cysts
Disease asymptomatic, not progressive

HEREDITARY NEPHRITIS

May be classified into two types
1. Angiokeratoma corporis diffusum (familial deposition of abnormal glycolipid deposition in glomerular epithelial cells, nervous system, heart, etc.)
    Proteinuria begins in second decade.
    Urine may contain lipid globules and foam cells.
    Uremia occurs by fourth or fifth decade.
2. Familial autosomal dominant disease associated with nerve deafness and lens defects
    Hematuria, gross or microscopic, is common; more marked after occurrence of unrelated infection.

ARTERIAL INFARCTION OF KIDNEY

Microscopic or gross hematuria is usual.
BUN is normal unless other renal disease is present.
In some cases, urine shows no albumin or abnormal sediment at time of analysis.
WBC, SGOT, SGPT are increased if area of infarction is large; peak by second day; return to normal by fifth day.
Serum and urine LDH may be increased markedly.
CRP and serum LDH peak on third day; return to normal by tenth day.
Changes in serum enzyme levels, WBC, CRP, ESR are similar in time changes to those in myocardial infarction.
Plasma renin activity may rise on second day, peak about 11th day and remain elevated for more than a month.

RENAL VEIN THROMBOSIS

Hematuria
Proteinuria
Oliguria and uremic death if bilateral
Laboratory findings due to underlying causative condition (e.g., hypernephroma, metastatic cancer, trauma, polyarteritis, papillary necrosis, amyloidosis)
See Nephrotic Syndrome, p. 361.

RENAL CHANGES IN BACTERIAL ENDOCARDITIS

There are three types of pathologic changes: diffuse subacute glomerulonephritis; focal embolic glomerulonephritis; microscopic or gross infarcts of kidney.
Laboratory findings due to bacterial endocarditis are noted (see p. 150).
Albuminuria is almost invariably present even when no renal lesions are found.
Hematuria (usually microscopic, sometimes gross) is usual at some stage of the disease, but repeated examinations may be required.
Renal insufficiency is frequent (15% of cases during active stage; 40% of fatal cases).
    BUN is increased—usually 25–75 mg/100 ml.
    Renal concentrating ability is decreased.

KIDNEY IN GOUT

Urate calculi occur in 15% of patients with gout; may occur in absence of arthritis.

Early renal damage is indicated by decreased renal concentrating ability, mild proteinuria, and decreased PSP excretion.

Later renal damage is shown by slowly progressive azotemia with slight albuminuria and slight or no abnormalities of urine sediment.

Arteriolar nephrosclerosis and pyelonephritis are usually associated.

Renal disease causes death in up to one-half of patients with gout.

KIMMELSTIEL-WILSON SYNDROME (DIABETIC INTERCAPILLARY GLOMERULOSCLEROSIS)

The disease usually occurs after associated diabetes mellitus has been present more than 10 years; it is not related to control of diabetes. Occasionally it is associated only with prediabetes.

Proteinuria is usual (may be earliest clinical clue) and may be marked (often more than 5 gm/day). Nephrotic syndrome is often associated.

Urine shows many hyaline and granular casts and double refractile fat bodies. Hematuria is rare.

Serum protein is decreased.

Azotemia develops gradually after several years of proteinuria.

Biopsy of kidney is diagnostic.

Laboratory findings are those due to frequently associated infections of the urinary tract.

See sections on diabetes mellitus, acidosis, papillary necrosis, urinary tract infection, diabetic neuropathy.

RENAL DISEASE IN POLYARTERITIS NODOSA

Renal involvement occurs in three-fourths of patients.

Azotemia is often absent or only mild and slowly progressive.

Albuminuria is always present.

Hematuria (gross or microscopic) is very common. Fat bodies are frequently present in urine sediment.

There may be findings of acute glomerulonephritis with remission or early death from renal failure.

Always rule out polyarteritis in any case of glomerulonephritis, renal failure, or hypertension that shows unexplained eosinophilia, increased WBC, or laboratory evidence of involvement of other organ systems.

NEPHRITIS OF SYSTEMIC LUPUS ERYTHEMATOSUS (SLE)

Renal involvement occurs in two-thirds of patients with SLE.

Nephritis of SLE may occur as acute, latent, or chronic glomerulonephritis, nephrosis, or asymptomatic albuminuria.

Urine findings are as in chronic active glomerulonephritis.

Azotemia or marked proteinuria usually indicates death in 1–3 years.

Signs of lupus (e.g., positive LE test) may disappear during active nephritis, nephrosis, or uremia.

RENAL DISEASE IN SCLERODERMA

Renal involvement occurs in two-thirds of patients; one-third die of renal failure.

Proteinuria may be minimal and is usually less than 2 gm/day; this may be the only finding for a long time.

Azotemia usually signals death within a few months.

Terminal oligura or anuria may occur.

TOXEMIA OF PREGNANCY

Proteinuria varies from a trace to very marked (up to 800 mg/100 ml, equivalent to 15–20 gm/day). More than 15 mg/100 ml may indicate early toxemia.

RBCs and RBC casts are not abundant; hyaline and granular casts are present.

BUN, renal concentrating ability, and PSP excretion are normal unless the disease is severe or there is a prior renal lesion. (*BUN usually decreases during normal pregnancy because of increase in glomerular filtration rate.*)

Serum uric acid is increased (decreased renal clearance of urate) in 70% of patients in absence of treatment with thiazides which can produce hyperuricemia independent of any disease.

Serum total protein and albumin commonly are markedly decreased.

There may be multiple clotting deficiencies in severe cases.

Biopsy of kidney can establish diagnosis; rules out primary renal disease or hypertensive vascular disease.

GFR and renal plasma flow are 10–30% less than in normal pregnancy but may appear normal, increased, or decreased compared to rates in nonpregnant women. (Normally GFR increases gradually to a maximum of 40% more than nonpregnant level by 32d week, then decreases slightly until term. Renal plasma flow is not so markedly increased. Therefore the filtration fraction—ratio of GFR:RPF—increases slightly.)

Tubular reabsorption of sodium, water, urea, and uric acid is increased (perhaps on account of decreased GFR). Sodium excretion is decreased up to 35%

Beware of associated or underlying conditions: *hydatidiform mole, twin pregnancy, prior renal disease.*

KIDNEY IN MULTIPLE MYELOMA

Renal function is impaired in more than half the patients: usually loss of renal concentrating ability and azotemia.

Proteinuria is very frequent and is due to albumin and globulins in urine; Bence Jones proteinuria may be intermittent.

There is severe anemia out of proportion to azotemia.

Occasional changes due to altered renal tubular function are the following:

> Renal glycosuria, aminoaciduria, decreased serum uric acid, renal potassium wasting
>
> Renal loss of phosphate with decreased serum phosphorus and increased alkaline phosphatase
>
> Nephrogenic diabetes insipidus
>
> Oliguria or anuria with acute renal failure precipitated by dehydration

Changes due to associated amyloidosis are found; see p. 433.
Changes due to associated hypercalcemia are found.
See Multiple Myeloma, pp. 274–275.

PRIMARY OR SECONDARY AMYLOIDOSIS OF KIDNEY

Variation is from mild proteinuria with or without hematuria up to severe proteinuria with nephrotic syndrome.
Vasopressin-resistant polyuria is present if the medulla alone is involved (rare).
See Amyloidosis, p. 433.

SICKLE CELL NEPHROPATHY

Gross and microscopic hematuria is common.
Early decrease of renal concentrating ability is evident even with normal BUN, glomerular filtration rate, and renal plasma flow; it occurs in sickle cell trait as well as disease. The decrease is temporarily reversed by transfusion in children but not in adults.

HYPERCALCEMIC NEPHROPATHY

Diffuse nephrocalcinosis is the result of prolonged increase in serum and urine calcium (due to hyperparathyroidism, sarcoidosis, vitamin D intoxication, multiple myeloma, carcinomatosis, milk-alkali syndrome, etc.).
Urine is normal or contains RBC, WBC, WBC casts; proteinuria is usually slight or absent.
Early findings are decreased renal concentrating ability and polyuria.
Later findings are decreased glomerular filtration rate, decreased renal blood flow, azotemia.
Renal insufficiency is insidious and slowly progressive; it may sometimes be reversed by correcting hypercalcemia.
See various primary causative diseases.

RADIATION NEPHRITIS

Latent period is more than 6 months.
Slight proteinuria is present.
Hematuria and oliguria are absent.
Refractory anemia is present.
Progressive uremia is found; may be reversible later.

LABORATORY CRITERIA FOR KIDNEY TRANSPLANTATION

Donor: Three successive urinalyses and cultures must be negative.
Donor and recipient must show
    ABO and Rh blood group compatibility
    Leukoagglutinin compatibility
    Platelet agglutinin compatibility

LABORATORY FINDINGS OF KIDNEY TRANSPLANT REJECTION

Total urine output is decreased.
Proteinuria is increased.
Cellular or granular casts appear.
Urine osmolality is decreased.
Blood urea nitrogen rises.
Hyperchloremic renal tubular acidosis may be an early sign of rejection or indicate smoldering rejection activity.
Renal clearance values decrease.
Sodium iodohippurate ^{131}I renogram is altered.
Biopsy of kidney shows a characteristic microscopic appearance.

LEUKOPLAKIA OF RENAL PELVIS

Cell block of urine shows keratin or keratinized squamous cells.

CARCINOMA OF RENAL PELVIS AND URETER

Hematuria is present.
Renal calculi are associated.
Urinary tract infection is associated.
Cytologic examination of urinary sediment for malignant cells is necessary.

HYPERNEPHROMA OF KIDNEY

Even in the absence of the classic loin pain, flank mass, and hematuria, hypernephroma should be ruled out in the presence of these *unexplained* laboratory findings:
>Abnormal liver function tests (in absence of metastases to liver).
>>E.g., increased serum alkaline phosphatase, thymol turbidity, prolonged prothrombin time, retention of BSP, altered serum protein values (decreased albumin, increased alpha$_2$ globulin)
>Occurs in 40% of these patients
>Hypercalcemia
>Polycythemia
>Leukemoid reaction
>Refractory anemia and increased ESR
>Amyloidosis
>Cushing's syndrome
>Salt-losing syndrome

For laboratory assistance in diagnosis
>Exfoliative cytology of urine for tumor cells
>Increased urine LDH level
>Radioisotope scan of kidney

Needle biopsy is not recommended.

RENIN-PRODUCING RENAL TUMORS
(hemangiopericytomas of juxtaglomerular apparatus)

Plasma renin activity is increased with levels significantly higher in renal vein from affected side.

Plasma renin activity responds to changes in posture but not to changes in sodium intake.

Plasma renin activity maintains circadian rhythm despite marked elevation.

Secondary aldosteronism is evident, with hypokalemia, etc. (see p. 337).

Laboratory changes (and hypertension) are reversed by removal of tumor.

BENIGN PROSTATIC HYPERTROPHY

Laboratory findings are those due to urinary tract obstruction and secondary infection.

PROSTATITIS

Most frequently due to
  Streptococcus faecalis
  Staphylococcus albus
  Escherichia coli
  Proteus mirabilis
  Pseudomonas
  Klebsiella

The acute form usually shows laboratory findings of infected urine (WBC in centrifuged sediment of last portion of voided specimen; culture).

In the chronic form, prostatic fluid usually shows more than 10–15 WBC (pus cells). Cultures are frequently positive (because of bacteria listed above).

Laboratory findings due to associated or complicating conditions (e.g., epididymitis) may be present.

CARCINOMA OF PROSTATE

Increased serum acid phosphatase indicates local extension or distant metastases. It is increased in 80% of patients with bone metastases, 20% of patients with extension into periprostatic soft tissue but without bone involvement, 5% of patients with carcinoma confined to gland. Occasionally it remains low despite active metastases. Increased serum acid phosphatase shows pronounced fall in activity within 3–4 days after castration or within 2 weeks after estrogen therapy is begun; may return to normal or remain slightly elevated; failure to fall corresponds to the failure of clinical response that occurs in 10% of the patients. Most patients with invasive carcinoma show a significant increase in serum acid phosphatase after massage or palpation; this rarely occurs in patients with normal prostate, benign prostatic hypertrophy, or in situ carcinoma, or in patients with prostate carcinoma who are receiving hormone treatment.

Alkaline phosphatase is increased in 90% of patients with bone metastases. Increases with favorable response to estrogen therapy or castration and reaches peak in 3 months, then declines. Recurrence of bone metastases causes new rise in alkaline phosphatase.

Anemia is present.

Carcinoma cells appear in bone marrow aspirates.

Fibrinolysins are found in 12% of patients with metastatic prostatic cancer; occur only with extensive metastases and are usually associated with hemorrhagic manifestations; and show fibrinogen deficiency and prolonged prothrombin time.

Urinary tract infection and hematuria occur late.

Needle biopsy of suspicious nodules in prostate is called for.

Cytologic examination of prostatic fluid is not generally useful.

CARCINOMA OF BLADDER

Hematuria is present.

Biopsy of tumor should be taken.

Cytologic examination of urine for tumor cells is useful. (It may be of most value in screening dye workers in chemical industry.)

Urinary LDH level may be particularly useful in screening studies to discover asymptomatic cases of neoplasm of GI tract.

Laboratory findings due to complications will stem from infection, or obstruction of ureter.

Laboratory findings due to preexisting conditions may be those of, e.g., schistosomiasis, stone, or infection.

RETROPERITONEAL FIBROSIS

ESR is increased.

Leukocytosis is present.

Occasionally eosinophilia occurs.

Serum protein and A/G ratio are normal; if the person is chronically ill, total protein may be decreased.

Gamma globulins may be increased.

Anemia is present.

Laboratory findings due to ureteral obstruction are made.

The condition may be primary, due to angiomatous lymphoid hamartoma, or secondary to administration of methysergide.

VULVOVAGINITIS

Due To

Bacteria, especially gonococcus; also *Haemophilus vaginalis* (gram stain of smear, culture)

Fungi, especially *Candida albicans*, diagnosed by culture on Nickerson's or Sabouraud's medium and also by identification on Papanicolaou smears

Trichomonas, diagnosed by hanging drop preparation; often seen in routine urinalysis on microscopical examination

CARCINOMA OF UTERUS

Carcinoma of the Corpus

Cytologic examination (Pap smear) is positive in about 70% of cases; a false negative occurs in 30% of cases. Therefore a negative Pap smear does not rule out carcinoma.

Pap smear from aspiration of endometrial cavity is positive in 95% of cases. Endometrial biopsy may be helpful, but a negative result does not rule out carcinoma.

Diagnostic curettage is the only way to rule out carcinoma of the endometrium.

Carcinoma of the Cervix

Pap smear for routine screening in the general population may be positive for carcinoma of the cervix in approximately 6 of every 1000 women (prevalence); only 7% of these lesions are invasive. The prevalence rate is greatest in certain groups:

Age 21–35 years with peak in 31st to 35th year

Black and Puerto Rican compared to Caucasian

Use of oral steroid rather than diaphragm for contraception

Earlier onset or greater duration of sexual activity

Vaginal pool Pap smear has an accuracy rate of about 80% in detecting carcinoma of the cervix. Smears from a combination of vaginal pool, exocervical, and endocervical scrapings have an accuracy rate of 95%.

After an initial abnormal smear, the follow-up smear taken in the next few weeks or months may not always be abnormal; there is no clear explanation for this finding. Biopsy shows important lesions of the cervix in some of these patients. Therefore an abnormal initial smear requires further investigation of the cervix regardless of subsequent cytologic reports.

Late Cases

Laboratory findings due to obstruction of ureters with pyelonephritis, azotemia, etc., may be present.

General effects of cancer are found.

RUPTURED TUBAL PREGNANCY

Increased WBC usually returns to normal in 24 hours. Persistent increase may indicate recurrent bleeding. Half of the patients have normal WBC; three-quarters of the patients have WBC < 15,000/cu mm. Persistent WBC over 20,000/cu mm may indicate pelvic inflammatory disease.

Anemia is present but often precedes the tubal pregnancy in impoverished populations. Progressive anemia may indicate continuing bleeding into hematoma. Absorption of blood from hematoma may cause increased serum bilirubin.

Pregnancy tests are positive in about half the patients.

ALTERED LABORATORY TESTS DURING PREGNANCY

Hemoglobin decreases slightly to as low as 10 gm/100 ml with corresponding decrease of hematocrit.

RBC is decreased as much as 10–15% because of increased plasma volume.

Blood volume is increased as much as 45%, and plasma volume is decreased by 25–55% by 32d week.

WBC is increased during late pregnancy and labor.

Increased ESR is due to increased fibrinogen.

Serum iron is decreased and TIBC is increased during last half of pregnancy.

Serum albumin is decreased about 1 gm/100 ml during last 2 trimesters.

Serum alpha₁ globulin is markedly increased in last 2 trimesters.

Serum alpha₂ globulin is increased in last 2 trimesters.

Serum beta globulin is slightly increased in second trimester.

Serum gamma globulin may decrease slightly in last trimester.

Blood fibrinogen is moderately increased by fourth month; increased one-third by term.

Serum ceruloplasmin, copper, and transferrin alpha₁ antitrypsin are increased in last trimester.

Serum glucose is occasionally decreased.

Glucose tolerance is decreased during last trimester.

Blood urea nitrogen and NPN decrease about 25%, especially during first 2 trimesters.

Serum cholesterol increases after 8th week to maximum by 30th week.

Serum PBI is increased throughout pregnancy.

Serum T-3 uptake is decreased and T-4 is increased. Free thyroxine factor (T-3 times T-4) is normal. TBG is increased. BMR is moderately increased, especially in last trimester.

In late pregnancy, Factor XI is decreased and Factors II, VII, VIII, IX, and X are increased.

Serum CPK may be decreased during 8th to 20th week (maximum at 12th week). CPK is frequently definitely increased during last few weeks. Serum LDH is occasionally slightly increased.

At parturition there is a significant increase in serum of CPK with a smaller increase of LDH and SGOT. Levels become normal in 2–5 days.

In toxemia of pregnancy, serum SGOT and SGPT are increased; more marked increases occur with greater severity of toxemia.

Serum alkaline phosphatase is increased (2–3 times) and serum ICD is increased in third trimester. In toxemia, rise in serum alkaline phosphatase is greater. Alkaline phosphatase falls with intrauterine fetal death.

Serum leucine aminopeptidase (LAP) may be moderately increased throughout pregnancy.

Abnormal BSP retention occurs during last month.

Occasionally cold agglutinins may be positive and osmotic fragility increased.

Urine volume may increase up to 25% in last trimester.

Proteinuria is common.

Glycosuria is common with decreased glucose tolerance.

Urine porphyrins may be increased.

Urinary gonadotropins (HCG) are increased (see "Pregnancy" Test, p. 99).

Urine estrogens increase from 6 months to term (up to 100 μg/24 hours).

Urine 17-ketosteroids rise to upper limit of normal at term.

Gastric HCl and pepsin may be decreased.

ALTERED LABORATORY TESTS DURING MENSTRUATION

Platelet count is decreased by 50–70%; returns to normal by fourth day.

Hemoglobin is unchanged.

Fibrinogen is increased.

Serum cholesterol may increase just before menstruation.

Serum PBI may decrease slightly after menstruation.

Urine volume, sodium, and chloride decrease premenstrually and increase postmenstrually (diuresis).

Urine protein may increase during premenstrual phase.

Urine porphyrins increase.

Urine estrogens decrease to lowest level 2–3 days after onset.

34

Infectious Diseases

PNEUMOCOCCAL INFECTIONS

Pneumonia

Increased WBC (usually 12,000–25,000/cu mm) with shift to the left; normal or low WBC in overwhelming infection, in aged patients, or with other causative organisms (e.g., Friedländer's bacillus)

Blood culture positive for pneumococci in one-fourth of cases during first 3–4 days in untreated patients

Gram stain of sputum—many polynuclear leukocytes, many gram-positive cocci in pairs and singly; direct pneumococcus typing using Neufeld capsular swelling method rarely done now

Pleural effusion in about 5% of patients

Laboratory findings due to complications (endocarditis, meningitis, peritonitis, arthritis, empyema, etc.)

Endocarditis

See p. 150.

Meningitis

See p. 210.

Laboratory findings due to associated or underlying conditions—pneumococcal pneumonia, endocarditis, otitis, sinusitis, multiple myeloma

Peritonitis

Positive blood culture

Increased WBC

Ascitic fluid—identification of organisms by gram stain and culture
See section on laboratory findings in body fluids, p. 122.

STREPTOCOCCAL INFECTIONS

Group A streptococci showing beta hemolysis
   Upper respiratory infection
   Scarlet fever

WBC is usually increased (14,000/cu mm) early. It becomes normal by end of first week. (*If still increased, look for complication, e.g., otitis.*) Increased eosinophils appear during convalescence, especially with scarlet fever.

Urine may show transient slight albumin, RBCs, casts, without sequelae.

ASO titer (see p. 102)

See sections on rheumatic fever and acute glomerulonephritis, pp. 148–149, 359–360.

Group A streptococci are the most frequent type of streptococci causing

Otitis media, mastoiditis, sinusitis, meningitis, cerebral sinus thrombosis

Pneumonia, empyema, pericarditis

Bacteremia, suppurative arthritis

Puerperal sepsis

Lymphangitis, lymphadenitis, erysipelas, cellulitis

WBC is markedly increased (up to 20,000–30,000/cu mm).

Streptococci appear in smears and cultures from appropriate sites.

Blood culture may be positive.

Streptococcus viridans (alpha hemolytic streptococci)
    Subacute bacterial endocarditis (see p. 150)
Streptococcus faecalis (enterococcus; group D streptococci)
    Bacterial endocarditis
    Urinary tract infection
Anaerobic streptococci
    Associated with coliform bacilli, clostridia, *Bacteroides*
        Compound fractures and soft-tissue wounds
        Puerperal and postabortal sepsis
        Visceral abscesses (e.g., lung, liver, brain)
    Associated with *Staphylococcus aureus*
        Gangrenous postoperative abdominal incision
    Without associated bacteria
        Burrowing skin and subcutaneous infection

STAPHYLOCOCCAL INFECTIONS

Pneumonia—often secondary to measles, influenza, mucoviscidosis, debilitating diseases such as leukemia and collagen diseases
    WBC is increased (usually more than 15,000/cu mm).
    Sputum contains very many leukocytes with intracellular gram-positive cocci.
    Bacteremia occurs in less than one-fifth of patients.
Acute osteomyelitis—due to hematogenous dissemination
    Bacteremia occurs in more than half of early cases.
    WBC is increased.
    Anemia develops.
    Secondary amyloidosis occurs in long-standing chronic osteomyelitis.
Endocarditis—occurs in valves without preceding rheumatic disease and showing little or no previous damage; causes rapid severe damage to valve, producing acute clinical course of mechanical heart failure (rupture of chordae tendineae, perforation of valve, valvular insufficiency) plus results of acute severe infection

Metastatic abscesses occur in various organs.
Anemia develops rapidly.
WBC is increased (12,000–20,000/cu mm); occasionally is normal or decreased.

From 1 to 13% of cases of bacterial endocarditis are due to coagulase-negative Staphylococcus albus; *bacterial endocarditis due to* Staphylococcus albus *is found following cardiac surgery in one-third and without preceding surgery in two-thirds of patients.*

WBC is increased.
Bacteremia is common.
Food poisoning—due to enterotoxin
Culture of staphylococci from suspected food (especially custard and milk products and meats)

MENINGOCOCCAL INFECTIONS

Meningococcemia
Meningitis (see p. 210)
Waterhouse-Friderichsen syndrome (see p. 340)
Increased WBC (12,000–40,000/cu mm)
Gram-stained smears of body fluids
Tissue fluid from skin lesions
Buffy coat of blood
Cerebrospinal fluid (*Pyogenic meningitis in which bacteria cannot be found in smear is more likely to be due to meningococcus than other bacteria.*)
Nasopharynx
Culture (*use chocolate agar incubated in 10% CO_2*)—blood, spinal fluid, skin lesions, nasopharynx, other sites of infection
Urine—may show albumin, RBCs; occasional glycosuria
Cerebrospinal fluid (see Table 23, p. 202)
Markedly increased WBC (2500–10,000/cu mm), almost all polynuclear leukocytes
Increased protein (50–1500 mg/100 ml)
Decreased glucose (0–45 mg/100 ml)
Positive smear and culture

GONOCOCCAL INFECTIONS

Genital infection
Gram stain of smear from involved site, especially urethra, prostatic secretions, cervix, pelvic inflammatory disease, etc. (*Smear may become negative within hours of antibiotic therapy.*)
Bacterial culture (*Use special media such as Thayer-Martin.*)
Fluorescent antibody test on smear of suspected material

Beware of concomitant inapparent venereal infection which may be suppressed but not adequately treated by antibiotic therapy of gonorrhea.

Proctitis
Gram-stained smears are not sufficiently reliable.
Bacterial culture on special media (e.g., Thayer-Martin) is required for confirmation.

Rectal biopsy shows mild and nonspecific inflammation. In a few cases, gram stain of tissue section may reveal small numbers of gram-negative intracellular diplococci after prolonged examination.

(*Rectal gonorrhea accompanies genital gonorrhea in 20–50% of women and is found without genital gonorrhea in 6–10% of infected women. Therefore rectal cultures for gonococcus should be taken in all suspected cases of gonorrhea.*)

Arthritis
  Synovial fluid (see p. 235)
        Variable; may contain few leukocytes or be purulent
        Gonococci identified in about one-third of patients
  Gonococcal complement-fixation test for differential diagnosis of other types of arthritis. Not a reliable test in urethritis but may rarely be helpful in arthritis, prostatitis, and epididymitis. Becomes positive at least 2–6 weeks after onset of infection, remains positive for 3 months after cure. If test is negative, it should be repeated; two negative tests help to rule out gonococcus infection. False positive test may occur after gonococcus vaccine has been used. Test is of limited value and is seldom used.
  Associated nonbacterial ophthalmitis in up to one-fifth of patients
Rarely other sites
  Ophthalmitis of newborn
  Acute bacterial endocarditis (toxic hepatitis common) (see p. 150). (*Gonococcus is the most common bacteria infecting tricuspid or pulmonic valves.*)
  Bacteremia—resembles meningococcemia
  Peritonitis and perihepatitis following spread from pelvic inflammatory disease

INFECTIONS WITH COLIFORM BACTERIA
(*Escherichia coli, Enterobacter-Klebsiella* group, paracolon group)

Bacteremia
    Secondary to infection elsewhere; occasionally due to transfusion of contaminated blood
    Secondary to debilitated condition in one-fifth of patients (e.g., malignant lymphoma, irradiation or anticancer drugs, steroid therapy, cirrhosis, diabetes mellitus)

    Gram-negative shock occurs in one-fourth of patients.
        Azotemia
        Increased serum potassium
        Decreased serum sodium
        Metabolic acidosis
        Increased SGOT (decreased hepatic perfusion)
        Increased serum amylase (decreased renal perfusion)
        Other findings due to shock

Urinary tract infection, three-fourths of cases due to *E. coli*
Infections of intestinal tract and biliary tree (e.g., appendicitis, cholecystitis)
Wound infections, abscesses, etc.

Gastroenteritis in young children and infants—identification of specific strains by fluorescent antibody technique

Pneumonia—1% of primary bacterial pneumonias due to *Klebsiella* (Friedländer's bacilli), especially in alcoholics

WBC is often normal or decreased.

Sputum is very tenacious; is brown or red. Smear shows encapsulated gram-negative bacilli. (*Gram stain of sputum in lobar pneumonia allows prompt diagnosis of this organism and appropriate therapy.*) Bacterial culture confirms diagnosis.

Laboratory findings due to complications (lung abscess, empyema) are present.

Rarely chronic lung infection due to Friedländer's bacilli simulates tuberculosis.

PROTEUS INFECTIONS

Proteus infections usually follow other bacterial infections.

Indolent skin ulcers (decubital, varicose ulcers)
Burns
Otitis media, mastoiditis
Urinary tract infection
Bacteremia

Characteristic spreading growth on culture plate may obscure associated bacteria since Proteus *infection frequently is part of mixed infection; antibiotic sensitivity testing may not be possible.*

PSEUDOMONAS INFECTIONS

Pseudomonas infections occur in various different sites.

Due To
Replacement of normal bacterial flora or initial pathogen because of antibiotic therapy (e.g., urinary tract, ear, lung)
Burns
Debilitated condition of patient (e.g., premature infants, the aged, patients with leukemia)

Decreased WBC during bacteremia in patients with leukemia or burns is more frequently due to Pseudomonas *than to other gram-negative rods.*

GRAM-NEGATIVE BACTEREMIC SHOCK

Two-thirds of cases are due to gram-negative bacteria.

Shock is most frequently from urinary tract, gastrointestinal tract, uterus, lung, in that order.

E. coli is the most frequent organism and causes the lowest mortality (45%) and the lowest incidence of shock. *Pseudomonas aeruginosa* has the highest mortality (85%). *Klebsiella-Enterobacter*, paracolon bacilli, and *Proteus mirabilis* are intermediate with 70% mortality.

BACTEROIDES INFECTION

This is usually a component of mixed infection with coliform bacteria, aerobic and anaerobic streptococci or staphylococci.

Local suppuration or systemic infection is secondary to disease of the female genital tract, intestinal tract, or tonsillar region.

Laboratory findings due to complications (e.g., thrombophlebitis, endocarditis, metastatic abscesses of lung, liver, brain, joint) are present.

Laboratory findings due to underlying conditions (e.g., recent surgery, cancer, arteriosclerosis, diabetes mellitus, alcoholism, prior antibiotic treatment, and steroid, immunosuppressive, or cytotoxic therapy) are present.

TYPHOID FEVER
(due to *Salmonella typhosa*)

WBC is decreased: 4000–6000/cu mm during first 2 weeks, 3000–5000/cu mm during next 2 weeks; 10,000/cu mm or more suggests perforation or suppuration.

Normocytic anemia is frequent; with bleeding, anemia becomes hypochromic and microcytic.

Blood cultures are positive during first 10 days of fever in 90% of patients, and during relapse; less than 30% are positive after third week.

Stool cultures are positive after tenth day with increasing frequency up to fourth or fifth week. Positive stool culture after 4 months indicates a carrier.

Urine culture is positive during second to third week in 25% of patients even if blood culture is negative.

Widal reaction. H and O agglutinins appear in serum after 7–10 days, increase to peak in third to fifth week, then gradually fall for several weeks; there is no increase during relapse. O appears before H and is usually higher at first; during convalescence H titer becomes higher than O. Positive Widal test may occur on account of typhoid vaccination or previous typhoid infection; nonspecific febrile disease may cause this titer to increase (anamnestic reaction). Rising titer (especially of O) on serial determinations may be necessary for proper evaluation. Usual criteria for serologic diagnosis in unvaccinated patients is fourfold increase in O titer or O titer $> 1:50$ or $1:100$ in a single specimen or during first 2–3 weeks of illness. Up to 5% of healthy unvaccinated individuals may have O titer of $1:50$.

Early treatment with chloramphenicol or ampicillin may cause titer to remain negative or low.

Increase in O titer may reflect infection with any organism in the group D salmonellae (e.g., *S. enteritidis*, *S. panama*) and not just *S. typhosa*.

Because of differences in commercially manufactured antigens, there may be a twofold to fourfold difference in O titers on the same sample of serum tested with antigens of different manufacturers

H titer is very variable and may show nonspecific response to other infections; it is therefore of little value in diagnosis of typhoid fever.

Laboratory findings due to complications

Intestinal hemorrhage is occult in 20% of patients, gross in 10%;

it occurs usually during second or third week. It is less frequent in treated patients.

Intestinal perforation occurs in 3% of untreated patients.

Relapse occurs in up to one-fifth of patients. Blood culture becomes positive again; Widal titers are unchanged.

Secondary suppurative lesions (e.g., pneumonia, parotitis, furunculosis) are found.

INFECTIONS DUE TO OTHER *SALMONELLA* ORGANISMS

Enteritis
> Stool culture remains positive for 1–4 weeks, occasionally longer.
> WBC is normal.

Paratyphoid fever—usually due to *S. paratyphi A* or *B* or *S. choleraesuis*
> Cultures of blood and stool and decreased WBC show same values as indicated in section on Typhoid Fever.

Bacteremia—especially due to *S. choleraesuis*
> Blood cultures are intermittently positive.
> Stool cultures are negative.
> WBC is normal. It increases (up to 25,000/cu mm) with development of focal lesions (e.g., pneumonia, meningitis, pyelonephritis, osteomyelitis).

Local infections
> Meningitis, especially in infants
> Local abscesses with or without preceding bacteremia or enteritis

One-third of patients are predisposed by underlying disease (e.g., malignant lymphoma, disseminated lupus erythematosus). Bacteremia and osteomyelitis are more common in patients with sickle hemoglobinopathy. Bacteremia is more common in patients with acute hemolytic *Bartonella* infection.

Agglutination tests on sera from acute and convalescent cases are often not useful unless present in high titer (1:560 or greater) or rising titer is shown.

BACILLARY DYSENTERY
(due to *Shigella* species)

Stool culture is positive in more than three-fourths of patients.
> Rectal swab can also be used.

Microscopy of stool shows mucus, RBCs, and leukocytes.
Serologic tests are not useful.
WBC is normal.
Blood cultures are negative.
Laboratory findings due to complications
> Marked loss of fluid and electrolytes
> Intestinal bleeding
> Relapse (in 10% of untreated patients)
> Carrier state
> Acute arthritis—especially untreated disease due to *S. shigae* (culture of joint fluid negative)

CHOLERA
(due to *Vibrio comma*)

Stool culture is positive. One may also identify organism in stool using immunofluorescent techniques.
Laboratory findings due to marked loss of fluid and electrolytes
      Loss of sodium, chloride, and potassium
      Hypovolemic shock
      Metabolic acidosis
      Uremia

INFECTIONS WITH *VIBRIO FETUS*

Clinical types
      Occasional cases of subacute bacterial endocarditis, septic arthritis, meningoencephalitis, etc.; *seen especially in cases of thrombophlebitis of all limbs*
Culture of infected material from appropriate sites (Incubate blood culture under 10% CO_2.)
Complement-fixation test positive during active phase

HAEMOPHILUS INFLUENZAE INFECTIONS
(due to *Haemophilus influenzae*)

Clinical types
      Upper respiratory infections
      Lower respiratory infections
      Otitis media
      Meningitis
Increased WBC (15,000–30,000/cu mm) and polynuclear leukocytes
Positive blood culture in about half of patients with meningitis

PERTUSSIS (WHOOPING COUGH)
(due to *Bordetella pertussis*)

Marked increase in WBC (up to 100,000/cu mm) and up to 90% mature lymphocytes
Negative blood cultures
Positive cultures from nasopharynx or cough plate

CHANCROID
(due to *H. ducreyi*)

Biopsy of genital ulcer or regional lymph node is helpful.
Smear of genital ulcer or regional lymph node stained with Unna-Pappenheim method shows bacteria.
Smear of lesion for Donovan bodies is negative.
Dark-field examination of lesion for treponemae is negative.
Serologic tests for syphilis are negative.
Cultures of lymph node aspirate are more frequently positive than cultures from lesion. Culture is of limited practical value.

BRUCELLOSIS

Agglutination reaction becomes positive during second to third week of illness; 90% of patients have titers of 1:320 or more. Rising titer is of diagnostic significance. False negatives are rare.

False positive may occur with tularemia or cholera or with cholera vaccination or after brucellin skin test. In chronic localized brucellosis, titers may be negative or up to 1:200. They may remain positive long after infection has been cured.

Multiple blood cultures should be performed. (Br. abortus *requires 10% CO_2 for culture.*) They are more likely to be positive with high agglutination titer.

Bone marrow culture is occasionally positive when blood culture is negative. It may show microscopic granulomas

Opsonophagocytic test and complement-fixation test are not generally useful.

WBC is usually less than 10,000/cu mm with a relative lymphocytosis. Decreased WBC occurs in one-third of patients.

ESR is increased in less than one-quarter of patients and usually in nonlocalized type of brucellosis.

Anemia appears in less than one-tenth of patients and usually with localized type of disease.

Biopsy of tissue may show nonspecific granulomas suggesting a diagnosis of brucellosis. Tissue may be used for culture.

TULAREMIA
(due to *Pasteurella tularensis*)

Clinical types
> Typhoidal
> Ulceroglandular
> Glandular
> Pneumonic
> Rarely oculoglandular, gastrointestinal, endocarditis, meningitis, osteomyelitis, etc.

Agglutination reaction becomes positive in second week of infection. Significant titer is 1:40; usually it becomes 1:320 or more by third week.

Culture and animal inoculation (positive with 5 or more organisms) of suspected material from appropriate site are performed. (Positive blood culture is rare; regional lymph node and mucocutaneous lesions are usually positive.)

WBC is usually normal.

ESR may be increased in severe typhoidal forms; it is normal in other types.

Biopsy of involved lymph node shows a characteristic histologic picture.

PLAGUE
(due to *Pasteurella pestis*)

Clinical types
> Bubonic
> Primary septicemic
> Pneumonic

Identify bacteria by smear, culture, fluorescent antibody technique, or animal inoculation of suspected material from appropriate site (e.g., lymph node aspirate, blood, sputum).

Serum hemagglutination antibodies are present.

WBC is increased (20,000–40,000/cu mm), with increased polynuclear leukocytes.

INFECTIONS WITH *PASTEURELLA MULTOCIDA*

Clinical types
> Localized suppurative infections (e.g., osteomyelitis, cellulitis)
> Bacteremia with endocarditis, meningitis, etc.
> Respiratory tract infection

Gram stain and culture of bacteria from appropriate sites are performed (e.g., blood, skin, spinal fluid).
WBC is increased

GLANDERS
(due to *Malleomyces mallei*)

Clinical types
> Acute fulminant
> Chronic disseminated granulomas and abscesses in skin, respiratory tract, etc.

Culture or animal inoculation of infected material from appropriate sites is performed.
Agglutination and complement-fixation tests are positive in chronic disease.
WBC is variable.

MELIOIDOSIS
(due to *Pseudomonas pseudomallei*)

Clinical types
> Acute febrile
> Chronic febrile with abscesses in bone, skin, viscera

> *Infection is occasionally transmitted among narcotic addicts using common needles.*

Culture or animal inoculation of infected material from appropriate sites is performed (e.g., pus, urine, blood, sputum).
Agglutination test is positive in chronic disease; an occasional false positive test occurs.
WBC is normal or increased.

INFECTIONS WITH *MIMA-HERELLEA*

Clinical types
> Bacteremia, bacterial endocarditis, meningitis, pneumonia, etc.

> *Often associated with intravenous catheters or cutdowns*

Bacteria are isolated from appropriate sites (e.g., blood, spinal fluid, sputum).

GRANULOMA INGUINALE
(due to Donovan body)

Wright-stained or Giemsa-stained smears of lesions show intracytoplasmic Donovan bodies in large mononuclear cells in acute stage; they may be present in chronic stages.
Biopsy of lesion shows suggestive histologic pattern and is usually positive for Donovan bodies in acute stage.

Serologic tests for syphilis are negative unless concomitant infection is present.

Dark-field examination for syphilis is negative.

LISTERIOSIS
(due to *Listeria monocytogenes*)

Especially in newborn from antepartum infection of mother
> Findings due to meningitis or disseminated abscesses of viscera are made.
> WBC is increased, and other evidence of infection is found.
> Gram stain of meconium shows gram-positive bacilli. *This should be done whenever mother is febrile before or at onset of labor.*

Infection of adult nonpregnant patients is associated with debilitation (e.g., alcoholism, diabetes mellitus, adrenocorticoid therapy).
> Laboratory findings due to bacteremia, endocarditis, skin infection, etc., are present.

ANTHRAX
(due to anthrax bacillus)

Identification of gram-positive bacillus in material by gram stain, culture, and animal inoculation from site of involvement (fluid from cutaneous lesions; sputum and pleural fluid from patients with pulmonary disease; stool or vomit from patients with intestinal disease; blood from patients with bacteremia)

WBC and ESR normal in mild cases; increased in severe cases

With meningeal involvement
> CSF bloody
> Smear and culture positive for bacilli

Precipitin antibodies with high or increasing titer sometimes useful in pulmonary or intestinal disease

DIPHTHERIA
(due to *Corynebacterium diphtheriae*)

WBC is increased (up to 15,000/cu mm). If more than 25,000/cu mm are found, there is probably a concomitant infection (e.g., hemolytic streptococcus).

Smear from involved area stained with methylene blue is positive in more than three-fourths of patients.

Culture from involved area is positive within 12 hours on Loeffler's medium (more slowly on blood agar). *If there has been prior antibiotic therapy, culture may be negative or take several days to grow.* Penicillin G eliminates *C. diphtheriae* within 12 days; without therapy organisms usually disappear after 2–4 weeks.

Fluorescent-antibody staining of material from involved area is done.

Laboratory findings of peripheral neuritis (see p. 217) are present in 10% of cases, usually during second to sixth week. Increased CSF protein may be of prolonged duration.

Laboratory findings of myocarditis (which occurs in up to two-thirds of patients) are present.

Albumin is frequently present in urine.

Hemagglutination titer assays antitoxin titer of patient's serum. Fourfold increase in titer in acute and convalescent sera confirms diagnosis.

TETANUS
(due to *Clostridium tetani*)

WBC is normal.

Urine is normal.

CSF is normal.

Identification of organism in local wound is difficult and not usually helpful.

BOTULISM
(due to *Clostridium botulinum*)

CSF is normal.

Usual laboratory tests are not abnormal or useful.

Diagnosis is made by injecting suspected food intraperitoneally into mice, which will die in 24 hours unless protected with specific antiserum.

CLOSTRIDIAL GAS GANGRENE, CELLULITIS, AND PUERPERAL SEPSIS
(due to *Clostridium perfringens*, *C. septicum*, *C. novyi*, etc.)

WBC is increased (15,000 to more than 40,000/cu mm).

Platelets are decreased in half the patients.

In postabortal sepsis, sudden severe hemolytic anemia is common. Hemoglobinemia, hemoglobinuria, increased serum bilirubin, spherocytosis, increased osmotic and mechanical fragility, etc., may be associated.

Protein and casts are often present in urine.

Renal insufficiency may progress to uremia.

Smears of material from appropriate sites show gram-positive rods, but spores are not usually seen and other bacteria are often also present.

Anaerobic culture of material from appropriate site is positive. *Clostridia are frequent contaminants of wounds caused by other agents. Other bacteria may cause gas formation within tissues.*

LEPTOSPIROSIS
(most frequently due to *Leptospira icterohaemorrhagiae*, *L. canicola*, and *L. pomona*)

Normochromic anemia is present.

WBC may be normal or up to 40,000/cu mm in Weil's disease.

ESR is increased.

Urine is abnormal in three-fourths of patients: proteinuria, WBCs, RBCs, casts.

Liver function tests are abnormal in half the patients.

Increased serum bilirubin

Increased alkaline phosphatase

Reversed A/G ratio
Abnormal flocculation tests
CSF is abnormal in cases with meningeal involvement (up to two-thirds of patients)
Increased cells (up to 500/cu mm), chiefly mononuclear type
Increased protein (up to 80 mg/100 ml)
Glucose and chloride normal
Blood culture is positive during first 3 days of disease in up to 90% of cases.
Urine cultures may be positive only intermittently and are difficult because of contamination and low pH. They are rarely positive after the fourth week.
Of the serologic tests the hemolysis test is most useful. Agglutination, complement fixation, and hemolysis antibodies reach peaks in 4–7 weeks and may last for many years. An increasing titer is diagnostic. An individual titer of 1:300 is suggestive.

RELAPSING FEVER
(due to *Borrelia recurrentis, B. novyi, B. duttonii*)

Identification of organism by
Wright or Giemsa stain or dark-field microscopy of peripheral blood smear or buffy coat
Intraperitoneal injection of rats
Agglutination of *Proteus* OX-K
Biologic false positive serologic test for syphilis in up to one-fourth of patients
Increased WBC (10,000–15,000/cu mm)
Protein and mononuclear cells sometimes increased in CSF.
Laboratory findings due to complications (e.g., hemorrhage, rupture of spleen, secondary infection)

INFECTIONS WITH *STREPTOBACILLUS MONILIFORMIS* (RAT-BITE FEVER, HAVERHILL FEVER, ETC.)

Clinical types
Rat-bite fever
Febrile rash with multiple joint type of arthritis
Isolation of bacteria from appropriate sites (e.g., blood, pus, joint fluid) during acute febrile stage
Agglutination antibodies in serum during second to third week; rising titer significant

INFECTIONS WITH *BARTONELLA BACILLIFORMIS*

Oroya Fever
Sudden very marked anemia is found.
Blood smears may show gram-negative bacilli in up to 90% of RBCs (Giemsa stain); they are also present in monocytes. Bacteria are also present in phagocytes of reticuloendothelial system.
Blood culture is positive. (*Use special enriched media.*)

Beware of secondary Salmonella *infection.*

Verruga Peruana
Moderate anemia is found.
Blood smears and blood cultures are positive for bacilli.

SYPHILIS
(due to *Treponema pallidum*)

Primary Syphilis
Dark-field examination of genital lesion is made; if it is negative, regional lymph node aspirate may be used. *Examination will be negative if there has been recent therapy with penicillin or other treponemicidal drugs.*
Serologic test shows rising titer with or without positive dark-field examination. VDRL does not become positive until 7–10 days after appearance of chancre.
Biopsy of suspected lesion is done for histologic examination.

Secondary Syphilis
Dark-field examination of mucocutaneous lesions is positive.
Serologic tests are almost always positive in high titer.

Latent Syphilis
A positive serologic test is the only diagnostic method.

Congenital Syphilis
Dark-field examination of mucocutaneous lesions is positive.
Serologic tests are positive and show rising or very high titer. *The serologic test may be positive because of maternal antibodies but without congenital syphilitic infection.* Rising infant's titer or titer higher than mother's establishes diagnosis of congenital syphilis. If mother has been adequately treated, infant's titer falls steadily to nonreactive level in 3 months. If mother acquires syphilis late in pregnancy, infant may be seronegative and clinically normal at birth and then manifest syphilis 1–2 months later.

Late Syphilis
CNS
　　Meningitis
　　　　Up to 2000 lymphocytes/cu mm
　　　　Positive serologic test in blood and spinal fluid
　　Meningovascular disease
　　　　Increased cell count
　　　　Increased protein
　　　　Positive serologic test in blood and spinal fluid
　　　　Laboratory findings due to cerebrovascular thrombosis
　　Tabes dorsalis
　　　　Early—increased cell count and protein and positive serologic test in blood and spinal fluid (titer may be low)
　　　　Late—about 25% of patients may have normal spinal fluid and negative serologic tests in blood and spinal fluid
　　General paresis (spinal fluid always abnormal in untreated patients)
　　　　Increased cells and protein
　　　　Positive serologic test (titer usually high)

Asymptomatic CNS lues
> May have negative blood and positive spinal fluid serologic test
> Increased cell count and protein is index of activity

Cardiovascular syphilis-VDRL—usually reactive but titer often low
Gummatous lesions-VDRL—almost always reactive, usually in high titer
Cardiovascular, liver, etc., involvement
Biopsy of skin, lymph node, larynx, testes, etc.

Adequately treated primary and secondary syphilis usually becomes serologically nonreactive; late syphilis rarely becomes nonreactive although titers may fall steadily over a long period.
If late syphilis of any type is suspected, always do FTA-ABS even if VDRL is nonreactive.
One-third of patients with only weakly reactive VDRL are reactive with more sensitive test (e.g., TPI); weakly reactive VDRL should always be confirmed with FTA-ABS.
VDRL may be nonreactive in undiluted serum in presence of an actual high titer ("prozone" phenomenon) in 1% of patients with secondary syphilis.
See Serologic Tests for Syphilis, p. 101.

YAWS (due to *Treponema pertenue*), PINTA (due to *T. carateum*), BEJEL (due to treponema indistinguishable from *T. pallidum*)

Positive serologic tests for syphilis
Positive dark-field demonstration of treponema from appropriate lesions

TUBERCULOSIS

Acid-fast stained smears and cultures (and occasionally guinea pig inoculation) of concentrates of suspected material from involved sites (e.g., sputum, gastric fluid, effusions, urine, CSF, pus) should be performed on multiple specimens. If negative, guinea pig inoculation of this material may be needed.
WBC is usually normal. Granulocytic leukemoid reaction may occur in miliary disease. Active disseminated disease is suggested by more monocytes (10–20%) than lymphocytes (5–10%) in peripheral smear.
ESR is normal in localized disease; increased in disseminated or advanced disease.
Moderate anemia may be present in advanced disease.
Characteristic histologic pattern appears in random biopsy of lymph node, liver, bone marrow (especially in miliary dissemination), or other involved sites (e.g., bronchus, pleura).
Urine. Rule out renal tuberculosis in presence of hematuria (gross or microscopic) or pyuria with negative cultures for pyogenic bacteria.
Laboratory findings due to extrapulmonary tuberculosis
> Tuberculous meningitis
>> CSF shows
>>> 100–1000 WBC/cu mm (mostly lymphocytes)
>>> Increased protein
>>> Decreased glucose (less than half of blood glucose)
>>> Decreased chloride

Increased tryptophan

Acid-fast smear and culture from pellicle

Serum sodium may be decreased (110–125 mEq/L) especially in aged; may also occur in overwhelming tuberculous infection.

Tuberculous pleural effusion (see p. 122)

Sputum is positive on culture in 25% of patients; pleural fluid is positive on culture in 25% of patients.

Fluid is an exudate with increased protein (more than 3 gm/100 ml) and increased lymphocytes.

Lymph nodes

Culture is important to rule out infection due to other mycobacteria (atypical or anonymous).

Laboratory findings due to complications (see appropriate separate sections)

Amyloidosis

Addison's disease

Etc.

LEPROSY (HANSEN'S DISEASE)
(due to *Mycobacterium leprae*)

Mild anemia is found. Sulfone therapy frequently causes anemia, which indicates dosage change is needed.

Serum albumin is decreased, and serum globulin is increased.

ESR is increased.

Serum cholesterol is slightly decreased.

Serum calcium is slightly decreased.

False positive serologic test for syphilis occurs in up to 40% of patients.

Acid-fast bacilli are found in smear or tissue biopsy from nasal scrapings or lepromatous lesions. Acid-fast diphtheroids are not infrequently found in nasal septum smears or scrapings in normal persons, and *M. leprae* is not found here in two-thirds of early lepromatous cases. Therefore nasal smear may have very limited diagnostic value. Bacilli may show a typical granulation and fragmentation that precedes the clinical improvement due to sulfone therapy. Larger, more nodular lesions are more likely to be positive. During lepra reactions, enormous numbers·of bacilli may be present in skin lesions and may be found in peripheral blood smears. Bacilli are usually very difficult to find in skin lesions of tuberculoid leprosy.

Histologic pattern of the lesions is used for classification of type of leprosy.

Laboratory findings due to complications are made.

Amyloidosis occurs in 40% of patients in the United States.

Other diseases (e.g., tuberculosis, malaria, parasitic infestation) may be present.

Sterility due to orchitis is very frequent.

SWIMMING-POOL DISEASE
(due to *Mycobacterium balnei*)

Histologic pattern of ulcerated skin lesions on extremities is that of nonspecific granuloma containing acid-fast bacilli.

Cultures from these lesions must be incubated at 31° rather than 37° C.

ANTIBIOTIC TABLES

These represent a general guide in the selection of appropriate
   antibiotics when a specific organism is suspected. However, a
   sensitivity test for the organism cultured in that particular case is
   usually performed because the widespread use of antibiotics has
   resulted in many strains of resistant organisms and because
   various strains of some bacteria may have different susceptibility
   to antibiotics. The clinician must also consider other causes of
   antibiotic treatment failures, such as a mixed bacterial culture
   only one organism of which is susceptible to the administered
   antibiotics, lack of adequate drainage, etc.

A number of different tables related to the selection of antibiotic
   drugs are presented to answer the variety of problems faced by the
   clinician in initiating treatment and to illustrate various approaches to solving these problems.

Table 55. Usual Antibiotic Susceptibility of More Common Bacteria

Bacteria	Penicillin G and V	Ampicillin	Methicillin IV and IM, Staphcillin	Cloxacillin and Oxacillin	Nafcillin	Erythromycin	Tetracycline	Chloramphenicol	Cephalothin IM	Vancomycin and Ristocetin IV	Kanamycin IM	Polymyxin B and Colistin	Lincomycin	Streptomycin IM
Staph. aureus (penicillinase-producing)	R	R	S	S	S	S	R	V	S	S	S	R	S	R
Staph. aureus (non-penicillinase-producing)	S	S	V	S	S	S	S	S	S	S	S	R	S	R
Streptococcus (Diplococcus) pneumonia	S	S	V	V	S	S	V	S	S	S	R	R	S	R
Strept. pyogenes	S	S	V	V	S	S	V	R	S	S	R	R	S	R
Corynebacterium diphtheriae	S	S	R	R	R	S	S	R	R	S	R	R	S	R
Clostridium welchii	S	S	R	R	R	S	S	S	R	S	R	R	R	R
Neisseria meningitidis	S	S	R	R	R	S	S	S	S	R	R	R	R	R
Neisseria gonorrhoeae	S	S	R	R	R	S	S	S	S	R	S	R	R	S
Haemophilus influenzae	V	S	V	V	V	S	S	S	V	R	R	S	R	S
Bordetella pertussis	V	S	V	V	R	S	S	S	R	R	R	S	R	R
Brucella	R	S	R	R	R	S	S	R	R	R	R	R	R	S
Enterococci	S	S	R	R	R	R	S	R	S	R	R	R	R	S
Escherichia coli	R	S	R	R	R	S	S	V	R	S	S	S	R	S
Enterobacter aerogenes	R	R	R	R	R	V	V	V	R	R	S	S	R	R
Klebsiella pneumoniae	R	V	R	R	R	S	S	S	S	R	S	S	R	S
Pseudomonas aeruginosa	R	R	R	R	R	R	R	R	R	R	R	S	R	R
Proteus species	R	S	R	R	R	R	S	S	R	R	V	S	R	S
Salmonella	R	S	R	R	R	R	S	S	R	R	S	R	R	R
Shigella	R	S	R	R	R	R	S	S	S	R	S	S	R	R

S = susceptible; R = resistant; V = variable; IV = intravenous; IM = intramuscular.

Table 56. Summary of Some Common Microorganisms *Uniformly** Sensitive to Chemotherapeutic Agents

Bacteria	All Penicillins	Ampicillin	Penicillin G	Methicillin	Cloxacillin	Cephalothin	Erythromycin	Vancomycin	Tetracycline	Chloramphenicol	Sulfonamide	Polymyxin, Colistin, Gentamicin
Staph. aureus				+	+	+		+				
Streptococcus (Diplococcus) pneumoniae	+					+	+	+				
Strept. pyogenes	+					+	+	+				
Haemophilus influenzae and Bordetella pertussis		+	+						+	+		
Neisseria meningitidis		+	+									
Neisseria gonorrhoeae			+				+					
Brucella									+			
Pseudomonas aeruginosa												+
Clostridium perfringens	+					+			+			
Corynebacterium diphtheriae			+				+					
Actinomyces israelii			+									
Nocardia asteroides											+	

* Therefore gram stain of infected material may provide immediate guide to chemotherapy until results of culture and antibiotic sensitivity are available.

Table 57. Summary of Some Common Bacteria with Usual but Variable Sensitivity to Chemotherapeutic Agents

Bacteria	Ampicillin	Tetracycline	Cephalothin	Chloramphenicol	Kanamycin	Polymyxin	Penicillin G	Erythromycin	Sulfonamide	Nitrofurantoin
Escherichia coli	+	+	+	+	+	+			+	+
Enterobacter aerogenes		+		+	+	+				+
Klebsiella pneumoniae		+	+	+	+	+				+
Proteus vulgaris		+		+	+					+
Salmonella	+	+	+	+	+	+				
Shigella	+	+	+		+	+				
Listeria monocytogenes				+			+	+	+	

Table 58. Chemotherapy of Infection

Chemotherapeutic Agent	Treatment of Choice	Indicated In	Not Indicated In
Oral penicillin G	Only in rheumatic fever for infections	**Prevention of group A streptococcal infections**	Other infections
Oral penicillin V or phenethicillin	Moderately severe infections with susceptible bacteria (including subacute bacterial endocarditis and chronic osteomyelitis with sufficiently high doses)		
Erythromycin	Diphtheria Carriers of *Corynebacterium diphtheriae*	Penicillin substitute (e.g., penicillin allergy) for gram-positive coccal infections, gonorrhea, syphilis *Mycoplasma* pneumonia	Severe staph infections
Ampicillin		*Haemophilus influenzae* and other gram-negative bacillary infections (e.g., urinary tract; pulmonary) Acute otitis media (unless due to *Staph. aureus*) *Salmonella-Shigella* infections (except typhoid) Meningitis due to *H. influenzae*, pneumococci, meningococci	
Tetracycline	**Mixed infections from GI tract**	*Mycoplasma* pneumonia, rickettsial and viral (psittacosis, lymphogranuloma) infections, brucellosis Urinary tract infections, putrid lung abscess, infections in patients with chronic pulmonary disease	Conditions with bacteria that frequently develop resistant strains: *Staph. aureus*, group A beta-hemolytic streptococci, sometimes *Streptococcus (Diplococcus) pneumoniae*
Cephalothin		Acute sepsis due to staph infections with penicillinase-producing staphylococci Sepsis of unknown etiology (possibly due to staph or to gram-negative bacilli)	

Continued on next page

Table 58 (continued)

Chemotherapeutic Agent	Treatment of Choice	Indicated In	Not Indicated In
Chloramphenicol	*Salmonella* infections (especially typhoid fever), rickettsioses Sepsis of unknown etiology		Situations in which less toxic agent is available.
Kanamycin	Gram-negative bacillary infections (e.g., *E. coli, Enterobacter aerogenes, Klebsiella pneumoniae, Proteus; Pseudomonas* when in vitro sensitivity is demonstrated) *Always check renal function (e.g., BUN) because of renal toxicity.*		Gram-positive coccal infections
Lincomycin		Less serious gram-positive coccal infections; in serious staph infections, only as substitute for other agents (e.g., penicillin allergy; cephalothin and vancomycin cannot be used)	
Polymyxin B and colistin		Prevention and treatment of *Pseudomonas aeruginosa* infection	
Neomycin		Useful for topical infections. Orally, only for pathogenic *E. coli* or for carriers of *Salmonella-Shigella*	
Streptomycin	Tuberculosis Plague, tularemia Granuloma inguinale	May be combined with penicillin for treatment of subacute bacterial endocarditis (SBE) May be combined with tetracycline for treatment of brucellosis	Rarely indicated for other infections

[396]

Novobiocin		Rare instances in which preferable drug is not available (because of high frequency of adverse reactions)
Amphotericin B		IV or IM therapy of coccidioidomycosis, histoplasmosis, cryptococcosis, blastomycosis, disseminated candidiasis
Griseofulvin		Topical therapy of *Microsporum, Trichophyton*
Idoxuridine		Local therapy of herpes simplex keratoconjunctivitis

Table 59. Antibiotics in Pulmonary Infections

Infection	Chemotherapeutic Agent
Pneumococcal pneumonia (is most frequent cause of bacterial pneumonia)	Penicillin G is treatment of choice. With penicillin hypersensitivity, erythromycin or cephalothin may be used. Not tetracycline.
Staphylococcal pneumonia (occurs in aged, young, debilitated, postoperative cases, during influenza epidemics)	Penicillinase-resistant penicillins (e.g., methicillin, oxacillin, cloxacillin, nafcillin); may be combined with kanamycin in mixed infections or in overwhelming staph infection. With penicillin hypersensitivity, cephalothin may be used; if patient unable to take either drug, vancomycin may be used.
Beta-hemolytic streptococcal pneumonia	Penicillin G is treatment of choice. With penicillin hypersensitivity, erythromycin or cephalothin may be used. Do not use tetracycline.
Klebsiella pneumonia (occurs in aged, debilitated, alcoholic)	Kanamycin combined with tetracycline or cephalothin
Haemophilus influenzae pneumonia (in adults with chronic obstruction of airways and in children)	Ampicillin or tetracycline
Undiagnosed severe pneumonia (pending results of bacterial cultures)	Penicillin combined with methicillin and kanamycin, or nafcillin combined with kanamycin. With penicillin hypersensitivity, cephalothin combined with kanamycin may be used.
Aspiration pneumonia	Penicillin combined with kanamycin. With penicillin hypersensitivity, cephalothin may be used instead.
Pneumonia due to *Mycoplasma pneumoniae* (Eaton agent)	Tetracycline is treatment of choice. Erythromycin has also been used.
Psittacosis pneumonia	Tetracycline is treatment of choice.
Acute tracheobronchitis, bronchitis, and bronchiolitis (frequently due to *H. influenzae* and *S. pneumoniae*).	Tetracycline or ampicillin is empiric treatment of choice.
Primary lung abscess	Penicillin; may be combined with tetracycline + kanamycin. Depending on sensitivity studies, one may use cephalothin, colistin, penicillinase-resistant penicillins.
Pulmonary tuberculosis (original treatment)	Combinations of isoniazid, PAS, and streptomycin

With failure to respond, rule out underlying bronchogenic carcinoma, tuberculosis, fungus infection, or systemic disease (e.g., diabetes mellitus, collagen disease, lymphoma).

Because of toxicity, use chloramphenicol only for pneumonia associated with typhoid fever or melioidosis.

Table 60. Prophylactic Chemotherapy of Infections

Condition	Drug
Group A beta-hemolytic streptococcus infection	Penicillin G, erythromycin, sulfadiazine
Meningococcus infection	Penicillin G, sulfonamide
Pneumococcus or streptococcus infections with decreased patient resistance	Penicillin G
Subacute bacterial endocarditis; dental extraction in presence of known valvular heart disease	Penicillin G, erythromycin, vancomycin
Gonorrhea	Penicillin G
Clostridial infections in traumatic wounds	Penicillin, tetracycline
Open-heart surgery	Penicillin G + methicillin
Positive tuberculin reactors on adrenal steroid therapy	Isoniazid
Pseudomonas aeruginosa infection	Polymyxin B and colistin
Congenital syphilis – treatment of the mother	Penicillin

Table 61. Antibiotic Combinations

Infection	Combination
Tuberculosis	Streptomycin-isoniazid-PAS
Bacterial endocarditis due to enterococci	Penicillin-streptomycin
Brain abscess	Penicillin-tetracycline
Klebsiella pneumonia	Cephalothin-kanamycin
Enterobacter pneumonia	Chloramphenicol-kanamycin
Anaerobic lung abscess	Penicillin-tetracycline
Bacteremia due to unknown agents especially in patients with decreased resistance	Cephalothin-kanamycin Cephalothin-kanamycin-polymyxin B Cephalothin-polymyxin B Penicillin G-chloramphenicol-polymyxin B
Mixed infection, e.g., during bowel surgery With streptococci and *E. coli* or *Klebsiella*	Penicillin-streptomycin or penicillin-kanamycin
With streptococci and *Bacteroides*	Penicillin-tetracycline or penicillin-chloramphenicol

RICKETTSIAL DISEASES

Weil-Felix reaction. See Table 62, p. 401.

Complement-fixation or agglutination tests are positive in most cases when group-specific and type-specific rickettsial antigens are used. These tests permit differentiation of various rickettsial diseases. No test is available for trench fever. Rising titer during convalescence is the most important criterion. Early antibiotic therapy may delay appearance of antibodies for additional 1–4 weeks, and titers may not be as high as when treatment is begun later.

Guinea pig inoculation—scrotal reaction following intraperitoneal injection of blood into male guinea pig

Marked in Rocky Mountain spotted fever and endemic typhus

Moderate in boutonneuse fever

Slight in epidemic typhus and Brill-Zinsser disease

Negative in scrub typhus, Q fever, trench fever, and rickettsial-pox

Test is not often used at present.

Microscopical examination of organisms following animal inoculation; test is not often used.

In less severe cases, blood findings are not distinctive.

In *severe cases,* the following changes are found:

Early in disease WBC is decreased and lymphocytes are increased (usually 4000–6000/cu mm; as low as 1200/cu mm in early scrub typhus). Later it increases to 10,000–15,000/cu mm with shift to the left and toxic granulation. If count is higher, rule out secondary bacterial infection or hemorrhage.

Mild normochromic normocytic anemia (as low as Hg = 9 gm/100 ml) appears around tenth day.

ESR is increased.

Total protein and serum albumin are decreased.

BUN may be increased (prerenal).

Serum chloride may be decreased.

Urine shows slight increase in albumin; granular casts.

CSF is normal despite symptoms of meningitis.

Blood cultures for bacteria are negative (to rule out other tickborne diseases, e.g., tularemia).

Laboratory findings due to specific organ involvement (e.g., pneumonitis, hepatitis) or due to complications (e.g., secondary bacterial infection, hemorrhage) are present.

Acute glomerulonephritis occurs in 78% of patients with epidemic typhus, 50% of patients with Rocky Mountain spotted fever, and 30% of patients with scrub typhus.

VIRAL PNEUMONIA DUE TO EATON AGENT (*MYCOPLASMA PNEUMONIAE*)

WBC is slightly increased (in one-fourth of cases) or normal.

ESR is increased in two-thirds of cases.

Increased cold agglutination occurs late in course in half the patients (up to 90% in severe illness).

Increased *Streptococcus* MG agglutination occurs in one-fourth of patients; higher titer in more severe illness.

Viral serologic tests

Show fourfold increase in titer in complement-fixation and hemagglutination tests

Fluorescent antibody test is useful.

UPPER RESPIRATORY VIRAL INFECTION

Due to rhinoviruses, ECHO viruses

WBC may be slightly increased.

ESR is increased in about one-third of patients.

Due to adenovirus

WBC is slightly decreased after about 7 days.

ESR is increased.

Due to respiratory syncytial virus

ESR may be increased in children

Due to parainfluenza virus

WBC is variable at first; later becomes normal or decreased.

Table 62. Weil-Felix Reaction

Disease	Rickettsia	Proteus OX-19	Proteus OX-2	Proteus OX-K	Comments
Spotted fevers Rocky Mountain spotted fever	R. rickettsii	1 to 4+	1 to 4+	0	
Boutonneuse fever	R. conorii	1 to 4+	2 to 3+	0	OX-19 is frequently positive only in low titer.
Other spotted fevers	E.g., R. australis, R. sibirica	1 to 4+	2 to 3+	0	
Rickettsialpox	R. akari	0	0	0	
Typhus Group Endemic (murine) typhus	R. mooseri	3 to 4+	Usually 0 or 1+	0	
Epidemic typhus	R. prowazekii	3 to 4+	Usually 0 or 1+	0	
Brill-Zinsser disease (recrudescent latent epidemic typhus)	R. prowazekii	Usually negative, or positive only in very low titer	0	0	
Scrub typhus	R. tsutsugamushi	0	0	3+	OX-K appears late in second week. Positive in about 1/2 of patients.
Q fever	R. burnetii	0	0	0	Usually pneumonitis. Icteric hepatitis in 1/3 of severe cases. Occasional cases of subacute endocarditis.
Trench fever	R. quintana	0	0	0	Can be grown on blood agar.

Weil-Felix reaction: Rise in titer by comparison of acute and later serum samples is most useful diagnostic procedure. Agglutinins appear in 5–8 days, reach peak in 1 month, then decrease to negative by 5–6 months. Reaction will not detect Q fever and rickettsialpox and is usually negative in Brill-Zinsser disease. May not differentiate epidemic and endemic typhus and spotted fever. Thus, is not useful for *early* diagnosis.

INFLUENZA

WBC is usually normal (5000–10,000/cu mm) with relative lymphocytosis. Leukopenia occurs in half the patients. WBC over 15,000/
cu mm suggests secondary bacterial infection.

Influenza virus antibody (hemagglutination inhibition, complement-
fixation) titer shows fourfold increase in sera taken during acute
phase and 2–3 weeks later.

PSITTACOSIS

WBC may be normal or decreased in acute phase and increases
during convalescence.

ESR is increased or frequently is normal.

Cold agglutination is negative.

Albuminuria is common.

Sputum smear and culture shows normal flora.

Viral serologic tests. Positive complement-fixation test in early stage
is presumptive but is not conclusive because of cross-reaction with
lymphogranuloma venereum and false positive in presence of
some other infections (e.g., brucellosis, Q fever). Rising complement-fixation titer is seen between acute-phase and convalescent-
phase sera.

COXSACKIE AND ECHO VIRUS INFECTIONS
**(e.g., epidemic pleurodynia, "grippe," meningitis, myocarditis, herpan-
gina, etc.)**

Laboratory findings are not specific.

CSF
>   Cell count is up to 500/cu mm, occasionally up to 2000/cu mm;
>   predominantly polynuclear leukocytes at first, then predomi-
>   nantly lymphocytes.
>   Protein may increase up to 100 mg/100 ml.
>   Glucose is normal.

WBC varies but is usually normal.

Viral serologic tests show increasing titer of neutralizing or complement-fixing antibodies between acute-phase and convalescent-
phase sera.

VIRAL GASTROENTEROCOLITIS
(especially ECHO virus)

Identified by exclusion by negative tests for other causes of the
symptoms (e.g., failure to find *Entamoeba histolytica*, *Shigella*,
Salmonella)

POLIOMYELITIS

CSF
>   Cell count is usually 25–500/cu mm; rarely is normal or up to
>   2000/cu mm. At first most are polynuclear leukocytes; after
>   several days most are lymphocytes.
>   Protein may be normal at first; later increased (usually 50–200
>   mg/100 ml).
>   Glucose is usually normal.

GOT is always increased but does not correlate with serum

GOT; reaches peak in 1 week and returns to normal by 4 weeks; level of GOT does not correlate with severity of paralysis.

CSF findings are not diagnostic but may occur in many CNS diseases due to viruses (e.g., Coxsackie, mumps, herpes), bacteria (e.g., pertussis, scarlet fever), other infections (e.g., leptospirosis, trichinosis, syphilis), CNS tumors, multiple sclerosis, etc.

Blood shows early moderate increase in WBC (up to 15,000/cu mm) and polynuclear leukocytes; normal within 1 week.

Laboratory findings of associated lesions (e.g., myocarditis) or complications (e.g., secondary bacterial infection, stone formation in GU tract, alterations in water and electrolyte balance due to continuous artificial respiration) are present. Increased SGOT in 50% of patients is due to the associated hepatitis.

Viral serologic tests show fourfold increase in neutralizing antibody titer between acute-phase and convalescent-phase (after 3 weeks) sera.

Virus may be cultured from stool up to early convalescence (done by U.S.P.H.S. Communicable Disease Center (CDC) at Chamblee, Georgia).

LYMPHOCYTIC CHORIOMENINGITIS

WBC is slightly decreased at first; normal with onset of meningitis.
CSF
> Cell count is increased (100–3000 lymphocytes/cu mm, occasionally up to 30,000).
> Protein is normal or slightly increased.
> Glucose is usually normal.

Viral serologic tests show increasing titer between acute-phase and convalescent-phase sera in complement-fixing (after 2 weeks) and neutralizing (after 6-8 weeks) antibodies.

Viral isolation by animal inoculation is not routinely performed.

EASTERN AND WESTERN EQUINE ENCEPHALOMYELITIS

Marked decrease occurs in WBC with relative lymphocytosis.
CSF findings. See Table 23, p. 202.

RABIES (HYDROPHOBIA)

WBC is increased (20,000–30,000/cu mm), with increased polynuclear leukocytes and large mononuclear cells.

Urine shows hyaline casts; reaction for albumin, sugar, and acetone may be positive.

CSF is usually normal or has a slight increase in protein and an increased number of mononuclear cells (usually less than 100/cu mm).

Brain of suspected animal shows Negri bodies (absent in more than 10% of animals with virus isolated from brain).

Suspected animal dies within 7–10 days.

ENCEPHALOMYELITIS (VIRAL AND POSTINFECTIOUS)

CSF
> Early (first 2–3 days)
>> Cell count is usually increased (up to 100/cu mm), mostly

polynuclear leukocytes (higher total count and more polynuclear leukocytes in infants).

Protein is usually normal.

Glucose and chloride are normal.

Later (after third day)

Increased cell count is more than 90% lymphocytes.

Protein gradually increases after first week (up to 100 mg/100 ml).

Glucose and chloride remain normal.

Viral serologic tests are for specific virus identification (fourfold increase from acute-phase sera to convalescent-phase sera in hemagglutination-inhibition, neutralization, or complement-fixation titers).

For additional laboratory tests see

Cytomegalic inclusion disease (following section)

Mumps (below)

Rabies (preceding section)

Psittacosis (p. 402)

Etc.

CYTOMEGALIC INCLUSION DISEASE
(limited to salivary gland involvement in 10% of infant autopsies; disseminated in 1–2% of childhood autopsies)

Intranuclear inclusions in epithelial cells in urine sediment and liver biopsy (more useful in infants than adults)

Hemolytic anemia with icterus and thrombocytopenic purpura in infants

Complement-fixation test on acute-phase and convalescent-phase sera

Evidence of damage to liver, kidney, brain

Laboratory findings due to predisposing or underlying conditions (e.g., malignant lymphoma, leukemia, refractory anemia, after renal transplant); may be associated with pneumocystis pneumonia in adults

May cause a syndrome of heterophil-negative infectious mononucleosis in immunologically competent adults characterized by

Normal or decreased WBC during first week followed by increase to 15,000–20,000/cu mm with 60–80% lymphocytes, many of which are Downey cell type

Slightly increased ESR

Rise in cold agglutinin titer (same as in heterophil-positive infectious mononucleosis)

Slight increase of SGOT and thymol; more marked with clinical hepatitis in some cases

Rise in complement-fixing titer in 2–3 weeks to levels of 1:64 to 1:256

Same syndrome may follow immunosuppressive drug therapy and multiple blood transfusions as in open-heart surgery, hemodialysis, etc.

MUMPS

Uncomplicated salivary adenitis

WBC and ESR are normal; WBC may be decreased, with relative lymphocytosis.

Serum amylase is increased.

Serum lipase is normal.

Serologic tests

> Serum neutralization test becomes positive by fifth day. It is the most reliable and specific index of immunity but also the most cumbersome and time-consuming.

> Complement-fixation test becomes positive during second week and remains elevated more than 6 weeks; paired sera showing a fourfold increase in titer confirm recent infection. High titer suggests recent infection. Test correlates well with neutralization test.

> Hemagglutination-inhibition reaction develops later and persists longer (several months) than complement-fixation test. It is possibly useful for screening only at high titers and is less sensitive and specific than neutralization.

Complications of mumps

> Orchitis (in one-fifth of postpubertal males)

>> WBC is increased, with shift to left. ESR is increased.

>> Sperm are decreased or absent after bilateral atrophy.

> Pancreatitis (p. 196). Serum amylase and lipase are increased. Patient may have hyperglycemia and glycosuria.

> Meningitis or meningoencephalitis (p. 202). Mumps causes more than 10% of cases of aseptic meningitis. The disease may be clinically identical with mild paralytic poliomyelitis. WBC is usually normal. Serum amylase may be increased even if no abdominal symptoms are present. CSF contains 0–2000 mononuclear cells.

> Thyroiditis, myocarditis, arthritis, etc.

MEASLES (RUBEOLA)

WBC shows slight increase at onset, then falls to about 5000/cu mm with increased lymphocyte count. Increased WBC with shift to the left suggests bacterial complication (e.g., otitis media, pneumonia, appendicitis).

Wright's stain of sputum or nasal scrapings shows measles multinucleated giant cells especially during prodrome and early rash.

Viral serologic tests. Neutralizing antibody, complement-fixation, and antihemagglutinating tests become positive one week after onset, evidencing infection.

Measles encephalitis. CSF may show slightly increased protein and up to 500 mononuclear cells/cu mm.

Measles may cause remission in children with nephrosis.

RUBELLA (GERMAN MEASLES)

It is important to identify exposure to rubella infection and susceptibility status in pregnant women because infection in the first trimester of pregnancy is associated with congenital abnormalities, abortion, or stillbirth in about 30% of patients; during first month, up to 80% of patients show this association.

Viral serologic tests: hemagglutination inhibition (HAI), complement-fixation, neutralization

Screening of pregnant women shows lack of susceptibility (i.e., previous rubella infection) if HAI titer is more than 1:10–1:20 or if complement-fixation test is positive.

Change in HAI titer from acute-phase to convalescent-phase sera is the most useful technique to demonstrate a rise in antibody titer.

With rubella rash, diagnosis is established if acute sample titer is more than 1:10 or if convalescent-phase serum taken 7 days after rash shows a fourfold increase in titer.

If no rash develops in a patient exposed to rubella, a convalescent-phase serum specimen taken 14–28 days after exposure that shows a fourfold increase in titer compared to the earlier sample indicates rubella infection.

Complement-fixation antibodies appear early (within 1 week after rash); therefore acute-phase serum must be collected promptly or the rise in titer may not be detected. They may last for from 8 months up to some years. A positive test is useful to indicate recent infection or postinfection immunity. Rate of false positive test is less than 2%.

Neutralization antibodies appear within 1–3 days after rash and reach maximum in 2 weeks, and test may remain positive for more than 20 years; titer of 1:8 or more indicates past infection and therefore present immunity. A titer of 1:32 suggests recent infection. In infants with congenital abnormalities, a high neutralization antibody titer establishes the diagnosis. Test is technically difficult to perform and requires 7–10 days.

WBC is inconstantly decreased before the rash; during the rash, lymphocytes are increased, and some of them may be abnormal.

Decreased platelet count may be marked.

EXANTHEMA SUBITUM (ROSEOLA INFANTUM)

WBC is increased during fever, then decreased during rash.

ERYTHEMA INFECTIOSUM (FIFTH DISEASE)

WBC is normal. Some patients have slight increase in eosinophils.

CHICKENPOX (VARICELLA)

Microscopical demonstration of very large giant epithelial cells with intranuclear inclusion in fluid or base of vesicle

(*Similar giant cells may occur in herpes simplex and herpes zoster.*)

WBC is normal; increased with secondary bacterial infection.

Serum electrophoresis may show decreased albumin with increased beta and gamma globulin.

SMALLPOX (VARIOLA)

Microscopical finding of elementary bodies (Guarnieri bodies) in skin lesions

Fluorescent antibody staining of virus from skin lesion

Viral serologic tests

Increased titer of neutralizing antibody in acute-phase and convalescent-phase (2–3 weeks later) sera

Rapid technique using vesicular fluid in hemagglutination, precipitation, or complement-fixation tests

WBC decreased during prodrome, increased during pustular rash

VACCINIA
(vaccine virus skin infection during vaccination against smallpox)

Guarnieri bodies (cytoplasmic inclusions) in skin lesions

Complications

> Progressive vaccinia. *Rule out malignant lymphoma, chronic lymphatic leukemia, neoplasms, hypogammaglobulinemia, and dysgammaglobulinemia.*
> Superimposed infection (e.g., tetanus)
> Postvaccinal encephalitis

HERPES SIMPLEX

WBC normal

Intranuclear inclusions in cells in skin lesions or vesicle fluid

Findings of encephalitis if this complication occurs

HERPES ZOSTER (SHINGLES)
(reactivation of latent varicella virus)

Skin lesions may show intranuclear inclusions in degenerated epithelial cells or multinucleated giant cells.

Forty percent of patients show increased cells (up to 300 mononuclear/cu mm) in CSF.

LYMPHOGRANULOMA VENEREUM

WBC is normal or increased up to 20,000/cu mm. There may be relative lymphocytosis or monocytosis.

ESR is increased.

Slight anemia may be present.

Serum globulin is increased with reversed A/G ratio during period of activity.

Biologically false positive reaction for syphilis appears in one-fifth of patients which becomes negative in a few weeks. *If titer increases, beware of concomitant syphilitic infection.*

Biopsy of regional lymph node shows stellate abscesses.

High complement-fixation titer (more than 1:80) and increasing titers or conversion of negative to positive indicate recent infections. Fall in titer evidences therapeutic success in acute stage. Persistent negative in the presence of disease is rare.

CAT-SCRATCH DISEASE

Microscopical examination of excised lymph node should be done.

Culture of involved lymph nodes is sterile.

ESR is usually increased.

WBC is usually normal but occasionally is increased up to 13,000/cu mm; eosinophils may be increased.

Frei test is negative.
Skin test with cat-scratch antigen is positive.

YELLOW FEVER

Decreased WBC is most marked by sixth day, associated with decreased leukocytes and lymphocytes.
Proteinuria occurs in severe cases.
Laboratory findings are those due to GI hemorrhage, which is frequent; there may be associated oliguria and anuria.
Liver function tests are abnormal, but serum bilirubin is only slightly increased.
Biopsy of liver is taken for histologic examination.
Serum is positive by intracerebral mouse inoculation up to the fifth day; serum during convalescence protects mice.

DENGUE

WBC decreased (2000–5000/cu mm) with toxic granulation of leukocytes in early stage; often increased during convalescence
Children commonly have decreased platelets.

VIRAL EPIDEMIC HEMORRHAGIC FEVER

WBC is increased, with shift to the left.
Platelet count is decreased (less than 100,000/cu mm) in half of the patients.
Laboratory findings due to renal damage
 Proteinuria
 Oliguria with azotemia and hemoconcentration and abnormal electrolyte concentrations

 Return of normal tubular function may take 4–6 weeks.

Other viral hemorrhagic fevers (e.g., Philippine, Thailand, Singapore, Argentinian, Bolivian, Crimean, Omsk, Kyasanur Forest) show much less severe renal damage and WBC is normal (Philippine, Thailand) or decreased.

COLORADO TICK FEVER

WBC is decreased (2000–4000/cu mm). The number of polynuclear leukocytes is decreased, but with shift to the left.
Viral serologic tests show an increase in complement-fixation and neutralizing antibodies in sera taken during acute and convalescent phases.
Blood should be inoculated into suckling mice.

PHLEBOTOMUS FEVER (SANDFLY FEVER)

Decreased WBC and lymphocytes with shift to the left of polynuclear leukocytes are most marked when fever ends.
CSF is normal.
Liver function tests are normal.
Urine is normal.

CRYPTOCOCCOSIS
(due to *Cryptococcus neoformans*)

Serologic tests

> Latex slide agglutination on serum and spinal fluid detects specific cryptococcal *antigen*. Use for screening of suspected cryptococcosis, since it is more sensitive than India ink smears of spinal fluid. Serum or cerebrospinal fluid is positive in most cases; when negative, agglutination test may be positive.

> Use whole yeast cell agglutination test for presence of *antibodies* in serum and cerebrospinal fluid. It is positive only in early CNS disease or no CNS involvement, may become positive only after institution of therapy. Rising titer may be a favorable prognostic sign.

Culture of cerebrospinal fluid for *Cryptococcus neoformans* on Sabouraud's medium becomes positive in 1–2 weeks (positive in 97%) followed by mouse inoculation. One may also get a positive culture from blood (25%), urine (37%), stool (20%), sputum (19%), and bone marrow (13%).

India ink slide of cerebrospinal fluid is positive in about half the cases.

Cerebrospinal fluid cell count is almost always increased up to 800 cells (more lymphocytes than leukocytes). Protein is increased in 90% (up to 500 mg/100 ml). Sugar is moderately decreased in about 55% of patients. Relapse is less frequent when increase in protein and cells is marked rather than moderate.

In biopsy material, mucicarmine stain is positive; it is also positive on intraperitoneal injection of white mice.

There is evidence of coexisting disease in about half the patients (especially diabetes mellitus, Hodgkin's, prior steroid therapy, lymphosarcoma, leukemia).

COCCIDIOIDOMYCOSIS
(due to *Coccidioides immitis*)

Serologic tests

> Precipitin antibodies appear early, decrease after the third week, are uncommon after the fifth month. They occur at some stage of the disease in three-quarters of the patients and usually indicate early infection. In primary infection, they are the only demonstrable antibodies in 40% of cases. If tests are negative, repeat at intervals of 1–2 weeks 3 times. *Beware of occasional cross-reaction with primary histoplasmosis and cutaneous blastomycosis.*

> Complement-fixing antibodies appear later (positive in 10% of cases in first week), and the number rises with increasing severity. Antibodies decrease after 4–8 months but may remain positive for years. The titer is useful for following the course of the disease; a titer greater than 1:16 suggests dissemination; a fall in titer suggests effective therapy. Less than a third of cases are positive in the first month; most positive reactions occur between the fourth and fifth weeks. The antibodies are usually present in disseminated disease.

> Latex particle agglutination test shows 6% false positive reactions. Chief value is for screening purposes for detection of precipitin antibodies. A positive result should be confirmed

with complement-fixation and precipitin antibody tests. A negative test does not rule out coccidioidomycosis.

Agar immunodiffusion test parallels latex particle agglutination test but is somewhat less sensitive. Its chief value is for screening purposes.

Smear (wet preparation in 20% KOH) and culture are taken from sputum, gastric contents, cerebrospinal fluid, exudate, skin scrapings, etc., on Sabouraud's medium or intraperitoneal injection of mice.

Biopsy of skin lesions and affected lymph nodes is made.

Cerebrospinal fluid in meningitis shows 100–200 WBC/cu mm (mostly mononuclear), increased protein, frequently decreased glucose.

Eosinophilia is up to 35%; over 10% in one-fourth of patients.

WBC and ESR are increased.

HISTOPLASMOSIS
(due to *Histoplasma capsulatum*)

Culture is made (may be difficult) of skin and mucosal lesions, sputum, gastric washings, blood, bone marrow (Sabouraud's medium at room temperature; blood agar at 37°C not specific). Mouse inoculation, especially from sputum, may give a positive subculture from spleen on Sabouraud's in 1 month. A positive skin test can cause conversion of serologic titers within 1 week.

Complement-fixation titers are positive in 90% of chronic cases and in 50% of acute pulmonary cases. Positive titers persist for months or years if disease remains active. They appear during the third to sixth week. A low titer in known cases may indicate a poor prognosis. Titers may be negative in severe disease.

Latex agglutination titers become positive in 2–3 weeks and revert to negative in 5–8 months even with persistent disease. There are few false positives. A titer of 1:32 or more indicates active or very recent disease.

Biopsy is made of skin and mucosal lesions, bone marrow, reticuloendothelial system.

Anemia and leukopenia are nonspecific.

ACTINOMYCOSIS
(due to *Actinomyces israelii*)

Recognition of organism in material (e.g., sinus tracts, abscess cavities, empyema fluid; *may be found normally in sputum*) from sites of involvement (especially jaw, lung, cecum)

Sulfur granules show gram-positive bacilli or filaments.

No growth is seen on Sabouraud's medium.

Anaerobic growth on blood agar shows small colonies after 4–6 days.

Animal inoculation is negative.

Anaerobic culture methods (e.g., Brewer's thioglycollate medium) are positive.

Histologic examination is suggestive; the diagnosis may be confirmed if a "ray fungus" is seen.

Serologic tests are not useful.

WBC is normal or slightly increased (to 14,000/cu mm); high WBC indicates secondary infection.

ESR is usually increased.

Normocytic normochromic anemia is mild to moderate.

Table 63. Summary of Laboratory Findings in Fungus Infections

Disease	Causative Organism	Source of Material												Diagnostic Methods							
														Microscopical Examination				Serologic Tests			
		Blood	Cerebrospinal Fluid	Stool	Urine	Nasopharynx, Throat	Sputum, Lung	Gastric Washings	Vagina, Cervix	Exudates, Lesions, Sinus Tracts, Etc.	Skin, Nails, Hair	Bone Marrow	Lymph Node	Fresh Unstained Material	Stained Material	Culture	Animal Inoculation	Complement-Fixation	Agglutination	Precipitin	Histologic Examination
Cryptococcosis	*Cryptococcus neoformans*	+	+	+	+		+				+	+		+	+	+	+		+		+
Coccidioidomycosis	*Coccidioides immitis*		+		+		+	+			+			+	+	+	+	+		+	+
Histoplasmosis	*Histoplasma capsulatum*	+					+	+			+	+	+			+	+	+		+	+
Actinomycosis	*Actinomyces israelii*									+				+	+	+					+
Nocardiosis	*Nocardia asteroides*						+			+				+	+	+	+				+
North American blastomycosis	*Blastomyces dermatitidis*						+			+	+		+	+		+	+	+			+

Continued on next page

[411]

Table 63 (continued)

Disease	Causative Organism	Blood	Cerebrospinal Fluid	Stool	Urine	Nasopharynx, Throat	Sputum, Lung	Gastric Washings	Vagina, Cervix	Exudates, Lesions, Sinus Tracts, Etc.	Skin, Nails, Hair	Bone Marrow	Lymph Node	Fresh Unstained Material	Stained Material	Culture	Animal Inoculation	Complement-Fixation	Agglutination	Precipitin	Histologic Examination
														Microscopical Examination				Serologic Tests			
South American blastomycosis	*Paracoccidioides brasiliensis*	+				+					+		+	+		+		+			+
Moniliasis	*Candida albicans*					+			+		+				+	+					+
Aspergillosis	*Aspergillus fumigatus*, others						+							+		+					+
Geotrichosis	*Geotrichum candidum*						+									+					+
Chromoblastomycosis	*Phialophora pedrosi, compactum*, etc.										+			+		+					+
Sporotrichosis	*Sporotrichum schenckii*									+						+	+	+	+	+	+
Rhinosporidiosis	*Rhinosporidium seeberi*					+															+

[412]

NOCARDIOSIS
(due to *Nocardia asterides*)

Clinical types
  Lung abscess; metastatic brain abscesses in one-third of patients
  Maduromycosis
Recognition of organism
  Direct smear—gram-positive and acid-fast (*may be over-decolorized by Ziehl-Neelsen stain for tubercle bacilli*)
  Positive culture on Sabouraud's media and blood agar (*Beware of inactivation by concentration technique for tubercle bacillus.*)
  Positive guinea pig inoculation

May be saprophytic in sputum or gastric juice.

Rule out underlying pulmonary alveolar proteinosis, Cushing's syndrome.

BLASTOMYCOSIS
(North American due to *Blastomyces dermatitidis*; South American due to *Paracoccidioides brasiliensis*)

Clinical types
  South American—involvement of nasopharynx, lymph nodes, cecum
  North American—involvement of skin and lungs
  Later, visceral involvement may occur in both types.
Recognition of organism in material (e.g., pus, sputum, biopsied tissue)
  Wet smear preparation in 20% KOH
  Positive culture on Sabouraud's medium at room temperature and blood agar at 37°C; slow growth of *P. brasiliensis* on blood agar up to 1 month
  Negative animal inoculation
Complement-fixation test is positive in high titer with systemic infection.
WBC and ESR are increased.
Serum globulin is slightly increased.
Mild normochromic anemia is present.
Alkaline phosphatase may be increased with bone lesions.

MONILIASIS
(due to *Candida albicans*)

Positive culture on Sabouraud's medium and on direct examination of suspected material

In vaginitis, rule out underlying diabetes mellitus.
In skin and nail involvement in children, rule out congenital hypoparathyroidism.
In septicemia with endocarditis, rule out narcotic addiction.
In GI tract overgrowth, rule out chemotherapy suppression of normal bacterial flora.
Positive blood culture is rare: rule out serious underlying disease (e.g., malignant lymphoma), multiple therapeutic antibiotics, and plastic intravenous catheters.

Table 64. Summary of Laboratory Findings in Protozoan Diseases

Disease	Causative Organism	Source of Material										Diagnostic Procedures								Other Significant Laboratory Abnormalities									
		Blood	Cerebrospinal Fluid	Stool	Urine	Vagina	Urethra	Exudates, Ulcers, Skin Lesions	Bone Marrow	Spleen	Lymph Node Aspirate	Fresh Unstained Material	Stained Material	Culture	Animal Inoculation	Xenodiagnosis	Complement-Fixation	Others	Histologic Examination	Anemia	WBC Decreased	Monocytosis	Serum Globulin Increased	Cerebrospinal Fluid Abnormalities	Renal Function Abnormalities	Liver Function Abnormalities	Skeletal Muscle Abnormalities	Cardiac Abnormalities	Others
Malaria	Plasmodium species	+											+					+	+	+	+	+	+	+	+	+			
Trypanosomiasis																													
Acute sleeping sickness	T. rhodesiense	+	+						+		+		+	rare	+					+		+	+	+					
Chronic sleeping sickness	T. gambiense	+	+						+		+		+	rare	+		+			+		+	+	+					
Chagas' disease	T. cruzi	+											+	+		+	+		*					+			+	+	
Leishmaniasis																													
Kala-azar	L. donovani	+							+	+	+		+	+				+		+			+						
American mucocutaneous	L. braziliensis							+					+	+						+					+				
Oriental sore	L. tropica							+					+	+															
Toxoplasmosis	T. gondii	+									+		+		+		+	†	‡				+					+	

			§
Interstitial plasma cell pneumonia	Pneumocystis carinii		+
Amebiasis	Entamoeba histolytica	+	+ + ||
Giardiasis	G. lamblia	+#	+
Balantidiasis	B. coli	+	+
Coccidiosis	Isospora hominis or belli	+	+
Trichomoniasis	T. vaginalis	+ + +	

• Liver, lymph node; † hemaglutination Sabin-Feldman dye test; ‡lymph node, muscle; §special stains; ||rectum; #also duodenal washings

ASPERGILLOSIS
(due to *Aspergillus fumigatus* and other species)

Recognition of organism in material (especially sputum) from sites
of involvement (especially lung; also brain, sinuses, orbit, ear)
Positive culture on most media at room temperature or 35° C.

*Organisms occur as saprophytes in sputum and mouth. Confirm by
staining organisms in biopsy specimens.*

Laboratory findings due to underlying or primary disease
Superimposed on lung cavities caused by tuberculosis, bronchiectasis, carcinoma
Underlying disease (e.g., malignant lymphoma, irradiation,
steroid and antibiotic therapy)

GEOTRICHOSIS
(due to *Geotrichum candidum*)

Recognition of organisms from material (sputum) from sites of
involvement (respiratory tract; possibly colon)
Positive culture on Sabouraud's medium (room temperature).
Organisms occur as saprophytes in pharynx and colon.
Visualization of organisms in biopsy material

CHROMOBLASTOMYCOSIS
(due to *Phialophora pedrosi, P. compactum, etc.*)

Recognition of organism from sites of involvement (usually skin;
rarely brain abscess)
Wet smear preparation in 10% KOH
Positive culture on Sabouraud's medium (slow growth)
Biopsy of tissue

SPOROTRICHOSIS
(due to *Sporotrichum schenckii*)

Recognition of organism in skin pus or biopsy
Positive culture on Sabouraud's medium from unbroken pus-
tule. Intraperitoneal mouse inoculation of these colonies or of
fresh pus produces organism-containing lesions.
Direct examination is usually negative.
Serum agglutinins, precipitins, and complement-fixation (titer of
1:16 or higher) antibodies can be demonstrated in extracutaneous
disease (e.g., pulmonary, disseminated).

RHINOSPORIDIOSIS
(due to *Rhinosporidium seeberi*)

Recognition of organism in biopsy material from polypoid lesions of
nasopharynx or eye (*cannot be cultured*)

MUCORMYCOSIS
(due to *Mucorales fungi*)

Clinical types
Cranial (acute diffuse cerebrovascular disease and ophthalmo-
plegia in uncontrolled diabetes mellitus with acidosis)

Pulmonary (findings due to pulmonary infarction)

In abdominal blood vessels (findings due to hemorrhagic infarction of ileum or colon)

Mycologic cultures from brain and spinal fluid are negative; may be positive from infected nasal sinuses or turbinate.

Laboratory findings of underlying disease (e.g., diabetes mellitus with acidosis, leukemia, irradiation or cytotoxic drugs, uremic acidosis) are present.

Laboratory findings due to complications (e.g., visceral infarcts) are present.

MALARIA
(due to *Plasmodium vivax, P. malariae, P. falciparum, P. ovale*)

Identification of organism is made in thin or thick smears of peripheral blood or bone marrow.

Anemia (average 2.5 million RBC/cu mm in chronic cases) is usually hypochromic; may be macrocytic in severe chronic disease. Reticulocyte count is increased.

Monocytes are increased in peripheral blood; there may be pigment in large mononuclear cells occasionally.

WBC is decreased.

There is increased serum indirect bilirubin and other evidence of hemolysis.

Bone marrow shows erythroid hyperplasia, RBCs containing organisms, and pigment in RE cells. Marrow hyperplasia may fail in chronic phase. Agranulocytosis and purpura may occur late.

Serum globulin is increased (especially euglobulin fraction); albumin decreased.

ESR is increased.

Biologic false positive test of syphilis is frequent.

Osmotic fragility of RBCs is normal.

Acute hemorrhagic nephritis due to *P. malariae*

Albuminuria

Hematuria

Blackwater fever (massive intravascular hemolysis) due to *P. falciparum*

Severe acute hemolytic anemia (1–2 million RBCs/cu mm) with increased bilirubin, hemoglobinuria, etc.

May be associated with acute tubular necrosis with hemoglobin casts, azotemia, oliguria to anuria, etc.

Parasites absent from blood

Laboratory findings due to involvement of organs

Liver—vary from congestion to fatty changes to malarial hepatitis or central necrosis; moderate increase in SGOT, SGPT, and alkaline phosphatase

Pigment stones in gallbladder

Cerebral malaria

Serologic tests (performed in special reference laboratories, e.g., CDC, Atlanta, Ga.)

Indirect fluorescent antibody test shows high sensitivity and specificity and is useful for diagnostic purposes.

Indirect hemagglutination can detect antibody many years after infection and is useful for prevalence studies.

TRYPANOSOMIASIS

Sleeping sickness
> Acute (Rhodesian) due to *Trypanosoma rhodesiense*
> Chronic (Gambian) due to *T. gambiense*
>> Identification of organism in appropriate material (blood, bone marrow, lymph node aspirate, cerebrospinal fluid) by thick or thin smears or concentrations, animal inoculation, rarely culture
>> Anemia
>> Increased serum globulin producing increased ESR, positive flocculation tests, etc.
>> Increased monocytes in peripheral blood
>> Cerebrospinal fluid
>>> Increased number of cells (mononuclear type)
>>> Increased protein (use as index to severity of disease and to therapeutic response)
>> Complement-fixation test specific for *T. gambiense*

Chagas' disease (American trypanosomiasis) due to *T. cruzi*
> Identification of organism
>> Blood concentration technique during acute stage
>> Biopsy of lymph node or liver (shows leishmanial forms)
>> Culture on blood broth at 28°C from lymph node aspirate
>> Xenodiagnosis (laboratory-bred bug fed on patient develops trypanosomes in gut in 2 weeks)
> Complement-fixation test positive in half of acute cases; specific and positive in over 90% of chronic cases. In the acute infection the indirect hemagglutination test is more reliable.
> Laboratory findings due to organ involvement (e.g., heart, central nervous system, skeletal muscle)

LEISHMANIASIS

Kala-azar (due to *L. donovani*)
> Organism identified in stained smears from spleen, bone marrow, peripheral blood, liver biopsy, lymph node aspirate
> Culture (incubate at 28°C) from same sources
> Complement-fixation test usually positive but also positive in tuberculosis
> Anemia
> Leukopenia
> Thrombocytopenia
> Increased serum globulin with decreased albumin and reversed A/G ratio
> Increased ESR, abnormal cephalin flocculation, etc., due to increased serum globulin
> Frequent urine changes
>> Proteinuria
>> Hematuria
> Laboratory findings due to amyloidosis in chronic cases

American mucocutaneous leishmaniasis (due to *L. braziliensis*)
> Organisms identified by direct microscopy, culture, or histologic examination in scrapings from lesions
> Anemia sometimes present

Oriental sore (cutaneous leishmaniasis) (due to *L. tropica*)
> Organisms identified by direct microscopy and culture in scrapings from lesion

TOXOPLASMOSIS
(due to *T. gondii*)

Recognition of organism in appropriate material (cerebrospinal fluid, lymph node, muscle)
> Smears stained with Wright's or Giemsa stain
> Mouse inoculation
> Histologic examination of tissue (e.g., lymph node, muscle)

Serologic tests are sensitive and specific except for false positive indirect fluorescent antibody tests in patients with antinuclear antibodies. See Table 64a, p. 420.

Adult patients
> WBC varies from leukopenia to leukemoid reaction; atypical lymphocytes may be found.
> Anemia is present.
> Serum gamma globulins are increased.
> Heterophil agglutination is negative.
> Laboratory findings are those due to involvement of various organ systems.
>> Lymph node shows marked hyperplasia associated with identification of organism or concomitant malignant lymphoma.
>> Central nervous system shows CSF changes and identification of organism in smear of sediment.

PNEUMOCYSTIS PNEUMONIA
(due to *Pneumocystis carinii*)

There are no specific laboratory tests.

No culture techniques are available.

No serologic techniques are available.

Lung biopsy is necessary to make a definite diagnosis. The organism is rarely found in sputum or bronchial washings.

Organisms are found in postmortem histologic preparations. The morphology of the lung lesions suggests the diagnosis. *Organism does not stain with routine H & E stains; requires special stains (e.g., Giemsa, Schiff).*

Laboratory findings are those of associated diseases (especially cytomegalic inclusion disease) or of underlying diseases (malignant lymphoma, leukemia, tuberculosis, cryptococcosis; premature or debilitated infants; immunoglobulin defects), administration of cytotoxic drugs and corticosteriods. These are present in one-fourth of patients who die after renal transplant.

AMEBIASIS
(due to *Entamoeba histolytica*)

Microscopical examination of stool for *E. histolytica*. (*Beware of interfering substances in feces, e.g., bismuth, kaolin, barium sulfate, enema solutions of soap or hypertonic salt, antacids and laxatives, sulfonamides, antibiotic and antiprotozoal and antihelmintic agents.*)

Biopsy of rectum for *E. histolytica*

Serologic tests
> Indirect hemagglutination test is sensitive and specific; associated with current or previous infection. A negative test is unlikely if amebic infection (especially hepatic) is present. Significant titer is 1:128 or more.

Continued on page 421.

Table 64a. Serologic Tests for Toxoplasmosis

Test	Titer Indicating Possible Recent Infection*	Titer Strongly Suggests Recent or Present Infection†	Time of Rise of Titer	Duration of Rise of Titer
Sabin-Feldman dye	256	4096	Earliest 10–28 days	Indefinite 20–30 years
Complement fixation	8	32	14–28 days	Short-lived 2–4 years
Indirect fluorescent antibody	256	4096	Earliest 10–28 days	Indefinite 20–30 years
Indirect hemagglutination	256	4096	14–28 days	Indefinite 20–30 years

*Titer present in up to 10% of apparently healthy individuals. Therefore, perform serial titers at weekly intervals.
†Titers present in less than 1% of apparently healthy individuals.

Indirect fluorescent antibody test gives results comparable to Sabin-Feldman dye test but has greater laboratory ease of performance and safety.

Indirect hemagglutination and complement-fixation tests may be negative in congenital toxoplasmosis and therefore are not recommended in this condition.

Sabin-Feldman dye and indirect fluorescent antibody test titers are usually the same in the newborn and in the mother for the first 30 days of the infant's life. In diagnosis of congenital toxoplasmosis, these tests are useful when a persistently elevated or rising titer is found in the infant 2–3 months after birth.

Presence of antibodies before pregnancy probably assures protection against congenital toxoplasmosis in the child.

Complement-fixation test is usually positive only during active (especially hepatic) disease. Usually reverts to normal 6 months after cure. Significant titer is 1:16 or more.

Agar-gel diffusion test parallels complement-fixation test.

Height of titer above significant levels or changing titers are not clinically significant.

Liver abscess
Liver scanning
Leukocytosis
Increased ESR
Animal inoculation of liver biopsy
See chapter on liver disease, p. 177.

GIARDIASIS
(due to *Giardia lamblia*)

Recognition of organism is achieved in stools or duodenal washings stained with iodine. Chronic infection may cause malabsorption syndrome.

BALANTIDIASIS
(due to *Balantidium coli*)

Recognition of organisms in stool (*Intermittent appearance requires repeated examinations.*)

COCCIDIOSIS
(due to *Isospora hominis* or *I. belli*)

Recognition of organism in $ZnSO_4$-concentrated stool specimens

TRICHOMONIASIS
(due to *Trichomonas vaginalis*)

Recognition of organism in material from vagina (occasionally from male urethra)
Hanging-drop preparation of vaginal fluid freshly examined frequently found in routine urinalysis frequently found in routine Papanicolaou smears. *The organism is often not identified but may be associated with characteristic concomitant cytologic changes.*

ASCARIASIS
(due to *Ascaris lumbricoides*)

Stools contain ova.
Eosinophils are increased during symptomatic phase, especially pulmonary phase.

TRICHURIASIS
(due to whipworm—*Trichuris trichiura*)

Stools contain ova.
Increased eosinophils, leukocytosis, and anemia may be present.

PINWORM INFECTION
(due to *Enterobius vermicularis*)

Ova and occasionally adults are found on Scotch tape swab of perianal region. *Swab should be taken on first arising early in morning.*

Stool is usually negative for ova and adults.
Eosinophil count is usually normal.

VISCERAL LARVA MIGRANS
(due to *Toxocara canis* or *T. cati*)

WBC is increased; increased eosinophils are vacuolated and contain
  fewer than normal granules.
Serum gamma globulin is increased.
Indirect hemagglutination and bentonite flocculation tests may be
  insensitive and nonspecific.
Disease may cause Loeffler's syndrome.

Table 65. Identification of Parasites

Organism	Stool	Other Body Sites
Nematodes		
Ascaris lumbricoides	O, A	Rarely, L in sputum early
Trichuris trichiura	O	
Enterobius vermicularis	Usually neg.; A after enema	Scotch tape, perianal region – O and A
Strongyloides stercoralis	L	Occasional L in sputum and duodenal contents
Ancylostoma duodenale	O, rarely L	
Necator americanus	O, rarely L	
Trichinella spiralis	Occasionally A and/or L	
Wuchereria bancrofti or *W. malayi*	None	Microfilariae in blood
Loa loa	None	Microfilariae in blood; adult under conjunctiva
Onchocerca volvulus	None	Adult in subcutaneous nodules
Dracunculus medinensis	None	L in fluid from ulcer
Cestodes		
Taenia solium	G, O, S; A after treatment	
Taenia saginata	G, O, S	Scotch tape, perianal region – O
Hymenolepis nana, H. diminuta	O	
Diphyllobothrium latum	O	
Echinococcus multilocularis	Not found	Histologic examination of biopsy specimen
Trematodes		
Schistosoma mansoni, S. japonicum	O	See pp. 424–425
Clonorchis sinensis	O	O in duodenal contents
Opisthorchis felineus	O	O in duodenal contents
Paragonimus westermani	O	O in sputum
Fasciola hepatica	O	
Fasciolopsis buski	O, occasionally A	

O = ova; A = adult; L = larvae; G = gravid segments; S = scolex.

TRICHOSTRONGYLOSIS
(due to *Trichostrongylus* species)

Stools contain ova. *Usually a concentration technique is required; worm may be mistaken for hookworm.*

There is an increase in WBC and eosinophils (up to 75%) when patient is symptomatic.

STRONGYLOIDIASIS
(due to *Strongyloides stercoralis)*

Stools contain larvae. Larvae may also be found in duodenal washings. Larvae appear in sputum with pulmonary involvement.

Increase in eosinophils and leukocytosis is common.

HOOKWORM DISEASE
(due to *Necator americanus* or *Ancylostoma duodenale*)

WBC is normal or slightly increased, with 15–30% eosinophils; in early cases up to 75% eosinophils.

Anemia due to blood loss is hypochromic microcytic. When anemia is more severe, eosinophilia is less prominent.

Stools contain hookworm ova. Stools are usually positive for occult blood. Charcot-Leyden crystals are present in more than half the cases.

Laboratory findings are those due to frequently associated diseases (e.g., malaria, beriberi)

TRICHINOSIS
(due to *Trichinella spiralis)*

Eosinophilia appears with values of up to 85% on differential count and 15,000/cu mm on absolute count. It occurs about 1 week after the eating of infected food and reaches maximum after third week. It usually subsides in 4–6 weeks but may last up to 6 months and occasionally for years. Occasionally it is absent; usually absent in fatal infections.

Stool may contain adults and larvae *only* during the first 1–2 weeks after infection (during the stage of enteritis and invasion).

Identification of larvae is made in suspected meat by acid-pepsin digestion followed by microscopical examination.

Muscle biopsy may show the encysted larvae beginning 10 days after ingestion. Direct microscopical examination of compressed specimen is superior to routine histologic preparation.

Serologic tests become positive 1 week after onset of symptoms in only 20–30% of patients and reach a peak of 80–90% of patients by fourth to fifth week. Rise in titer in acute- and convalescent-phase sera is diagnostic. Titers may remain negative in overwhelming infection, may remain positive for more than 2 years. False positive results may occur in polyarteritis nodosa, serum sickness, penicillin sensitivity, infectious mononucleosis, malignant lymphomas, and leukemia.

> *Trichinella* complement-fixation test becomes positive about 2 weeks after occurrence of eosinophilia. It may remain positive for 6 months.

> Bentonite flocculation test may remain strongly positive for 6 months; less strongly positive for another 6 months.

> Precipitin tests are also used.

Decrease in serum total protein and albumin occurs in severe cases between 2 and 4 weeks and may last for years.

Increased (relative and absolute) gamma globulins parallel titer of serologic tests and of thymol turbidity. The increase occurs between 5 and 8 weeks and may last 6 months or more.

ESR is normal or only slightly increased.

BSP is usually normal.

Decreased serum cholinesterase often lasts 6 months.

Some serum enzymes may be increased (e.g., aldolase).

Urine may show albuminuria with hyaline and granular casts in severe cases.

Cerebrospinal fluid. With meningoencephalitis, CSF may be normal or up to 300 lymphocytes/cu mm with increased protein.

FILARIASIS
(due to *Wuchereria bancrofti* or *W. malayi*)

Microfilariae appear in peripheral blood smear (Wright's or Giemsa stain) or wet preparation.

Eosinophils are increased.

Biopsy of lymph node may contain adult worms.

Complement-fixation test may not be reliable.

TAPEWORM INFESTATION

Due to *Taenia saginata* (beef tapeworm)
>In stool, ova cannot be distinguished from those of *T. solium.* Proglottids establish diagnosis. Stool examination is positive in one-half to three-quarters of cases.
>Scotch tape swab of perianal region is positive in up to 95% of cases.
>Eosinophils may be slightly increased.

Due to *Taenia solium* (pork tapeworm)
>Stool and Scotch tape swab of perianal region are examined.
>Eosinophils may be slightly increased.
>Cerebrospinal fluid may show increased eosinophils with cysticercal meningoencephalitis.

Due to *Hymenolepis nana* (dwarf tapeworm)
>Stool shows ova, occasionally proglottids, etc.

Due to *Diphyllobothrium latum* (fish tapeworm)
>Stool shows ova.
>Macrocytic anemia (see p. 243) occurs when worm is in proximal small intestine.

Due to *Echinococcus granulosus* (*multilocularis*)
>Cystic lesion appears, especially in liver (see Metastatic or Infiltrative Disease of Liver, p. 188).
>Identification of scolices and hooklets is made in cyst fluid and histologic examination.
>Eosinophils are occasionally increased.
>Stool examination is not helpful.

SCHISTOSOMIASIS
(due to *Schistosoma mansoni, S. japonicum, S. haematobium*)

Acute
>Eosinophilia occurs.
>ESR is increased.
>Serum globulin is increased.
>Cephalin flocculation is positive.

Chronic

Ova appear in stools.

Unstained rectal mucosa examined microscopically may show living or dead ova when stools are negative.

Serologic tests are particularly useful for chronic infections when stools contain no ova; they are not useful to assess chemotherapeutic cure.

Fluorescent antibody test requires additional standardization.

Cercarial slide flocculation test has some technical shortcomings and difficulties; some cross-reaction to other infestations.

Bentonite flocculation test is somewhat less sensitive than cercarial slide test; some cross-reaction to other infestations.

Complement-fixation test is the best serologic procedure (100% specific and 95% sensitive).

Circumoval precipitin test is particularly useful for testing spinal fluid since it is specific for involvement of central nervous system; intestinal involvement alone causes positive reaction with serum but negative reaction with spinal fluid.

Cercarienhullen reaction test is performed with living infectious cercariae and therefore is not useful as a routine procedure.

Indirect hemagglutination test is more often used for epidemiologic studies.

Rectal biopsy of mucosal fold may show parasites and granulomatous lesions.

Multiple granulomatous lesions appear in uterine cervix.

Changes appear that are secondary to clay pipestem fibrosis of liver with portal hypertension, esophageal varices, splenomegaly, etc. Liver function changes are quite minimal; increased serum bilirubin is rare even with advanced cirrhosis; abnormal BSP is infrequent. Increased serum globulin is frequent. Serum alkaline phosphatase is elevated in 50% of these cases.

Changes secondary to pulmonary hypertension are seen.

Ova appear in urine sediment and in biopsy of vesical mucosa in infection with *S. haematobium*.

CLONORCHIASIS
(due to *Clonorchis sinensis*)

Ova appear in stool or duodenal contents.
Complement-fixation test may be positive.

OPISTHORCHIASIS
(due to *Opisthorchis felineus*)

Ova appear in stool or duodenal contents.

FASCIOLIASIS
(due to *Fasciola hepatica*)

Ova appear in stool or duodenal contents.
Eosinophils are increased.
Liver function tests are abnormal.

FASCIOLOPSIASIS
(due to *Fasciolopsis buski*)

Ova appear in stool.

OPPORTUNISTIC INFECTIONS

Laboratory findings due to underlying diseases (e.g., malignant lymphoma and leukemia, diabetes mellitus, immunoglobulin defects, following renal transplant, uremia, hypoparathyroidism, hypoadrenalism)

Laboratory findings due to administration of drugs (antibiotics, corticosteroids, cytotoxic and immunosuppressive drugs)

Associated with other factors (e.g., plastic intravenous catheters, narcotic addiction)

Laboratory findings due to particular organism (see separate section)

    Candida albicans

    Aspergillus

    Mucor

    Staph. aureus

    Staph. albus, Bacillus subtilis, B. cereus, and other saprophytes

    Enteric bacteria (*Pseudomonas aeruginosa, Escherichia coli, Klebsiella-Enterobacter, Proteus*)

Table 66. Commonly Associated Pathogens in Patients with Immuno-suppression (for Organ Transplantation or Treatment of Malignancies)

Immune Response Depressed	Underlying Condition	Commonly Associated Pathogens
Humoral	Lymphatic leukemia	Pneumococci
	Lymphosarcoma	*Haemophilus influenzae*
	Multiple myeloma	Streptococci
	Congenital hypogamma-globulinemias	*Pseudomonas aeruginosa*
		Pneumocystis carinii
	Nephrotic syndrome	
	Treatment with cyto-toxic or antimetabolite drugs	
Cellular	Terminal cancers	Tubercle bacillus
	Hodgkin's disease	*Listeria*
	Sarcoidosis	*Candida* species
	Uremia	*Toxoplasma*
	Treatment with cyto-toxic or antimetabolite drugs or corticosteroids	*Pneumocystis carinii*
Leukocyte bactericidal	Myelogenous leukemia	Staphylococci
	Chronic granulomatous disease	*Serratia*
		Pseudomonas
	Acidosis	*Candida* species
	Burns	*Aspergillus*
	Treatment with corticosteroids	*Nocardia*
	Granulocytopenia due to drugs	

Table 67. Some Human Diseases That May Be Transmitted by Animal Pets

		Dogs	Cats	Birds	Farm Animals	Poultry	Rodents	Reptiles	Monkeys
BACTERIAL	*Salmonella* infections	+	+	+	+	+	+	+	+
	Bacillary dysentery								+
	Pasteurella infections	+	+		+	+	+		
	Anthrax	+			+				
	Brucellosis	+	+		+	+	+		
	Tularemia	+	+				+		
	Leptospirosis	+		+	+		+		
	Tuberculosis	+	+		+				
VIRAL	Rabies	+	+		+		+		
	Cat-scratch disease		+						
	Psittacosis			+		+			
	Encephalomyelitis			+	+				
	Lymphocytic choriomeningitis	+					+		
FUNGAL	Ringworm	+	+		+		+		
PARASITIC	Roundworm infestation	+	+						
	Tapeworm infestation	+	+		+				
	Visceral larva migrans	+	+						
	Cutaneous larva migrans	+	+						
	Scabies	+	+						
	Toxoplasmosis	+	+						

35

Miscellaneous Diseases

SYSTEMIC LUPUS ERYTHEMATOSUS (SLE)

LE test is positive in 75% or more of patients but may be intermittent and require repeated examinations. Other antinuclear and anticytoplasmic antibodies are often present. (See LE Cell Test and Serologic Tests for SLE, pp. 102–103.)

Moderate normochromic normocytic anemia is usual; it may be hemolytic with positive Coombs' test in 5% of patients.

Decreased WBC without neutropenia is usual; increased WBC occurs with secondary infections.

SLE may present as "idiopathic" thrombocytopenic purpura.

Serum gamma globulin is increased in half the patients; a continuing rise may indicate poor prognosis. Alpha$_2$ globulin is increased; albumin, decreased. Immunoglobulins may be abnormal on immunoelectrophoresis. Cephalin flocculation and thymol turbidity may be positive.

ESR and CRP are increased.

Abnormal serum proteins frequently occur.

Biologically false positive (BFP) test for syphilis is very common—occurs in up to one-fifth of patients. (*This may be the first manifestation of SLE and may precede other features by many months; 7% of asymptomatic individuals with BFP test for syphilis ultimately develop SLE.*)

Cryoglobulins, circulating anticoagulants, etc., are evident.

Tests for rheumatoid factor are positive in one-third of patients.

Laboratory findings reflecting specific organ involvement

Urine findings indicate acute nephritis, nephrotic syndrome, chronic renal impairment, secondary pyelonephritis. Patients with azotemia and marked proteinuria usually die in 1–3 years. Sediment is the same as in chronic active glomerulonephritis. With uremia, nephrotic syndrome, or active nephritis the LE test may become negative.

CSF findings are of aseptic meningitis (increased protein and pleocytosis are found in 50% of these patients). (*Rule out complicating tuberculosis and cryptococcosis.*)

Cardiovascular, pulmonary, etc., findings may be present.

Joint involvement occurs in 90% of patients.

Laboratory findings reflecting frequently associated diseases
    Hashimoto's thyroiditis (see p. 320)
    Sjögren's syndrome (see p. 237)
    Myasthenia gravis (see p. 219)
Tissue biopsy of skin, muscles, kidney, and lymph node may be useful.
Drug-induced lupus syndromes (see pp. 440, 457) are due to prolonged administration of
    Procainamide *Thorazine*
    Hydralazine
    Isoniazid
    Various anticonvulsants (e.g., Dilantin)
    Differ from spontaneous SLE by lower incidence of renal findings and of anemia and leukopenia. About two-thirds of patients receiving these drugs develop serologic abnormalities (see pp. 102–103) even though clinical findings and other laboratory changes are absent. May also occur as allergic reaction to certain drugs (e.g., sulfonamides, methyldopa, oral contraceptives).

POLYARTERITIS NODOSA

WBC is increased (up to 40,000/cu mm), and polynuclear leukocytes are increased. A rise in eosinophils takes place in 25% of patients, sometimes very marked; it usually occurs in patients with pulmonary manifestations.
ESR is increased.
Mild anemia is frequent; may be hemolytic anemia with positive Coombs' test.
Urine is frequently abnormal.
    Albuminuria in 60% of cases
    Hematuria in 40% of cases
    "Telescoping" of sediment (variety of cellular and noncellular casts)
Uremia occurs in 15% of patients.
Tissue biopsy
    Random skin and muscle biopsy is confirmatory in 25% of patients, most useful from area of tenderness; if no symptoms are present, pectoralis major is the most useful site.
    Testicular biopsy is useful when local symptoms are present.
    Lymph node and liver biopsies are usually not helpful.
    Renal biopsy is not specific; often shows glomerular disease.
Serum globulins are increased.
Abnormal serum proteins occasionally occur. BFP test occurs for syphilis, circulating anticoagulants, cryoglobulins, macroglobulins, etc.
Laboratory findings due to organ involvement by arteritis may be present: genitourinary system, nervous system, pulmonary, etc.

WEGENER'S GRANULOMATOSIS
(variant of polyarteritis)

Anemia is common.
Increased WBC is common; occasionally 50% of patients show increase in eosinophils.
Serum globulins are frequently increased.

Laboratory findings reflecting specific organ involvement

Kidney. Urine contains protein, RBCs, and RBC casts; frequent terminal uremia. Most patients develop renal insufficiency. There may be laboratory findings of nephrosis or chronic nephritis.

Central nervous system

Heart

Pulmonary

TEMPORAL ARTERITIS

WBC is usually slightly increased with shift to the left.

Usually moderate normocytic normochromic anemia is present.

Serum protein electrophoresis may show increased gamma globulins. Rouleaux may occur.

ESR is increased.

Laboratory findings reflecting specific organ involvement

Kidney

Central nervous system

Heart and great vessels

Biopsy of involved segment of temporal artery is diagnostic.

Intracerebral artery involvement may cause increased CSF protein.

SCLERODERMA

Laboratory findings reflect specific organ involvement.

Malabsorption syndrome due to small intestine involvement

Abnormal urinary findings, renal function tests, and uremia due to renal involvement

Myocarditis, pericarditis, secondary bacterial endocarditis

Pulmonary fibrosis, secondary pneumonitis

Etc.

Biopsy of skin, esophagus, intestine, synovia may establish diagnosis.

ESR is normal in one-third of patients, mildly increased in one-third of patients, markedly increased in one-third of patients.

Mild hypochromic microcytic anemia may be present in 10% of patients.

Serum gamma globulins are increased in 25% of patients (usually slight increase).

Abnormal serum proteins occasionally occur, as revealed by BFP test for syphilis (5% of patients), positive LE test, positive RA test (one-third of patients), cold agglutinins, cryoglobulins, etc.

Antinuclear antibodies in titer of 1:16 or higher are found in 60% of patients.

SCLEREDEMA

WBC, ESR, and other laboratory tests are usually normal.

WEBER-CHRISTIAN DISEASE (RELAPSING FEBRILE NODULAR NONSUPPURATIVE PANNICULITIS)

Biopsy is taken of involved area of subcutaneous fat.

WBC may be increased or decreased.

Mild anemia may occur.

DISCOID LUPUS

Some patients may show
> Decreased WBC
> Decreased platelet count
> Increased ESR
> Increased serum gamma globulins
> Positive LE cell test (less than 10% of patients)

SARCOIDOSIS

Kveim reaction (skin biopsy 4–6 weeks after injection of human sarcoid tissue shows histologic picture of sarcoid at that site) is positive in 80% of patients with sarcoidosis; many false negatives are seen in patients who are later proved to have sarcoidosis; a positive reaction is less frequent if there is no lymph node involvement, if the disease is of long standing and inactive, and during steroid therapy; false positive reactions occur in 2–5% of patients.

Tissue biopsy may be taken at several sites.
> Needle biopsy of liver shows granulomas in 75% of cases even if there is no impairment of liver function.
> Lymph node biopsy is likely to be positive if lymph node is enlarged.
> Muscle biopsy is likely to be positive if arthralgia or muscle pain is present.
> Skin lesions occur in one-third of cases.
> Other sites of biopsy are synovium, eye, lung, etc.

Serum globulins are increased in 75% of patients producing reduced A/G ratio and increased total protein (in 30% of patients).

Serum protein electrophoresis shows decreased albumin and increased globulin (especially gamma) with characteristic "sarcoid-step" pattern.

There is positive thymol turbidity, and other tests are affected by increased globulin.

WBC is decreased in 30% of patients. Eosinophilia occurs in 15% of patients.

Mild normocytic, normochromic anemia occurs.

ESR is increased.

Increased urine calcium occurs twice as often as hypercalcemia and may be found even with normal serum calcium. Increased frequency of renal calculi is found, and of nephrocalcinosis in some series of patients.

Serum calcium is increased in more than 16% of patients.

Serum and urine calcium abnormalities are frequently corrected by cortisone.

Increased sensitivity to vitamin D is often present.

Serum phosphorus is normal.

Increased serum uric acid may occur even with normal renal function in up to 50% of patients.

Laboratory findings reflect specific organ involvement.
> Liver. Serum alkaline phosphatase is increased. See pp. 188 ff.
> Spleen. Hypersplenism may occur (anemia, leukopenia, thrombocytopenia).
> Central nervous system. CSF may be normal or may show moderate to marked increase in protein and pleocytosis (chiefly lymphocytes). Sugar is sometimes decreased.

Pituitary. Diabetes insipidus is evident.
Kidney. Renal function is decreased (because of hypercalcemia or increased uric acid with resultant nephrocalcinosis or renal calculi).
Lung. pO_2 and pCO_2 are decreased.
Etc.

AMYLOIDOSIS

Biopsy of tissue may be done at several sites.
Gingival biopsy is positive in one-half to two-thirds of patients.
Rectal biopsy is positive in one-half to two-thirds of patients.
Needle biopsy of kidney is useful when gingival and rectal biopsies are not helpful and there is a differential diagnosis of nephrosis.
Needle biopsy of liver is often positive, but beware of intractable bleeding or rupture.
Skin biopsy is taken from sites of plague formation.
Other areas of involvement include GI tract, spleen, respiratory tract, etc.

One should use Congo red stain of tissue under polarized light (apple green birefringence) as well as transmitted light.

Congo red test is positive in one-third of patients with primary amyloidosis and approximately two-thirds of patients with secondary amyloidosis.
Evans blue dye is retained in serum.
Laboratory findings due to primary or associated diseases may occur.
Leprosy (one-third of patients)
Rheumatoid arthritis (one-fourth of patients)
Chronic infections (e.g., chronic osteomyelitis, paraplegia with infections of GU tract)
Tuberculosis
Multiple myeloma (10–20% of patients)
Neoplasms (e.g., renal carcinoma, lymphoma)
Familial types of amyloidosis
Familial Mediterranean fever
Other familial types
Laboratory findings associated with involvement of specific organs may be present.
Liver. See p. 188.
Thymol turbidity and cephalin flocculation, SGOT, LDH, serum bilirubin are usually normal.
BSP retention is increased in three-fourths of patients.
Prothrombin time is occasionally decreased.
Kidney. See p. 369.
Nervous system—peripheral neuropathy
Gastrointestinal system. See, for malabsorption, intestinal obstruction, hemorrhage.
Endocrine system. See Addison's disease, pp. 339–340.
Skin—petechiae, purpura
Increased serum globulin and decreased albumin with reversed A/G ratio are frequent. Serum protein electrophoresis shows decreased albumin and beta and gamma globulins. In familial primary amyloidosis there may be an abnormal peak between $alpha_2$ and beta globulins.

ESR is increased.
Moderate normochromic, normocytic anemia is present.
WBC is frequently increased (above 12,000/cu mm).

GAUCHER'S DISEASE

Gaucher's cells appear in bone marrow aspiration, needle biopsy, or aspiration of spleen, liver, or lymph nodes.
Serum acid phosphatase is increased (if substrate for test is different from that for prostatic acid phosphatase; i.e., use phenyl phosphate or p-nitrophenylphosphate instead of glycerophosphate). It may return to normal following splenectomy.
Serum cholesterol and total fats are normal.
Laboratory findings due to involvement of specific organs
> Spleen. Hypersplenism occurs with anemia (normocytic normochromic), leukopenia (with relative lymphocytosis; monocytes may be increased), and/or thrombocytopenia.
> Bone. Serum alkaline phosphatase may be increased.
> Liver. Serum SGOT may be increased.
> Spinal fluid. SGOT may be increased.

NIEMANN-PICK DISEASE

Foamy histiocytes may be found in bone marrow aspiration and may appear in peripheral blood terminally.
Peripheral blood lymphocytes and monocytes may be vacuolated (2–20% of cells). WBC is variable.
Rectal biopsy may show changes in ganglion cells of myenteric plexus.
Laboratory findings due to involvement of specific organs
> Anemia is due to hypersplenism or microcytic anemia associated with anisocytosis, poikilocytosis, and elliptocytosis.
> SGOT may be increased in serum and spinal fluid.
> Enzyme changes in CSF are same as in Tay-Sachs disease except that LDH is normal (see following section).
Acid phosphatase is increased (same as Gaucher's disease—see section above).
Serum aldolase is increased.
LDH is normal in serum and CSF.

INFANTILE AMAUROTIC IDIOCY (TAY-SACHS DISEASE)

SGOT and cerebrospinal fluid GOT are increased throughout course of disease and may even be increased before clinical symptoms are present; return to normal if patient lives 3 or 4 years. Similar changes in LDH and MDH in serum and cerebrospinal fluid with peak at second year are followed by gradual return to normal.
Serum aldolase is normal during first few months, then progressively rises to peak (of twice normal) at age 12–24 months correlating with skeletal muscle atrophy, then returns to normal in next 3–12 months.
Cerebrospinal fluid aldolase rises early and then declines slowly as disease progresses; does not parallel serum level since it originates from a different source.
Serum acid phosphatase is normal.

HISTIOCYTOSIS X

Letterer-Siwe disease
> Bone marrow aspiration or biopsy of lymph node may show characteristic histiocytes and histologic changes.
> Progressive normocytic normochromic anemia is present.
> Hemorrhagic manifestations (thrombocytopenia) occur.

Hand-Schüller-Christian disease
> Diabetes insipidus may occur.
> Histologic examination of skin, bone, etc., is diagnostic.
> Anemia may or may not be present.

Eosinophilic granuloma
> Biopsy of bone is diagnostic.
> Blood is normal; eosinophilia is unusual.

Development of leukopenia and thrombocytopenia suggests poorest prognosis.

SYSTEMIC MAST CELL DISEASE (MASTOCYTOSIS)

This is a rare condition of disseminated mast cell tumor with functional secretion or abnormal proliferation of tissue mast cells.

Progressive anemia and thrombocytopenia are present.
WBC may be increased or rarely is decreased.
Peripheral blood contains up to 10% mast cells.
Eosinophilia and occasionally basophilia may occur.
Histamine is increased in blood, urine, and tissues.
Gastric acid is increased; there is a higher incidence of peptic ulcer. Hypochlorhydria and achlorhydria have been reported.
Urinary 5-HIAA (hydroxyindole acetic acid) is normal.
Many mast cells appear in bone marrow smears and in metastatic sites.

BASAL CELL NEVUS SYNDROME

Rare disease that shows
> Multiple basal cell tumors of skin
> Odontogenic cysts of jaw
> Bone anomalies (especially of ribs, vertebrae, and metacarpals) and defective dentition
> Neurologic abnormalities (calcification of dura, etc.)
> Ophthalmologic abnormalities (abnormal width between the eyes, lateral displacement of inner canthi, etc.)
> Sexual abnormalities (frequent ovarian fibromas; male hypogonadism, etc.)
> Normal karyotyping by chromosomal analysis
> Hyporesponsiveness to parathormone (Ellsworth-Howard test)

Rule out presence or development of occult neoplasms (e.g., ovarian fibroma, medulloblastoma).

MALIGNANT NEOPLASMS

Hemorrhage
Anemia
Malnutrition

Hypoproteinemia
Development of autoantibodies, hemolytic anemia, increased ESR, etc.
Tumor cells in bone marrow, liver biopsy, etc.
Metastatic tumor masses (e.g., liver, brain)
Obstruction (e.g., ureters, bile ducts, intestine)
Functional changes due to metastases that interfere with endocrine secretion (e.g., adrenal, pituitary)
Secretion of active hormonal substances by nonendocrine tumors (e.g., bronchogenic carcinoma)
Diseases that occur with particular frequency in association with neoplasms (e.g., polymyositis)
Laboratory findings associated with specific tumors (e.g., carcinoid, thymoma, functioning endocrine tumors, leukemia, melanoma)

OCCULT NEOPLASIA   (E.g., Pheochromocytoma, Hypernephroma, Breast Carcinoma, Etc., and Various Benign Tumors)

Rule out presence or development of occult neoplasia in
    Neurofibromatosis
    Sturge-Weber syndrome
    Lindau-von Hippel disease
    Tuberous sclerosis
    Basal cell nevus syndrome
    Polymyositis
    Acanthosis nigricans

BREAST CANCER

Indications for administration of adrenal hormones
    Hypercalcemia
    Metastases
        To brain or liver
        Diffuse pulmonary

36
Conditions Due to Physical and Chemical Agents

NARCOTICS ADDICTION

Persistent absolute and relative lymphocytosis occurs, with lymphocytes often bizarre and atypical that may resemble Downey cells.

Liver function tests commonly show increased serum SGOT and SGPT and/or increased cephalin flocculation and thymol turbidity tests. Higher frequency of positive tests is evident on routine periodic repeat of these tests. (This probably represents a mild, chronic, intermittently active, usually anicteric serum hepatitis.) Serum protein electrophoresis is usually normal.

Laboratory findings due to preexisting glucose-6-phosphate dehydrogenase deficiency may be precipitated (by quinine, which is often used to adulterate the heroin).

Laboratory findings due to malaria transmitted by common syringes may occur. (*Malaria is not frequent; may be suppressed by quinine used for adulteration of heroin.*)

Laboratory findings due to tuberculosis, which develops with increased frequency in narcotics addicts, may be present.

Laboratory findings due to staphylococcal pneumonia or septic pulmonary emboli secondary to skin infections or bacterial endocarditis, which are more frequent in narcotics addicts, may be present.

Laboratory findings due to endocarditis

  Right-sided; usually *Staphylococcus aureus* affecting previously normal tricuspid valve

  Left-sided; may be due to *Candida* superimposed on previously damaged valve or may be *Streptococcus* or other bacteria superimposed on previously normal valve

Oral and IV glucose tolerance curves are often flat (explanation for this finding is not known).

Urinalysis is usually normal unless renal failure due to endocarditis occurs.

Laboratory findings due to syphilis, which occurs with increased frequency in narcotics addicts, may occur. BFP tests for syphilis also occur with increased frequency.

Laboratory findings due to tetanus, which occurs with increased

frequency in narcotics addicts because of "skin-popping," may occur. (*Tetanus causes 5–10% of addicts' deaths in New York City.*)
Laboratory findings due to concomitant use of sedative, especially alcohol, barbiturates, and glutethimide (Doriden), may occur.

ALCOHOLISM*
Laboratory findings due to major alcohol-associated illnesses (see appropriate separate sections)
> Fatty liver, alcoholic hepatitis, cirrhosis, esophageal varices, peptic ulcer, chronic gastritis, pancreatitis, malabsorption, vitamin deficiencies
> Head trauma, Korsakoff's syndrome, delirium tremens, peripheral neuropathy, myopathy
> Cardiac myopathy
> Various pneumonias, lung abscess, tuberculosis
> Associated addictions
> Others

Laboratory tests due to alcohol ingestion
> Direct
>> Blood alcohol level at any time of more than 300 mg/100 ml or level of more than 100 mg/100 ml in routine examination. (*Blood alcohol level over 150 mg/100 ml without gross evidence of intoxication suggests alcoholic patient's increased tolerance.*)
> Indirect
>> Serum osmolality (reflects blood alcohol levels): Every 22.4 increase over 200 mOsm/L reflects 50 mg/100 ml alcohol.
>> Results of alcohol ingestion
>>> Hypoglycemia
>>> Hypochloremic alkalosis
>>> Low magnesium level
>>> Increased lactic acid
>>> Transient increase of serum uric acid
>>> Potassium depletion
>> Thrombocytopenia
>> Anemia—most often due to folic acid deficiency; less frequently due to iron deficiency, hemorrhage, secondary to inflammation, etc.

SALICYLATE INTOXICATION
(due to aspirin, sodium salicylate, oil of wintergreen, methyl salicylate)

Increased serum salicylate
> More than 10 mg/100 ml when symptoms are present
> More than 40 mg/100 ml when hyperventilation is present
> At about 50 mg/100 ml, severe toxicity with acid-base imbalance and ketosis
> At 45–70 mg/100 ml, death

In older children and adults, serum salicylate level corresponds well with severity; in younger children, correlation is more variable. Gastric lavage may increase salicylate level as much as 10 mg/100 ml.

---

* Criteria Committee, National Council on Alcoholism. Criteria for the diagnosis of alcoholism. *Ann. Intern. Med.* 77 (August 1972): 249–258.

Early, serum electrolytes and CO_2 are normal.

Later, progressive decrease in serum sodium and pCO_2 occurs. There is combined respiratory alkalosis and metabolic acidosis; change in blood pH reflects the net result. (*Infants may show immediate metabolic acidosis with the usual initial respiratory alkalosis.*)

Hypokalemia accompanies the respiratory alkalosis. Dehydration occurs.

Urine shows paradoxic acid pH despite the increased serum bicarbonate.

> Ferric chloride test is positive on boiled as well as unboiled urine (thus differentiating from ketone bodies); it may have a false positive result on account of phenacetin.
>
> Tests for glucose (e.g., Clinistix), reducing substances (e.g., Clinitest), or ketone bodies (e.g., Ketostix) are positive.
>
> RBCs may be present.
>
> Number of renal tubular cells is increased because of renal irritation.

Hypoglycemia occurs, especially in infants on restricted diet and in diabetics.

Serum SGOT and SGPT may be increased.

Hypoprothrombinemia after some days of intensive salicylate therapy is temporary and occasional; rarely causes hemorrhage.

BMR is markedly increased.

Hydroxyproline is decreased in serum and urine.

DIFFERENTIATION OF ACIDOSIS IN SALICYLATE INTOXICATION AND DIABETES MELLITUS

Measurement	Salicylate Intoxication	Diabetes Mellitus
Ferric chloride test on urine	Remains positive after boiling	Becomes negative after boiling (volatile acetoacetic acid is removed)
Nitroprusside test for acetoacetic acid in urine	Negative	Positive
Urinary reducing substances	May be due to glucose or other reducing substances (e.g., salicylglucuronide)	Due to glucose
Serum ketone level	Usually less than 20 mg/100 ml.	Often more than 50 mg/100 ml.
Prothrombin time	Increased	Normal
Serum salicylate level	More than 40 mg/100 ml.	Negative or increased to nontoxic level

PHENACETIN—CHRONIC EXCESSIVE INGESTION

Laboratory findings due to increased incidence of peptic ulceration, especially of stomach, often with bleeding, may be present.

Laboratory findings associated with increased incidence of papillary necrosis and interstitial nephritis may be present.

> Proteinuria is slight or absent.
> Hematuria is often present in active papillary necrosis.
> WBC is increased in urine in absence of infection.
> Papillae are passed in urine.
> Creatinine clearance is decreased.
> Renal failure may occur.

Anemia is common and frequently precedes azotemia.

BROMISM

Bromism should always be ruled out in the presence of mental symptoms or psychosis.

Serum and urine bromide levels are increased.
CSF protein is increased in acute bromide psychosis.
Serum "chloride" is increased, as indicated by AutoAnalyzer.

(If result of chloride determination with AutoAnalyzer is increased out of proportion to result with Cotlove coulimetric titrator, bromism should be ruled out.)

SOME POSSIBLE SIDE-EFFECTS OF STEROID THERAPY THAT CAUSE LABORATORY CHANGES

Endocrine effects (e.g., adrenal insufficiency after prolonged use, suppression of pituitary or thyroid function, development of diabetes mellitus)

Increased susceptibility to infections

Gastrointestinal effects (e.g., peptic ulcer, perforation of bowel, infarction of bowel, pancreatitis)

Musculoskeletal effects (e.g., osteoporosis, pathologic fractures, arthropathy, myopathy)

Decreased serum potassium, increased WBC, glycosuria, ecchymoses, etc.

PROCAINAMIDE THERAPY

Procainamide therapy may induce the findings of systemic lupus erythematosus (SLE).

Positive serologic tests for SLE are very frequent, especially in dosage of 1.25 gm/day or more, and may precede clinical manifestations.

> LE cell tests become positive in one-half of cases.
> Anti-DNP (anti-deoxyribonucleoprotein) tests become positive in two-thirds of cases.
> Anti-DNA tests become positive in one-third of cases.
> One of these becomes positive in three-fourths of cases.

Perform serologic tests for lupus on all patients receiving this drug.

APRESOLINE REACTION
(for hypertension therapy)

Anemia and pancytopenia occur infrequently.

Prolonged use causes a syndrome resembling lupus erythematosus (microscopical hematuria, leukopenia, increased ESR, presence of LE cells, altered serum proteins with increased gamma globulin). After cessation of drug, remission is aided by administration of ACTH.

ENTERIC-COATED THIAZIDE POTASSIUM CHLORIDE

Laboratory findings due to small-intestine ulceration, obstruction, or perforation.

COMPLICATIONS OF DIPHENYLHYDANTOIN (DILANTIN) THERAPY

Megaloblastic anemia may occur. It is completely responsive to folic acid (even when Dilantin therapy is continued) but not always to vitamin B_{12}. This is the most common hematologic complication.

Rarely there may occur pancytopenia, thrombocytopenia alone, or leukopenia, including agranulocytosis.

Laboratory findings of hepatitis may be present.

Laboratory findings resembling those of malignant lymphomas may be present.

Laboratory findings resembling those of infectious mononucleosis may occur, but heterophil agglutination is not increased.

PBI is decreased, with increased T-3 intake, but ^{131}I uptake, PB ^{131}I, BMR, serum cholesterol, etc., are normal (because of competition for binding sites of thyroxin-binding globulin).

Dilantin therapy may induce a lupus-like syndrome.

LABORATORY CHANGES AND SIDE-EFFECTS FROM LIPID-LOWERING DRUGS

Nicotinic acid may cause
- Dramatic lowering (often) of blood triglyceride in Types II and IV and probably also in Types III and V
- Increased blood sugar
- Increased blood uric acid
- Abnormal liver function tests
- Jaundice (rarely)

Cholestyramine in the form of a chloride salt may cause
- Lowering of cholesterol in familial Type II hyperlipidemia
- Mild hyperchloremic acidosis

HYPERVITAMINOSIS A

Increased serum vitamin A level (up to 2000 μg/100 ml)

May also show
- Increased ESR
- Increased serum alkaline phosphatase

Decreased serum albumin
Increased serum bilirubin
Decreased hemoglobin
Slight proteinuria
Slightly increased serum carotene
Increased prothrombin time
Bromsulphalein (BSP) retention

CHRONIC ARSENIC POISONING
(from insecticides, rat poisons; therapeutic arsenic, e.g., Fowler's solution)

Increased arsenic appears in urine (usually more than 0.1 mg/L; in acute cases may be more than 1.0 mg/L).
Increased arsenic appears in hair (more than 0.1 mg/100 mg of hair).
Increased arsenic appears in nails.
Moderate anemia is present.
Moderate leukopenia occurs (2000–5000/cu mm), with mild eosinophilia.
Liver function tests show mild abnormalities.
Urine shows slight proteinuria.
Cerebrospinal fluid is normal.

Arsine gas (hydrogen arsenide) causes hemolysis with hemoglobinuria.

LEAD POISONING

Delta-aminolevulinic acid is increased in urine. Since it is increased in 75% of asymptomatic lead workers who have normal coproporphyrin in urine, it can be used to detect early excess lead absorption.
Increased coproporphyrin in urine is a reliable sign of intoxication and is often demonstrable before basophilic stippling (but one should rule out a false positive due to drugs such as barbiturates and salicylates).
Confirm diagnosis with determination of blood lead (less than 20 μg/100 ml is considered normal; 25–40 μg/100 ml evidences increased lead exposure; more than 50 μg/100 ml is a treatable level) and urine lead (normal for children is less than 80 μg/1000 ml and for adults is less than 150 μg/1000 ml).
Anemia (slightly hypochromic and microcytic) in chronic exposure may be of moderate degree or may be absent.
Stippled RBCs occur later.
Urine urobilinogen and uroporphyrin are increased.
Renal tubular damage occurs, with aminoaciduria and glycosuria.
CSF protein is increased, with normal cell count in encephalopathy.

MERCURY POISONING

Levels of mercury in serum, urine, and CSF are increased
Asymptomatic normal people (not exposed to mercury) have a urine value of less than 20 μg/L and blood level less than 3 μg/L in 95% of the cases. Urine and blood levels are nondiagnostic, in that they vary among patients with symptoms, and daily urine levels vary in the same patient. Thus in one epidemic, urine levels up to 1000 μg/L occurred in asymptomatic patients whereas other patients had symptoms at levels of 200 μg/L.

ACUTE IRON POISONING
(occurs in children who have ingested medicinal iron preparations)

Increased serum iron and TIBC
Poor prognostic sign when serum iron greatly exceeds TIBC. Blood
for these should be drawn within the first few hours.

ORGANIC PHOSPHATE (INSECTICIDES—PARATHION, MALATHION, ETC.) POISONING

Decreased RBC and plasma cholinesterase by 50% or more (due to
inhibition of cholinesterase by organic phosphate pesticides)

*For industrial exposure, worker should not return to work until these
values rise to 75% of normal. RBC cholinesterase regenerates at rate
of 1%/day. Plasma cholinesterase regenerates at rate of 25% in 7–10
days.*

MOTHBALLS (CAMPHOR, PARADICHLOROBENZENE, NAPHTHALENE) POISONING

Paradichlorobenzene inhalation may cause liver damage.
Naphthalene ingestion may cause hemolytic anemia in patients with
RBC deficient in G-6-PD (see p. 259).

YELLOW PHOSPHORUS POISONING
(rat poison ingestion)

Acute yellow atrophy of liver occurs.
Vomitus may glow in the dark.

PHENOL AND LYSOL POISONING

Severe acidosis often occurs.
Acute tubular necrosis may develop.

OXALATE POISONING
(due to ingestion of stain remover or ink eradicator containing oxalic acid)

Hypocalcemic tetany (due to formation of insoluble calcium oxalate)

METHYL ALCOHOL POISONING

Onset is 12–24 hours after ingestion.

Severe acidosis
Frequent concomitant acute pancreatitis

MILK SICKNESS ("TREMBLES")
(poisoning from goldenrod, snakeroot, richweed, etc., or from eating poisoned animals)

Acidosis
Hypoglycemia

Increased nonprotein nitrogen (particularly guanidine)
Acetonuria

HEAT STROKE

Uniformly increased SGOT (mean 20 times normal), SGPT (mean
10 times normal), and LDH (mean 5 times normal) reach peak on
third day and return to normal by 2 weeks. Very high levels are
often associated with lethal outcome.
Cerebrospinal fluid GOT, GPT, and LDH are normal.

DROWNING AND NEAR-DROWNING

Hypoxemia (decreased pO_2)
Metabolic acidosis (decreased blood pH)
In severe freshwater aspiration
    Decreased serum sodium and chloride
    Increased serum potassium
    Increased plasma hemoglobin
In severe seawater aspiration
    Hypovolemia
    Increased serum sodium and chloride
    Normal plasma hemoglobin

Above changes follow aspiration of very large amounts of water.
Electrolytes return toward normal within 1 hour following survival,
even without therapy.

In near-drowning in fresh water, often
    Normal serum sodium and chloride
    Variable serum potassium
    Increased free plasma hemoglobin
    Fall in RBC, hemoglobin, and hematocrit in 24 hours
In near-drowning in seawater, often
    Moderate increase in serum sodium and chloride
    Normal or decreased serum potassium
    Normal hemoglobin, hematocrit, and plasma hemoglobin

Blood count may appear normal even when considerable hemolysis is
present because usual methodology does not distinguish between
hemoglobin within RBC and free hemoglobin in serum. Fall in
hemoglobin and hematocrit may be delayed 1–2 days.

INJURY DUE TO ELECTRIC CURRENT

Increased WBC with large immature granulocytes
Albuminuria; hemoglobinuria in presence of severe burns
CSF sometimes bloody

BURNS

Decreased plasma volume and blood volume. This follows (therefore is not due to) marked drop in cardiac output. Greatest fall in
plasma volume occurs with the first 12 hours and continues at a
much slower rate for only 6–12 hours more. In a 40% burn,
plasma volume falls to 25% below preburn levels.

Infection
- Burn sepsis. Gram-positive organisms predominate until the third day, when gram-negative organisms become dominant. By fifth day, untreated infection is active. *Fatal burn-wound sepsis shows no noteworthy spread of bacteria beyond wound in half the cases. Before antibiotic therapy, this caused 75% of deaths due to burns; it now causes 10–15% of deaths.*
- Laboratory findings due to pneumonia, which now causes most deaths that result from infection. Two-thirds of pneumonia cases are airborne infections. One-third are hematogenous infections and are often due to septic phlebitis at sites of old cutdowns.
- Local and systemic infection due to *Candida* and *Phycomycetes.*

Laboratory findings due to renal failure. Reported frequency varies: 1.3% of total admissions to 15% of cases with burns involving more than 15% of body surface.

Laboratory findings due to Curling's ulcer. Occurs in 11% of burn patients. *Gastric ulcer is more frequent in general, but duodenal ulcer occurs twice as often in children as in adults. Gastric lesions are seen throughout the first month with equal frequency in all age groups, but duodenal ulcers are most frequent in adults during the first week and in children during the third and fourth weeks after the burns.*

Blood viscosity rises acutely; remains elevated for 4–5 days although hematocrit has returned to normal.

Fibrin split products are increased for 3–5 days.

Other findings that may occur in all types of trauma
- Platelet count rises slowly, lasting for 3 weeks. Platelet adhesiveness is increased.
- Fibrinogen falls during first 36 hours, then rises steeply for up to 3 months.
- Factors V and VIII may be 4–8 times normal level for up to 3 months.

CONVULSIVE THERAPY
(e.g., electric shock therapy)

Increased cerebrospinal fluid GOT and LDH peak (3 times normal) in 12 hours; return to normal by 48 hours.

SNAKEBITE

Pit vipers (rattlesnake, copperhead, water moccasin)
- Increased WBC (20,000–30,000/cu mm)
- Platelets decreased to approximately 10,000/cu mm within an hour; return to normal in about 4 hours
- Burrs on almost all RBCs
- Clotting caused by some venoms; normal coagulation prevented by others, which destroy fibrinogen
- Albuminuria

Elapidae (coral snakes, kraits, cobras)
- Hemolytic manifestations

SPIDER BITE

Black widow spider (*Latrodectus mactans*)
- Moderately increased WBC
- Findings of acute nephritis

Brown spider (*Loxosceles reclusa*)
    Hemolytic anemia with hemoglobinuria and hemoglobinemia
    Increased WBC
    Thrombocytopenia
    Proteinuria

INSECT BITES
(due to ticks, lice, fleas, bugs, beetles, ants, flies, bees, wasps, etc.)

No specific laboratory findings unless secondary infection occurs

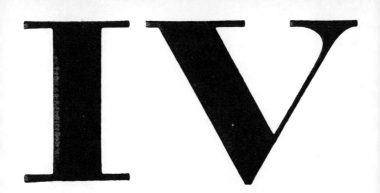

IV

*Effects of Drugs on
Laboratory Test Values*

37

Alteration of Laboratory Test Values by Drugs

With the coincident ingestion of a large number of drugs and the performance of many laboratory tests (many of which are unsolicited), test abnormalities may be due to drugs as often as to disease. Correct interpretation of laboratory tests requires that the physician be aware of all drugs that the patient is receiving. It is important to remember that patients often do not tell their physician about medications they are taking (prescribed by other doctors or by the patients themselves). In addition, there is environmental exposure to many drugs and chemicals.

The classes of drugs most often involved include the anticoagulants, anticonvulsants, antihypertensives, anti-infectives, oral hypoglycemics, hormones, and psychoactive agents.

The following lists of the more frequently performed laboratory test values that may be altered by commonly used drugs are only a general guide to the direction of increase or decrease, not an all-inclusive collection of such information. The selection and arrangement of data by clinical groups provide the most useful, most rapid, and simplest summary of a very complex subject. Only generic names for drugs are used.

The frequency of such modified laboratory test values is variable. A number of causative mechanisms may operate, sometimes simultaneously. Thus some changes are due to interference with the chemical reaction used in the testing procedure. Other changes reflect damage to a specific organ such as the liver or kidney. In some cases, specific metabolic alterations are induced such as accelerated or retarded formation or excretion of a specific chemical, competition for binding sites, stimulation or suppression of degradative enzymes, etc. Often the mechanism of these altered laboratory test values is not known.

DRUGS THAT MAY CAUSE FALSE POSITIVE ELEVATION OF URINE SPECIFIC GRAVITY

Dextran
Radiopaque contrast media

DRUGS THAT MAY ALTER URINE COLOR

Urine coloration due to drugs may mask other abnormal colors (e.g., due to blood, bile, porphyrins) as well as interfere with various chemical determinations (fluormetric, colorimetric, photometric).

Drugs	*Resulting Color*
Acetophenetidin	Hematuria or pink red due to metabolite
Aminosalicylic acid (PAS)	Discoloration abnormal but not distinctive
Amitriptyline	Blue green
Anisindione (indandione)	Orange (alkaline urine), pink-red-brown (acid urine)
Cascara	Brown (acid urine), yellow pink (alkaline urine), black on standing
Chloroquine	Brown
Chlorzoxazone (metabolite)	Purple, red, pink, rust
Cinchophen	Red brown
Dihydroxyanthraquinone	Pink to orange (alkaline urine)
Diphenylhydantoin	Pink, red, red-brown
Emodin	Pink to red to red-brown (alkaline urine)
Ethoxazene	Orange, red, pink, rust
Furazolidone	Brown
Iron sorbitol	Brown
Methocarbamol	Dark brown, black, blue or green on standing
Methyldopa	Red darkens on standing, pink or brown
Methylene blue	Greenish yellow to blue
Metronidazole (metabolite)	Dark brown
Nitrofurantoin and derivatives	Brown, yellow
Pamaquine	Brown
Phenazopyridine	Orange to red
Phenindione	Red-orange in alkaline urine
Phenolphthalein	Pink to red to magenta (alkaline urine), orange, rust (acid)
Phenothiazines	Pink, red, purple, orange, rust
Phensuximide	Pink, red, purple, orange, rust
Primaquine	Rust yellow to brown
Quinacrine (mepacrine)	Deep yellow on acidification
Quinine and derivatives	Brown to black
Rhubarb	Yellow-brown (acid), yellow-pink (alkaline), darkens
Riboflavin	Yellow
Rifampin	Red-orange
Salicylazosulfapyridine	Pink, red, purple, orange, rust
Sulfonamides	Rust, yellow, or brown
Thiazolsulfone	Pink, red, purple, orange, rust
Tolonium	Blue, green
Triamterene	Green, blue with blue fluorescence

DRUGS THAT MAY CAUSE FALSE POSITIVE TEST FOR URINE PROTEIN

Drugs with nephrotoxic effect, e.g., gold, arsenicals, antimony compounds
Drugs that may interfere with sulfosalicylic acid methods, e.g.,
 Cephaloridine
 Cephalothin
 Sulfamethoxazole
 Tolbutamide
Drugs that may cause false positive turbidity tests, e.g.,
 Chlorpromazine, promazine
 Penicillin (massive doses)
 Radiopaque contrast media (for up to 3 days)
 Sulfisoxazole
 Thymol
Drugs that react with Folin-Ciocalteu reagent of Lowry procedure, e.g.,
 Aminosalicylic acid (PAS)
 Dithiazine
Drugs that cause false positive reaction with Labstix because of high pH, e.g.,
 Sodium bicarbonate
 Acetazolamide

DRUGS THAT MAY CAUSE POSITIVE TEST FOR URINE GLUCOSE

Drugs that may cause hyperglycemia with secondary glycosuria, e.g., corticosteroids, indomethacin, isoniazid
Drugs that cause renal damage, e.g., degraded tetracycline
Vaginal powders that contain glucose, causing artifactual false positive, e.g., furazolidone
Drugs that cause false positive by reducing action with Benedict's solution and Clinitest but not with Clinistix or Testape
 Acetylsalicylic acid
 Aminosalicylic acid (PAS)
 Cephaloridine (abnormal dark color)
 Cephalothin (brown-black color)
 Chloral hydrate
 Cinchophen
 Etc.

DRUGS THAT MAY CAUSE FALSE NEGATIVE TEST FOR URINE GLUCOSE
(glucose oxidase method, e.g., Clinistix, Testape)

Ascorbic acid
Levodopa (with Clinistix but not Testape)
Phenazopyridine

DRUGS THAT MAY CAUSE FALSE POSITIVE URINE ACETONE TEST

Ketostix or Acetest Methods	*Labstix, Bili-Labstix, Etc.*
BSP	Levodopa
PSP	BSP
Inositol or methionine	
Metformin, phenformin	

DRUGS THAT MAY CAUSE FALSE POSITIVE URINE DIACETIC ACID TEST
(Gerhardt ferric chloride test; Phenistix)

Aminosalicylic acid (PAS)
Chlorpromazine
Phenothiazines
Levodopa
Salicylates

DRUGS THAT MAY CAUSE POSITIVE TEST FOR URINE AMINO ACIDS

ACTH and cortisone
Tetracyclines (degraded) and other nephrotoxic agents

DRUGS THAT MAY ALTER URINE TESTS FOR OCCULT BLOOD

Guaiac	*Benzidine*
False positive	False positive
Bromides	Bromides
Copper	Copper
Iodides	Iodides
Oxidizing agents	Permanganate

False negative
Ascorbic acid (high doses)

DRUGS THAT MAY CAUSE POSITIVE TESTS FOR HEMATURIA OR HEMOGLOBINURIA

Drugs that cause nephrotoxicity, e.g., amphotericin B, bacitracin
Drugs that cause actual bleeding, e.g., phenylbutazone, indometha-cin, coumarin
Drugs that cause hemolysis, e.g., acetylsalicylic acid, acetopheneti-din, acetanilid

DRUGS THAT MAY CAUSE POSITIVE TESTS FOR BILE IN URINE

Drugs that cause cholestasis
Drugs that are hepatotoxic
Drugs that interfere with testing methods
    Acriflavine (yellow color when urine is shaken)
    Chlorpromazine (interferes with Bili-Labstix)
    Ethoxazene (atypical red color with Bili-Labstix and Ictotest)
    Mefenamic acid
    Phenazopyridine (false positive with Bili-Labstix and Ictotest)
    Phenothiazines (may interfere with Bili-Labstix)
    Thymol (affects Hay's test for bile acids)

DRUGS THAT MAY CAUSE URINE UROBILINOGEN TO BE

Increased	*Decreased*
Drugs that interfere with testing methods	Drugs that cause cholestasis
Aminosalicylic acid (PAS)	Drugs that reduce the bacterial flora in the gastrointestinal tract (e.g., chloramphenicol)
Antipyrine	
Bromsulfalein (BSP)	
Cascara	
Chlorpromazine	
Phenazopyridine	
Phenothiazines	
Sulfonamides	
5-Hydroxyindoleacetic acid	
Bananas	
Drugs that cause hemolysis	

DRUGS THAT MAY CAUSE POSITIVE TESTS FOR URINE PORPHYRINS (FLUORMETRIC METHODS)

Drugs that produce fluorescence, e.g.,
    Acriflavine
    Ethoxazene
    Phenazopyridine
    Sulfamethoxazole
    Tetracycline
Drugs that may precipitate porphyria, e.g.,
    Antipyretics
    Barbiturates
    Phenylhydrazine
    Sulfonamides

DRUGS THAT MAY CAUSE URINE CREATINE TO BE

Increased	*Decreased*
Caffeine	Androgens and anabolic steroids
Methyltestosterone	
PSP	Thiazides

DRUGS THAT MAY CAUSE URINE CREATININE TO BE

Increased	*Decreased*
Ascorbic acid	Androgens and anabolic steroids
Corticosteroids	
Levodopa	Thiazides
Methyldopa	
Nitrofurans	
PSP	

DRUGS THAT MAY CAUSE URINE CALCIUM TO BE

Increased	*Decreased*
Androgens and anabolic steroids	Sodium phytate
Cholestyramine	Thiazides
Corticosteroids	
Dihydrotachysterol, vitamin D parathyroid injections	
Viomycin	

DRUGS THAT MAY CAUSE FALSE POSITIVE PSP TEST IN URINE

Kaolin
Magnesium
Methylene blue
Nicotinic acid
Quinacrine (mepacrine)
Quinidine
Quinine

SOME DRUGS THAT MAY CAUSE URINE 17-KETOSTEROIDS TO BE

Increased	*Decreased*
Chloramphenicol	Chlordiazepoxide
Chlorpromazine	Estrogens
Cloxacillin	Meprobamate
Dexamethasone	Metyrapone
Erythromycin	Probenecid

Ethinamate
Meprobamate
Nalidixic acid
Oleandomycin
Penicillin
Phenaglycodol
Phenazopyridine
Phenothiazines
Quinidine
Secobarbital
Spironolactone

Promazine
Reserpine

DRUGS THAT MAY CAUSE URINE 17-HYDROXYCORTICOSTEROIDS TO BE

Increased	*Decreased*
Acetazolamide	Estrogens and oral contraceptives
Chloral hydrate	Phenothiazines
Chlordiazepoxide	Reserpine
Chlorpromazine	
Colchicine	
Erythromycin	
Etryptamine	
Meprobamate	
Oleandomycin	
Paraldehyde	
Quinine and quinidine	
Spironolactone	

DRUGS THAT MAY INTERFERE WITH DETERMINATION OF URINE CATECHOLAMINES
(by producing urinary fluorescence)

Ampicillin
Ascorbic acid
Chloral hydrate
Epinephrine
Erythromycin
Hydralazine
Methenamine
Methyldopa
Nicotinic acid (large doses)
Quinine and quinidine
Tetracycline and derivatives
Vitamin B complex

DRUGS THAT MAY CAUSE URINE VMA (VANILMANDELIC ACID) TO BE

Increased	*Decreased*
Aspirin	(Values are usually not depressed to normal in patients with pheochomocytoma
Aminosalicylic acid (PAS)	
Bromsulfalein (BSP)	Clofibrate
Glyceryl guaiacolate	Guanethidine analogs
Mephenesin	

Methocarbamol
Nalidixic acid
Oxytetracycline
Penicillin
Phenazopyridine
PSP
Sulfa drugs

Imipramine
Methyldopa
Monoamine oxidase (MAO) inhibitors

DRUGS THAT MAY CAUSE URINE 5-HIAA (5-HYDROXYINDOLEACETIC ACID) TO BE

Increased	*Decreased*
Acetanilid	Chlorpromazine, promazine
Acetophenetidin	Imipramine
Glyceryl guaiacolate	Isoniazid
Mephenesin	MAO inhibitors
Methocarbamol	Methenamine
Reserpine	Methyldopa
	Phenothiazines
	Promethazine

DRUGS THAT MAY CAUSE URINE DIAGNEX BLUE EXCRETION TO BE

Increased	*Decreased*
Aluminum salts	Caffeine benzoate
Barium salts	
Calcium salts	
Iron salts	
Kaolin	
Magnesium salts	
Methylene blue	
Nicotinic acid	
Quinacrine (mepacrine)	
Quinidine, quinine	
Riboflavin	
Sodium salts	
Vitamin B	

DRUGS THAT MAY CAUSE A FALSE POSITIVE URINE PREGNANCY TEST

Chlorpromazine (frog, rabbit, immunologic)
Phenothiazines (frog, rabbit, immunologic)
Promethazine (Gravindex)

DRUG THAT MAY CAUSE A FALSE NEGATIVE URINE PREGNANCY TEST

Promethazine (DAP test)

DRUGS THAT MAY CAUSE THE ERYTHROCYTE SEDIMENTATION RATE (ESR) TO BE

Increased	*Decreased*
Dextran	Quinine (therapeutic effect)
Methyldopa	Salicylates (therapeutic effect)
Methysergide	Drugs that cause a high blood
Penicillamine	glucose level
Theophylline	
Trifluperidol	
Vitamin A	

SOME DRUGS THAT MAY CAUSE A POSITIVE DIRECT COOMBS' TEST

Acetophenetidin
Chlorpromazine
Chlorpropamide
Diphenylhydantoin
Dipyrone
Ethosuximide
Hydralazine
Isoniazid
Levodopa
Mefenamic acid
Melphalan
Oxyphenisatin
Phenylbutazone
Procainamide
Quinidine, quinine
Streptomycin
Sulfonamides
Tetracyclines

Illustrative information. For methyldopa, a positive direct Coombs' test occurs in 10–20% of patients on continued therapy. Occurs rarely in first 6 months of treatment. If not found within 12 months, is unlikely to occur. Is dose-related, with lowest incidence in patients receiving 1 gm daily or less. Reversal may take weeks to months after the drug is discontinued.

DRUGS THAT MAY CAUSE POSITIVE TESTS FOR LE CELLS AND/OR ANTINUCLEAR ANTIBODIES

Acetazolamide
Aminosalicylic acid (PAS)
Chlorprothixene
Chlorthiazide
Diphenylhydantoin
Griseofulvin
Hydralazine
Isoniazid
Methyldopa

Oral contraceptives
Penicillin
Phenylbutazone
Procainamide
Streptomycin
Sulfonamides
Tetracyclines
Thiouracil
Trimethadione

DRUGS THAT MAY CAUSE THE BLEEDING TIME TO BE INCREASED

Acetylsalicylic acid
Dextran
Pantothenyl alcohol and derivatives
Streptokinase-streptodornase

DRUGS THAT MAY CAUSE THE COAGULATION TIME TO BE

Increased	*Decreased*
Anticoagulants	Corticosteroids
Tetracyclines	Epinephrine

DRUGS THAT POTENTIATE COUMARIN ACTION (INCREASE PROTHROMBIN TIME)

Anabolic steroids
Chloral hydrate
Chloramphenicol
Clofibrate
Diphenylhydantoin
Glucagon
Indomethacin
Mefenamic acid

Neomycin
Oxyphenbutazone
Phenylbutazone
Phenyramidol
Quinidine
Salicylates
D-thyroxine

DRUGS THAT *MAY* POTENTIATE COUMARIN ACTION (INCREASE PROTHROMBIN TIME)

Acetaminophen
Allopurinol
Diazoxide
Disulfiram
Ethacrynic acid
Heparin
Mercaptopurine
Methyldopa
Methylphenidate

Monoamine oxidase (MAO) inhibitors
Nalidixic acid
Northriptyline
Sulfinpyrazone
Sulfonamides (long-acting)
Thyroid drugs
Tolbutamide

DRUGS THAT INHIBIT COUMARIN ACTION (DECREASE PROTHROMBIN TIME)

Barbiturates
Ethchlorvynol

Glutethimide
Griseofulvin
Heptabarbital

DRUGS THAT *MAY* INHIBIT COUMARIN ACTION (DECREASE PROTHROMBIN TIME)

Adrenocortical steroids
Cholestyramine
Colchicine
Meprobamate
Oral contraceptives
Rifampin

Patients on long-term coumarin treatment should not take: barbiturates, chloral hydrate, chloramphenicol, ethchlorvynol, glutethimide, phenylbutazone (or its congeners), phenyramidol, quinidine, salicylates. Patients on long-term coumarin treatment should not take any other drugs without consideration of possible drug interaction.

COLOR CHANGES IN STOOL

Alkaline antacids and aluminum salts	White discoloration or speckling
Anticoagulants (excess)	Due to bleeding
Bismuth salts	Black
Anthraquinones	Brown staining
Dithiazine	Green to blue
Iron salts	Black
Mercurous chloride	Green
Phenazopyridine	Orange red
Phenolphthalein	Red
Pyrvinium pamoate	Red
Rhubarb	Yellow
Salicylates	Due to bleeding
Santonin	Yellow
Senna	Yellow to brown
Tetracyclines in syrup (due to glucosamine)	Red

Table 68. Effects of Drugs on Laboratory Test Values

	Hepatotoxic and/or cholestatic	Nephrotoxic	Intestinal malabsorption	Serum iron	Serum TIBC	Serum folate (inhibit *L. casei*)	Creatinine	BUN	Uric acid	Calcium	Bilirubin	SGOT/SGPT	Glucose	Glucose tolerance	Cholesterol	PBI	T–3 uptake	T–4	¹³¹ I uptake	Amylase/lipase	Sodium	Potassium	Chloride	Prothrombin time	Comments
Antihistamines	+																							D	
Antimony compounds	+	+									D	I													
Arsenicals	+	+									I	I													
Caffeine													I	I											
Cholinergics												I								I					I – BSP. Changes due to spasm, sphincter of Oddi
Cinchophen	+								D			I													
Clofibrate	+								D			I			D									I	D – triglycerides, total lipids, LDH
Coumarins	+								D															I	
Cyclophosphamide	+																								
Dextran				I			I	I	I															I	I – protein
Diphenylhydantoin	+		+			D										D	I	D							D – IgA
Heparin			+							*							I	D							*Alters turbidity tests (e.g., thymol) and lipoprotein electrophoresis pattern. May interfere with BSP and calcium*

[460]

Drug	Markings	Notes
Levodopa	+	
Methotrexate	+	I; I*
Procainamide	+	
Propylthiouracil	+	I* — D D D; *SMA methodology
Quinacrine	+	I* — I – Diagnex blue
Quinine, Quinidine		I
Radiopaque contrast media	+	+ — I – BSP and protein. Serum protein electrophoresis pattern cannot be interpreted
Theophylline		I; D — I – ESR
Ascorbic acid	+	I I; I I I I — D – LDH
Nicotinic acid (large doses)		I; I I
VITAMINS		
Vitamin A		I; I
Vitamin D	*	I; I — *With hypervitaminosis D
Vitamin K		D
HORMONES		
ACTH	+	D; D D; I D; D D I I D D
Anabolic steroids and androgens		D; D I; D I
Corticosteroids		D D; I I; I D I
Estrogens	+	D; I D D I
Oral contraceptives (estrogens + progestin)	+	D; I D D I I I — D
D-Thyroxine		I; D I I I; I

See footnotes on page 465.

[461]

Table 68 *(continued)*

	Hepatotoxic and/or cholestatic	Nephrotoxic	Intestinal malabsorption	Serum iron	Serum TIBC	Serum folate (inhibit *L. casei*)	Creatinine	BUN	Uric acid	Calcium	Bilirubin	SGOT/SGPT	Glucose	Glucose tolerance	Cholesterol	PBI	T−3 uptake	T−4	131I uptake	Amylase/lipase	Sodium	Potassium	Chloride	Prothrombin time	Comments
ANTI-INFLAMMATORY, ANTI-GOUT, ANTI-ARTHRITIS																									
Allopurinol	+																							D*	*On coumarins
Colchicine	+		+													D*									*With some methods
Gold	+	+																						I	
Indomethacin	+																I							I	
Phenylbutazone	+																I		D						
Probenecid	+	+							D								I								
Salicylates	+	+							I								I	D							

[462]

							Remarks
PSYCHOACTIVE AGENTS	Chloral hydrate	+		I*			D *React with Neisler's reagent
	Chlordiazepoxide	+			D	D	D – VMA and 5-HIAA
	Imipramine	+			D		D
	Phenobarbital		D				
	Phenothiazines						
	Chlorpromazine	+		D	I	D	D – 5-HIAA. May cause false positive pregnancy test
	Chlorprothixene	+		D			
	Fluphenazine		D				
	Thiothixene	+					
NARCOTICS	Codeine			I	I	I	⎫
	Meperidine (Demerol)			I	I	I	⎬ I – LDH and BSP. Laboratory changes due to spasm of sphincter of Oddi
	Morphine (heroin)			I	I	I	⎪
	Marihuana		I	D		D	⎭
ANTI-DIABETIC (ORAL)	Acetohexamide (Sulfonylurea)	+		I			
	Chlorpropamide	+					
	Tolbutamide	+			I*		*SMA methodology
ANTI-HYPERTENSIVES	Guanethidine analogs		I	I	D	I	D – VMA
	Hydralazine	+		I	I		D – VMA, 5-HIAA
	MAO inhibitors	+		I	I		D – 5-HIAA
	Methyldopa	+		I		D	I – 5-HIAA
	Reserpine	+		I		D	I – 5-HIAA

[463]

Table 68 *(continued)*

	Hepatotoxic and/or cholestatic	Nephrotoxic	Intestinal malabsorption	Serum iron	Serum TIBC	Serum folate (inhibit *L. casei*)	Creatinine	BUN	Uric acid	Calcium	Bilirubin	SGOT/SGPT	Glucose	Glucose tolerance	Cholesterol	PBI	T–3 uptake	T–4	₁₃₁I uptake	Amylase/lipase	Sodium	Potassium	Chloride	Prothrombin time	Comments
DIURETICS																									
Acetazolamide									I																
Chlorthalidone		+											I	D										I	
Ethacrynic acid	+								I				I	D							D	D	D	I	
Furosemide	+							I	I				I	D							D	D	D		
Thiazides	+							I	I				I	D						I	D	D	D		D – PSP and creatinine tolerance
ANTIBIOTICS, ETC.																									
Aminosalicylic acid (PAS)	+					D																			
Amphotericin B	+	+																							
Ampicillin		+				D																			
Cephaloridine		+																							
Cephalothin		+																							
Chloramphenicol	+			I	D	D	I or D*																		*Depends on method
Colistin		+																							
Erythromycin	+					D						I*													*Colorimetric method
Gentamicin	+	+																							

[*464*]

ANTIBIOTICS, ETC. *(continued)*

					Notes
Griseofulvin	+	+			
Isoniazid	+	+	I*	D	*SMA method. D – 5-HIAA
Kanamycin	+	+	+		
Lincomycin	+			D	
Methicillin	+	*			
Nalidixic acid	+	*	I**		*Nitrogen retention **Copper reduction method.
Neomycin	+	+			
Nitrofurantoin	+	+			
Novobiocin	+				
Oleandomycin	+				
Oxacillin	+	+			
Penicillin			D	D	*With massive dosage D – PSP
Polymyxin B	+				
Rifampin	+	+			
Streptomycin	+				
Sulfonamides	+	+	I	D	D	I – PAH clearance
Tetracyclines	+	+		D	D	

+ = presence of laboratory test changes due to drug effect on organ.

I = values may be increased, elevated, or falsely positive.

D = values may be decreased, lowered, or falsely negative.

*and ** See last column on right.

Hepatotoxic refers to liver damage that may alter one or more laboratory tests of liver function, including the following: alkaline phosphatase, bilirubin, transaminase, cephalin flocculation, thymol turbidity, BSP retention, etc. When this column is marked with a + sign, the individual columns (e.g., bilirubin, SGOT) are not also marked with a + sign.

Nephrotoxic refers to renal damage that may cause changes in BUN, creatinine, urine protein, casts, or cells. When this column is marked with a + sign, the individual columns (e.g., BUN, creatinine) are not also marked with a + sign.

REFERENCES

Christian, D. G.   Drug interference with laboratory blood chemistry determinations. *Amer. J. Clin. Path.* 54: 118, 1970.

Elking, M. P., and Kabat, H. F.   Drug induced modifications of laboratory test values. *Amer. J. Hosp. Pharm.* 25: 485,1968.

Koch-Weser, J., and Sellers, E. M.   Drug interactions with coumarin anticoagulants. *New Eng. J. Med.* 285: 547, 1971.

Lubran, M.   The effects of drugs on laboratory values. *Med. Clin. N. Amer.* 53(1): 211,1969.

Rayfield, E. J., Cain, J. P., Casey, M. P., Williams, G. H., and Sullivan, J. M.   Influence of diet on urinary VMA excretion. *J.A.M.A.* 221: 704, 1971.

Sunderman, F. W., Jr.   Effects of drugs upon hematological tests. *Ann. Clin. Lab. Sci.* 2: 2, 1972.

Young, D. S., Thomas, D. W., Friedman, R. B., and Pestaner, L. C.   Effect of drugs on clinical laboratory tests. *Clin. Chem.* 18: 1041, 1972.

Bibliography

1. Bloodworth, J. M. B., Jr. *Endocrine Pathology*. Baltimore: Williams & Wilkins, 1968.
2. Bockus H. L. *Gastroenterology*, 2d ed. Philadelphia: Saunders, 1964.
3. Conn, H. F., and R. B. Conn, Jr. (Eds.). *Current Diagnosis 3*. Philadelphia: Saunders, 1971.
4. Davidsohn, I., and J. B. Henry (Eds.). *Todd-Sanford's Clinical Diagnosis by Laboratory Methods*, 14th ed. Philadelphia: Saunders, 1969.
5. Frankel, S., S. Reitman, and A. C. Sonnenwirth (Eds.). *Gradwohl's Clinical Laboratory Methods and Diagnosis*, 7th ed. St. Louis: Mosby, 1970.
6. Friedberg, C. K. *Diseases of the Heart*, 3rd ed. Philadelphia: Saunders, 1966.
7. Harrison, T. R., R. D. Adams, I. L. Bennett, W. H. Resnik, G. W. Thorn, and M. W. Wintrobe (Eds.). *Principles of Internal Medicine*, 6th ed. New York: Blakiston Div., McGraw-Hill, 1970.
8. Miale, J. B. *Laboratory Medicine: Hematology*, 4th ed. St. Louis: Mosby, 1972.
9. Popper, H., and F. Schaffner. *Liver: Structure and Function*. New York: Blakiston Div., McGraw-Hill, 1957.
10. Strauss, M. B., and L. G. Welt. *Diseases of the Kidney*, 2d ed. Boston: Little, Brown, 1971.
11. Wintrobe, M. M. *Clinical Hematology*, 6th ed. Philadelphia: Lea & Febiger, 1967.

Index

and diagnex blue excretion, 456
excretion of, urinary, 30
urine coloration from, 450
Richweed, poisoning from, 443
Rickets, 226–227, 321
alkaline phosphatase levels in, 46
and calcium in serum, 45
and calcium in urine, 111
phosphorus levels in, 46
renal, 321
phosphorus levels in, 46
vitamin D-resistant, 227
in Fanconi syndrome, 305
Rickettsial diseases, 399–400
monocytosis in, 84
myocardial disease with, 154
pneumonia in, 159
Weil-Felix reaction in, 401
Rickettsialpox, 400, 401
Rifampin
and laboratory test values, 465
and prothrombin time, 459
urine coloration from, 450
Riley bodies, in gargoylism, 226
Riley-Day syndrome, 313
RISA, in lung scanning, 133–134
Ristocetin, susceptibility of bacteria to, 393
Robinson-Power-Kepler water tolerance
test, in Addison's disease, 340
Rocky Mountain spotted fever, 399–400, 401
monocytosis in, 84
Rod myopathy, 224
Roseola infantum, 406
Rosettes, with LE cells, 103
Rotor syndrome, liver function tests in, 191
Rouleaux formation
in macroglobulinemia, 275
in multiple myeloma, 274
in temporal arteritis, 431
Rubella, 405–406
leukopenia in, 82
lymphocytes in, 83
plasma cells in, 84
Rubeola, 405. *See also* Measles
Rubidium-81, in spleen scanning, 135
Rumpel-Leede tourniquet test, in hemor-
rhagic conditions, 279–281

Sabin-Feldman dye test, 420
Sabouraud's medium
in actinomycosis, 410
in chromoblastomycosis, 416
in geotrichosis, 416
in moniliasis, 413
in sporotrichosis, 416
Salicylates. *See also* Acetylsalicylic acid;
p-Aminosalicylic acid
coma from, 200
and erythrocyte sedimentation rate, 457
and false positive urine diacetic acid
test, 452
intoxication from, 438–439
blood and urine changes in, 42
and laboratory test values, 462
and protein-bound iodine levels, 63
and prothrombin time, 98, 458
serum levels of, 11, 15
in salicylate intoxication, 438
stool coloration from, 459
and transaminase levels in serum, 147
and triiodothyronine uptake, 62
and uric acid levels, 40
and urine color, 110
Salicylazosulfapyridine, urine coloration
from, 450
Saliva
in cystic fibrosis of pancreas, 198
excretion of radioiodine in
in hyperthyroidism, 315
in hypothyroidism, 318
potassium and sodium in
in aldosteronism, 335
in Cushing's syndrome, 332

Salivary gland
amylase levels in diseases of, 49
cytomegalic inclusion disease of, 404
Salmonella species, 382
antibiotic susceptibility of, 393, 394
in blood, 127
in colon, 125
in gallbladder, 126
and osteomyelitis, 226
typhosa, 381
in urine, 128
Salmonellosis, and leukocytes in stools, 119
Salt-depletion syndrome, 291
Salt-dilution syndrome, 291
Sandfly fever, 408
Sanfilippo's syndrome, 309
Santonin, stool coloration from, 459
SAP. *See* Acid phosphatase, in serum
Sarcoidosis, 321, 432
calcium levels in, 45
corticoids affecting elevated serum calcium
in, 77
eosinophilia in, 85
liver disease with, 188
serum enzymes in, 182
marrow aspiration in, 95
monocytosis in, 84
myocardial disease with, 155
phosphorus levels in, 46
protein electrophoresis in, 57
protein gammopathy in, 58
thymol turbidity in, 62
and tubular reabsorption of phosphate, 77
uric acid levels in, 40
Sarcoma
Ewing, 229
lymphosarcoma. *See* Lymphosarcoma
osteogenic, 228
reticulum cell
of bone, 226
leukocyte alkaline phosphatase staining
reaction in, 85
Scanning
adrenal, 136
bone, 135
brain, 134
cardiac blood pool, 134
liver, 133
in metastatic disease, 188
lung, 133–134
in pulmonary embolism and infarction,
162
pancreas, 135–136
in carcinoma, 199
in chronic disease, 197
parathyroid, 136
parotid gland, 135
renal, 134
spleen, 135
thyroid, 133
in Hashimoto's thyroiditis, 320
Scarlet fever
antistreptococcal antibody titers in, 102
cold autohemagglutination in, 104
eosinophilia in, 84
oral manifestations of, 164
Schei syndrome, 309
valvular heart disease in, 149
Schilling test, 129
in malabsorption, 171
in pernicious anemia, 248
in vitamin B12 deficiencies, 249
Schistosoma mansoni, 422, 424
Schistosomiasis, 424–425
anemia in, 265
cirrhosis in, 186
gastrointestinal manifestations of, 164
liver in, 177
rectal biopsy in, 173
Schizophrenia, cerebrospinal fluid in, 201
Schmidt's syndrome, hyperglycemia in, 328
Schönlein's purpura, 284. *See also* Purpura,
Schönlein-Henoch

Little, Brown's Paperback Book Series

Basic Medical Sciences

Albers, Agranoff, Katzman, & Siegel	Basic Neurochemistry
Colton	Statistics in Medicine
Hine & Pfeiffer	Behavioral Science
Levine	Pharmacology
Peery & Miller	Pathology, 2nd Ed.
Selkurt	Physiology, 3rd Ed.
Sidman & Sidman	Neuroanatomy
Snell	Clinical Anatomy for Medical Students
Snell	Clinical Embryology for Medical Students, 2nd Ed.
Valtin	Renal Function
Watson	Basic Human Neuroanatomy

Clinical Medical Sciences

Clark & MacMahon	Preventive Medicine
Eckert	Emergency-Room Care, 2nd Ed.
Grabb & Smith	Plastic Surgery, 2nd Ed.
Green	Gynecology, 2nd Ed.
Judge & Zuidema	Methods of Clinical Examination, 3rd Ed.
Keefer & Wilkins	Medicine
MacAusland & Mayo	Orthopedics
Nardi & Zuidema	Surgery, 3rd Ed.
Thompson	Primer of Clinical Radiology
Ziai	Pediatrics, 2nd Ed.

Nursing Sciences

DeAngelis	Basic Pediatrics for the Primary Health Care Provider
Sana & Judge	Physical Appraisal Methods in Nursing Practice
Selkurt	Basic Physiology for the Health Sciences

Manuals and Handbooks

Arndt	Manual of Dermatologic Therapeutics
Children's Hospital Medical Center, Boston	Manual of Pediatric Therapeutics
Condon & Nyhus	Manual of Surgical Therapeutics, 3rd Ed.
Friedman & Papper	Problem-Oriented Medical Diagnosis
Massachusetts General Hospital	Manual of Nursing Procedures
Neelon & Ellis	A Syllabus of Problem-Oriented Patient Care
Spivak & Barnes	Manual of Clinical Problems in Internal Medicine: Annotated with Key References
Wallach	Interpretation of Diagnostic Tests, 2nd Ed.
Washington University Department of Medicine	Manual of Medical Therapeutics, 21st Ed.
Zimmerman	Techniques of Patient Care

Little, Brown and Company
34 Beacon Street
Boston, Massachusetts 02106